RENAL
MEDICINE

Guidelines in Medicine

VOLUME 2

RENAL MEDICINE

E. N. Wardle

MA, MD, MRCP
King's College Hospital
London

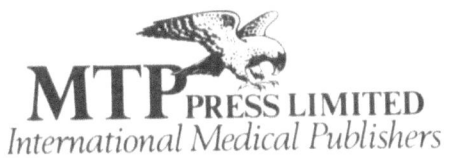

MTP PRESS LIMITED
International Medical Publishers

Published by
MTP Press Limited
Falcon House
Lancaster, England

British Library Cataloguing in Publication Data

Wardle, E. N.
  Renal medicine. – (Guidelines in medicine; vol. 3)
  1. Kidneys – Diseases
  I. Title   II. Series
  616.6'1   RC902
ISBN-13: 978-94-011-7205-9   e-ISBN-13: 978-94-011-7203-5
DOI: 10.1007/978-94-011-7203-5

Phototypesetting by Rainbow Graphics, Liverpool.

Contents

Foreword

Professor David Kerr
Royal Victoria Infirmary, Newcastle upon Tyne

Do we need another book on renal disease? There are few small books, particularly from this side of the Atlantic, which provide a really sound foundation of renal physiology, biochemistry and immunology. For two decades "The Kidney" by Hugh de Wardener has given a splendid background in renal physiology but I doubt if any author has brought to this subject as wide an experience and knowledge of basic science as Dr Wardle possesses. His researches have ranged over haematology, the role of intravascular coagulation in acute renal failure, the biochemistry of uremic metabolites, the immunology of glomerulonephritis, to hyperlipidemia in the genesis of arterial disease. In all these topics he has mastered the laboratory techniques as well as studying the patients personally. He therefore has a unique opportunity to show how renal disease can be illuminated by an understanding of the pathogenetic mechanism and to point the way to future treatment more logical than the crude and empirical methods we use today. This approach should appeal particularly to the young graduate whose memory of biochemistry and physiology is still reasonably fresh. I can also recommend it to the middle-aged physician who has long forgotten the little basic science he ever knew but who wishes to rejuvenate his knowledge and to stay on speaking terms with his Registrar and SHO.

1
The kidneys in health and disease: renal physiology and pathophysiology

Each kidney, weight 130 g, contains about one million glomeruli. The glomerulus is the filtering unit at the upper end of each nephron and consists of a tuft of glomerular capillaries which invaginate into an epithelial sac known as Bowman's capsule which joins with the actual renal tubule. Each of the one million nephrons then drains via coalescing collecting tubules into the renal pelvis, so that finally the urine enters the ureter en route to the bladder.

In embryogenesis, in fact, the system develops in reverse. The ureter, renal pelvis, calyces and collecting tubules sprout successively from a bud that originates from the mesonephric duct. The whole proliferating collecting system then unites with the Malpighian corpuscles (glomeruli) and their secretory ducts, which have differentiated meanwhile in the metanephros at the caudal end of the nephrogenic cord. As new orders of collecting ductules arise, each mass of metanephric tissue increases steadily in amount thus leading to the formation of a lobulated cortex. Then the Bowman's capsule of each glomerulus with its attached S-shaped secretory tubule finally establishes connection with the collecting tubules. In this way the definitive anatomy of the kidney is established (details are shown in Figure 1 overleaf).

Figure 1(a) indicates the major anatomical features. The nephrons are seen to join a system of collecting tubules which aggregate in the medullary

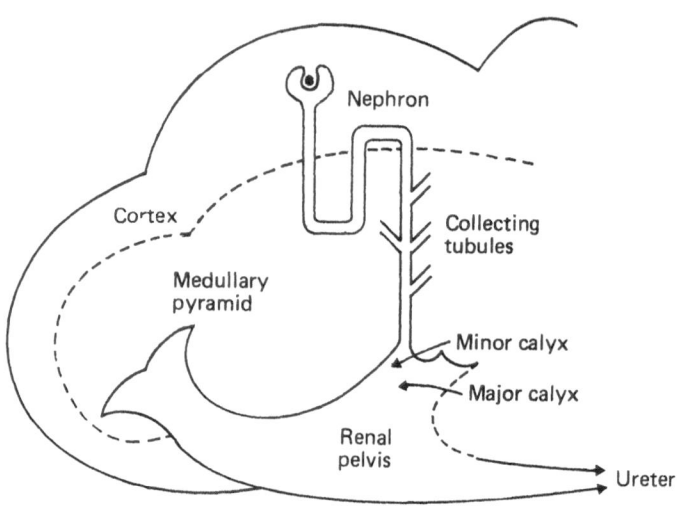

Figure 1. (a) **Anatomy of the kidney**

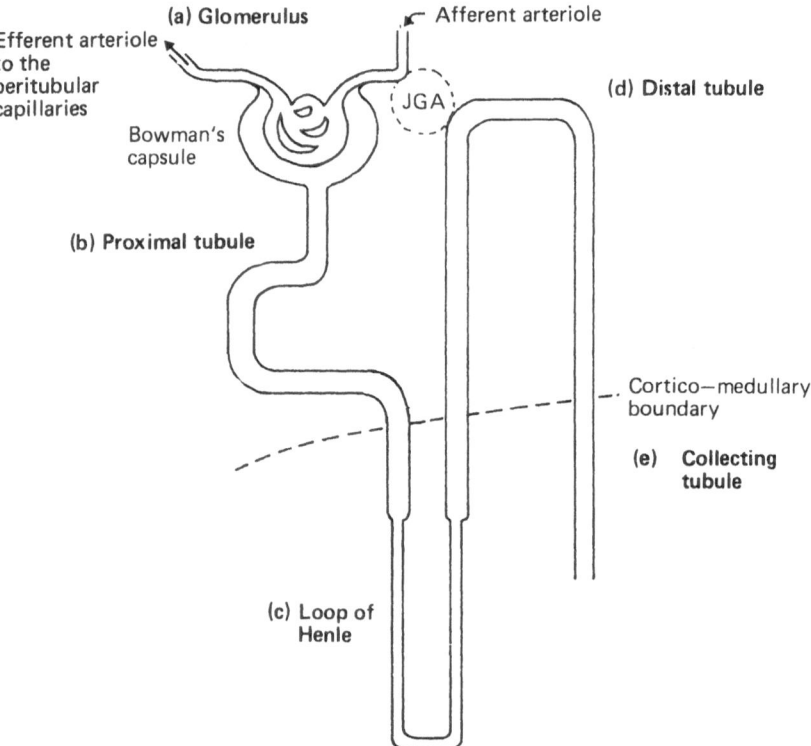

Figure 1. (b) **The parts of the nephron**

pyramid, where they lead into a minor calyx. Urine then flows on into the major calyx, the renal pelvis and then the ureter. Figure 1(b) shows a nephron in detail. Filtrate which is formed in the capillaries of the glomerulus (*a*) goes through into Bowman's capsule and from there passes into the proximal tubule (*b*) to the loop of Henle (*c*), the distal tubule (*d*) and the collecting tubule (*e*).

The functions of the nephron are best considered in terms of the separate segments, (see below).

Nephron structure and function

In the *glomerulus* there is filtration of plasma from the glomerular 'capillaries' (which in effect are arterioles) into Bowman's capsule (see also Figure 3).

In the *proximal tubule* there is reabsorption of 70% sodium and water, and of potassium, calcium, phosphate and bicarbonate, hexose sugars and urate so that the final fluid is still isotonic with plasma (see also Figure 4). At the same time hydrogen ions are secreted.

In the *loop of Henle* active sodium transport from the ascending limb together with the countercurrent system establishes a hypertonic renal medulla (see also Figure 5). The abstraction of sodium from the lumen of the tubule results in the entry of hypotonic fluid into the *distal tubule* (see also Figure 6), which is responsible for five functions:

(1)   Water is reabsorbed under the influence of antidiuretic hormone.
(2)   Sodium is reabsorbed, in exchange for the secretion of hydrogen ions and potassium, under the control of aldosterone.
(3)   Bicarbonate is reabsorbed.
(4)   Urate is secreted.
(5)   Ammonia is secreted.

In the *collecting duct* (see also Figure 7) water and urea are each reabsorbed so that concentrated early morning urine has a SG 1040 and an osmolality of 750 mosmol/kg.

THE RENAL CIRCULATION

The blood flow to the kidneys amounts to one-quarter of the cardiac output and is thus some 1300 ml/min. Each main renal artery splits into radial lobar and then lobular arteries. These feed arcuate arteries which run tangentially along the corticomedullary junction in the 'boundary zone'. From the latter arise interlobular arteries which run vertically towards the surface of the kidney and in so doing give off the afferent arterioles to the glomeruli. It is from the second capillary network that venules arise and eventually join to form the arciform veins.

The renal circulatory system is actually unique since there are two capillary beds (Figure 2). This is because the afferent arteriole which feeds each Malpighian unit splits into the glomerular 'capillaries' (*a*), which then reunite as the efferent arteriole, and in turn this goes on to form the peritubular capillaries (*b*), which surround those parts of the tubules in the cortex. From the deeper glomeruli, designated *juxtamedullary,* a further capillary bed forms the arteriae vasa rectae which supply the medullary loops, and these, together with the loops of Henle, constitute the *countercurrent* system of the medulla.

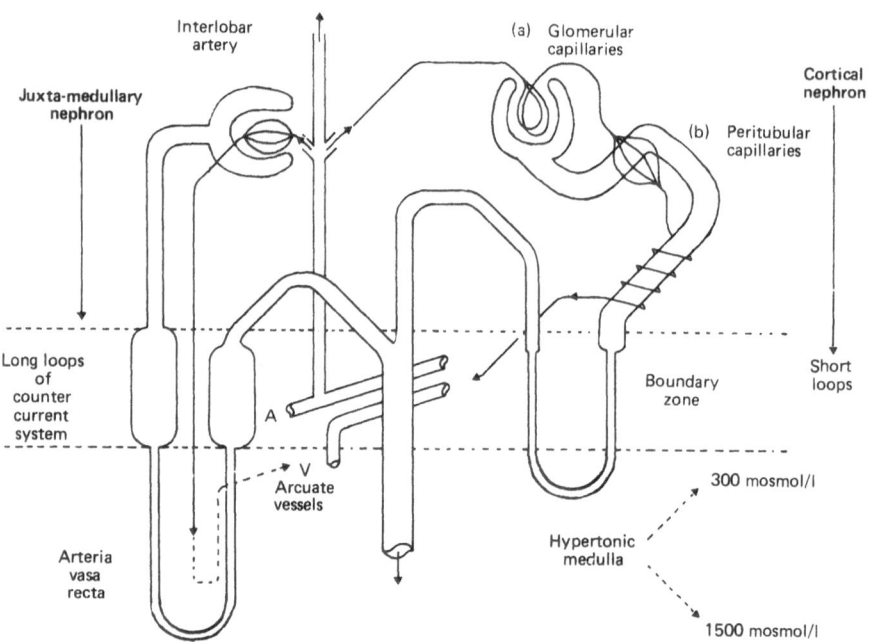

Figure 2. The renal circulation

Whereas the efferent arterioles of the cortical nephrons feed the peritubular capillaries of the proximal and distal tubules that are in the renal cortex, the efferents of the juxtamedullary nephrons form the vasa rectae of the renal medulla. The loop arrangement of the vasae rectae, in which there is both downflow and upflow of a slowly moving column of blood, ensures the maintenance of medullary hypertonicity (Figure 5(c)).

The cortical nephrons have short loops and therefore poor concentrating ability and sodium-retaining capacity. On the other hand the juxtamedullary nephrons have long loops with accordingly a greater concentrating capacity and ability to conserve sodium.

The renal cortex receives 90% of the renal blood flow to the extent of 5 ml/min per g of tissue, and the medulla only 0.5–1.5 ml/min per g. The pressure in the renal artery is at 100 mmHg but it falls to 75 mmHg in the afferent arteriole and thence to 22 mmHg in the peritubular capillaries. It is of consequence that changes of pressure in the first order peritubular capillaries are directly dependent on changes in the glomerular capillary pressure, because the efferent arteriole has no independent tone.

Normally, in fact, there is little activity of the nerves to the cortical blood vessels and flow is 'autoregulated' according to the myogenic response of the smooth muscle in the arteriolar walls. In effect this means that a high pressure applied to the arterioles results in an adaptive vasoconstriction so that blood flow distally remains the same, and of course the converse applies. If in addition sympathetic nervous activity is increased, then flow to the superficial cortex is reduced but rises through the juxtamedullary cortex and the medulla. It has to be emphasized, however, that there is no form of anatomical shunt from the cortical to the medullary vessels.

GLOMERULAR FILTRATION

Filtration through the capillaries of the glomeruli (Figure 3) obeys Starling's principles, so that the total glomerular filtration rate (GFR) of 130 ml/min is seen as the result of a normal balance of hydrostatic forces.

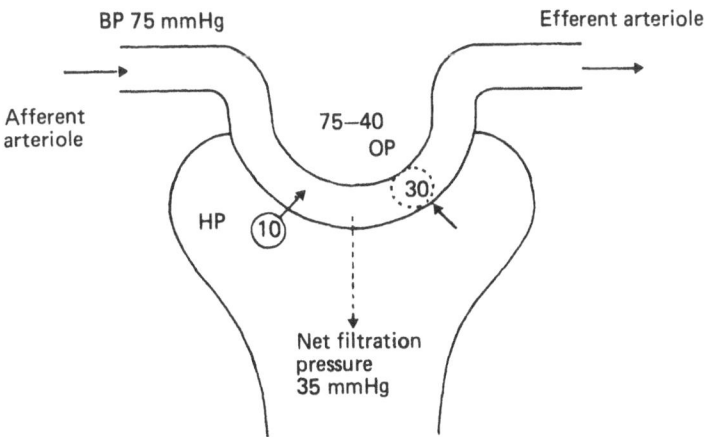

Figure 3. Hydrostatics of glomerular filtration

5

GFR – 130 ml/min = net filtration pressure x filtering area

$$= (BP - HP - OP) \times K_p$$

where the normal blood pressure driving filtration is 75 mmHg (BP) (Figure 3).

This haemofiltration pressure has to exceed (*a*) the hydrostatic pressure in Bowman's capsule (10 mmHg), and (*b*) the osmotic pressure of plasma proteins that retain fluid in the circulation (30 mmHg). Additionally the equation incorporates a factor K_p, the filtration constant, which represents the area of the filtration surface together with its porosity.

Clearly the osmotic pressure is determined by those molecules of high molecular weight, the proteins, which cannot be filtered. However, if the osmotic pressure is lowered due to hypoproteinaemia, as by an increase in glomerular permeability in the nephrotic syndrome, then the glomerular filtration rate will rise.

A fall in the hydrostatic pressure occurs in shock (by definition), and glomerular filtration will cease at a glomerular blood pressure of 40 mmHg.

The entire circulating plasma volume is filtered and reabsorbed twice an hour, so that in the course of a day the extracellular fluid volume is filtered some 12–15 times. We can assume that in a man weighing 70 kg there are 50 litres of water, of which 15 litres are in the extracellular space (3.5 litres plasma and 11.5 litres interstitial water) with 35 litres forming the intracellular water.

Consider then that:

(1)   the renal blood flow (RBF) is 1300 ml/min (one-quarter of the cardiac output);

(2)   the renal plasma flow (RPF) is 700 ml/min; and

(3)   the glomerular filtration rate is 130 ml/min.

Thus the fraction of the plasma filtered is given by GFR/RPF = 130/700 = 0.18–0.20. In all some 200 litres/day of water with solute will be filtered, and yet only 1000–1500 ml/day are lost in the urine. Hence over 99% of the water is reabsorbed, and this applies to sodium, chloride and bicarbonate. Glucose reabsorption actually achieves 100%, except when the blood glucose is raised or there is a tubular leak. A little potassium is lost (about 7% of that filtered, or 100 mmol) to compensate for that acquired in the diet. Of the 50 g/day urea filtered, some 60% is retained and 40% is excreted.

TUBULAR REABSORPTION

If so much fluid and solute has to be reabsorbed, the task is tremendous.

Reabsorption is in part passive (as a result of physical forces) and partly by active transport which requires chemical energy as adenosine triphosphate (ATP). These processes are summarized below.

Proximal tubule

The ultrafiltrate which enters the proximal tubule from Bowman's capsule is almost identical to plasma. As it passes down the proximal tubule some 70% is reabsorbed with no change in sodium or osmotic concentration (Figure 4).

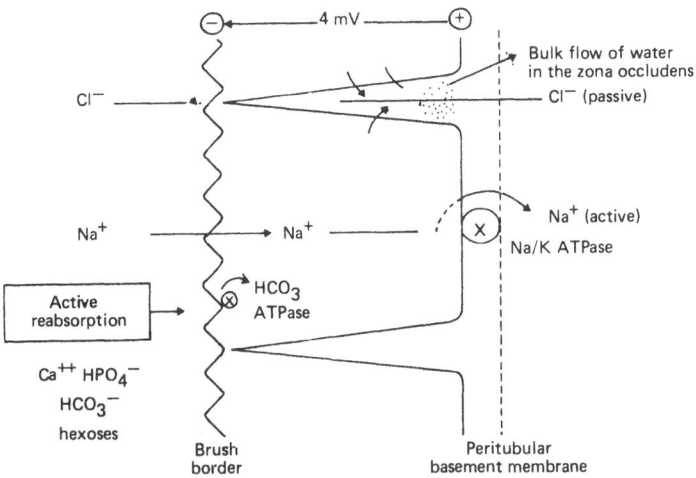

Figure 4. Re-absorption in the proximal tubule

Sodium reabsorption is an active energy-dependent process, the driving force for which is provided by the sodium–potassium-stimulated ATPase at the peritubular cell membrane. Chloride reabsorption follows passively. The isotonic reabsorption of water coincides with sodium reabsorption, and depends on the raised osmotic pressure of the plasma proteins in the peritubular capillaries. This arises as a result of the haemoconcentration following filtration in the glomeruli. Bicarbonate reabsorption is also an active process, since it depends on a bicarbonate-stimulated ATPase on the brush border. Similarly there is active transport reabsorption of d-glucose and amino acids, and of calcium and phosphate. In fact the appearance of phosphate in the urine is a classical marker for proximal tubular damage.

The energy source for glomerular filtration is essentially the work of the left ventricle. On the other hand the reabsorptive process depends on ATP

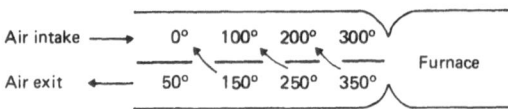

Figure 5(a)

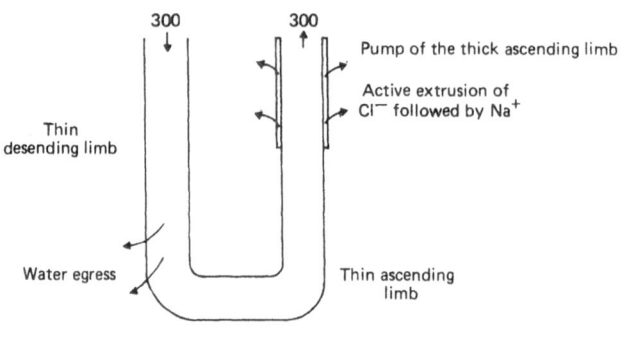

Figure 5(b)

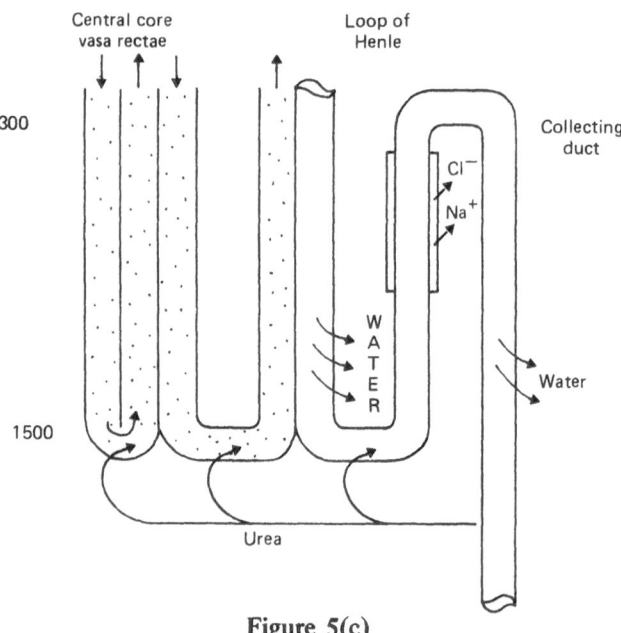

Figure 5(c)

Figure 5.   (a) Counter-current principle (b) the loop of Henle (c) counter-current multiplier. The figures are mosmoles

formed by oxidative phosphorylation in the mitochondria. An adaptive coupling, referred to as *glomerulotubular balance,* is the process whereby the rate of tubular reabsorption is geared to the filtration rate. The balance is probably regulated by the colloid osmotic pressure of the blood in the peritubular capillaries. Thus a fall of GFR will reduce the filtration fraction, and this in turn reduces the osmotic pressure of the blood which leaves the glomerulus, so that there is then a fall in reabsorption from the proximal tubule. Conversely, when the GFR rises the amount of fluid reabsorbed in the proximal tubule also rises, for then the oncotic pressure in the peritubular capillaries is raised.

Loop of Henle and the countercurrent system of urine concentration

The structure of the hairpin loops of Henle and the vasa rectae suggest that they operate on a 'countercurrent mechanism', which is the principle used to conserve heat in a furnace. The air in the intake pipe carrying cold air is warmed before it reaches the heater by being positioned adjacent to the air exit pipe which is carrying hot air (Figure 5a).

For the purpose of urine concentration a countercurrent 'exchanger' alone might be inadequate but when a further driving force is provided by the active transport of sodium chloride out of the ascending loop of Henle into the hypertonic medulla, the resulting countercurrent 'multiplier' is very efficient. In the loop of Henle fluid flows first down the thin *descending* limb, which has a high water permeability but a low permeability to sodium. In this way the hyperosmotic environment of the medulla causes water to move out of the descending limb, so that the osmolality of the urine content rises from 300 mosmol on entry to 1500 mosmol at the tip of the loop. The thin *ascending* limb, on the other hand, is relatively impermeable to water but reabsorbes sodium chloride. In the thick part of the ascending limb sodium chloride is actively reabsorbed by a most powerful mechanism. Indeed the interior of the thick ascending limb develops a positive potential as a result of active chloride transport. Thus sodium follows passively. Moreover the solute deposited in the medulla is trapped there, and contributes to the medullary hypertonicity (Figure 5b).

The thick limb thus serves two very important functions. First it generates hypotonic fluid in the lumen of the tube, and this fluid then moves on to the distal convoluted tubule. Second, since it adds sodium chloride to the medullary interstitium, it helps maintain the osmolarity of the medulla.

There is additionally a mechanism for trapping urea. The collecting duct is permeable to urea, which is then trapped in high concentration in the inner medulla by the countercurrent exchange mechanism. Naturally some will be

9

lost back into the loop of Henle, so that ultimately it appears in the urine in order to maintain the urea clearance.

The vasa rectae occupy a central vascular core and also contribute to the driving mechanism, as the ascending limb of the vasa recta is actually adjacent to the thin descending limb of the loop of Henle.

Hence the integrated system can be viewed as shown in Figure 5c.

The distal tubule

The distal tubule (Figure 6) starts at the corticomedullary boundary, at which level fluid enters with a tonicity of 200 mosmol/kg. The first part exhibits electrogenic sodium transport. After this comes the portion of the distal tubule adjacent to its own renal glomerulus. Here the tubular cells are small with prominent nuclei and are called the macula densa. Together with the adjacent wall of the afferent arteriole, they make up the juxtaglomerular apparatus (JGA in Figure 1b). Finally there is the distal 'exchange segment' in which active sodium reabsorption occurs with passive loss of hydrogen or potassium ions. In effect for every three atoms of sodium reabsorbed, two ions of potassium and one atom of hydrogen are lost into the urine. This segment is under the control of aldosterone, and yet normally only accounts for some 2% of the total sodium that is reabsorbed.

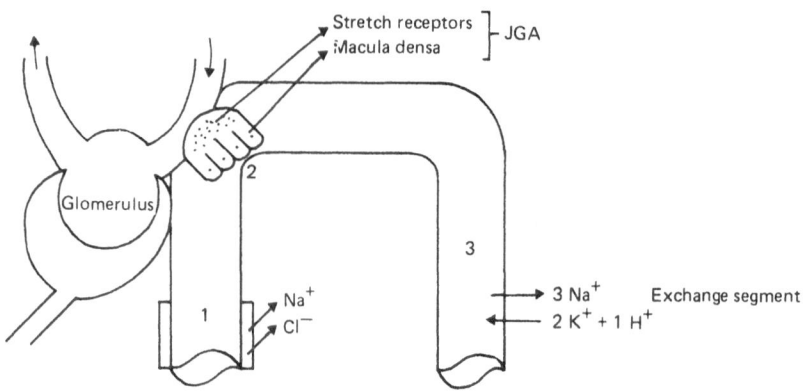

Figure 6.   The distal tubule

Two points should be emphasized here. First, this segment only works to full capacity if there is some reason why sodium is not being reabsorbed more proximally, for example when diuretics are being used. Second, the potassium excretion in this segment is essentially passive and depends on:

(1)   tubular flow rate and sodium content, and thus sodium reabsorption;
(2)   intracellular potassium stores;
(3)   intracellular pH;
(4)   the transepithelial potential difference;
(5)   luminal permeability.

The collecting ductules

The urine which enters these is now isotonic at 300 mosmol/kg as the tubule again crosses the corticomedullary boundary. The collecting duct system includes the cortical, medullary and papillary collecting duct segments. The fluid therein is thus exposed to those osmotic forces which operate from the cortex to the papilla, so this is the most important segment for reabsorption of water and final concentration of the urine. Under conditions of severe dehydration (*hydropenia*) the urine concentration attains the osmolality of the medullary tip, that is 1500 mosmol/kg. In fact this segment is not permeable to water in the absence of antidiuretic hormone (ADH). This fact explains the massive fluid loss in diabetes insipidus but with the help of ADH such maximal urine concentration can be achieved.

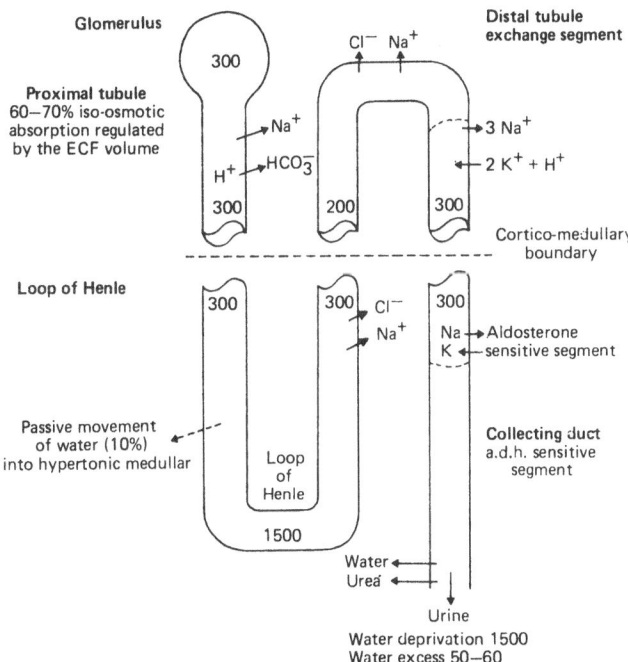

Figure 7.   Summary of the normal physiology of sodium and water reabsorption. Figures are mosmol/kg

As explained above the collecting duct is also the only segment distal to the thin ascending limb that is permeable to urea. In hydropenia, therefore, urea diffuses out of the papillary duct and into the interstitium and thin ascending limb, and thus accounts for urea recirculation and the ability of the papilla to maintain its hyperosmolarity.

TUBULAR ABSORPTION AND SECRETION

A substance like the polysaccharide inulin is filtered at the glomerulus, but at no point along the tubule is there any extra addition by secretion nor is there any reabsorption. It is therefore used to measure glomerular filtration rate (C_{in}). Glucose on the other hand is filtered at the glomerulus and then reabsorbed by the proximal tubule. Indeed all glucose in the tubule can be reabsorbed up to a tubular reabsorptive maximum (*Tm-G*) of 200 mg/min— this represents the 'threshold value', so that loads greater than this will result in the appearance of glucose in the urine. In fact this *Tm-G* tends to be exceeded whenever the blood glucose is above 180 mg/dl (which is twice the normal fasting value or 2×5 mmol/l). This means that normally glucose only appears in the urine of diabetics, or in those rare conditions in which the Tm-G glucose is reduced, resulting in a 'renal leak', or *renal glycosuria*.

The substance PAH (*p*-amino-hippuric acid) is filtered in the glomeruli and also secreted in the proximal tubules. There is no threshold for a substance secreted by the tubules, but a limit will be imposed by the renal plasma flow (see below), which PAH is used to measure.

These facts are worth expressing in mathematical form in order to clarify some concepts that will be used later. Thus the amount of inulin that appears in the urine will be given by:

$$[U]_I \times V = [P]_I \times C_{in} \tag{1}$$

where U and P are the urine and plasma concentrations respectively and the clearance of inulin·(C_{in}) we know is equal to the glomerular filtration rate.

In the case of glucose where a large part is reabsorbed:

$$[U]_g \times V = [P]_g \times C - Tm_G \tag{2}$$

And in the case of PAH which is in part secreted:

$$[U]_H \times V = [P]_H \times C + Tm_{PAH} \tag{3}$$

$$(Tm_{PAH} = 80 \text{ mg/min}).$$

These equations appear in visual form in Figure 8.

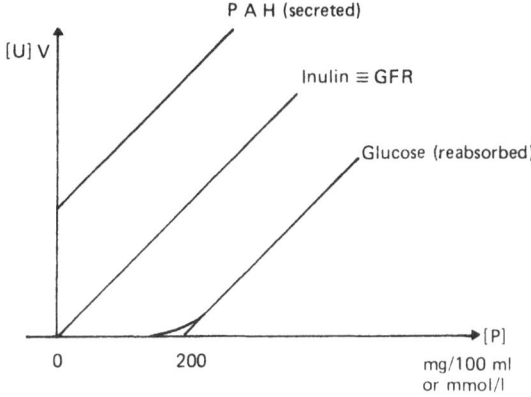

Figure 8. Substances used for the evaluation of renal tubular function

It is usual to express a 'clearance' as that volume of plasma/min which would have to be cleared to account for the amount of a given substance in the urine.

Thus

$$\text{Clearance (ml/min)} = \frac{[U] \times \text{Vol}}{[P]}$$

If the above equations are converted by dividing by the plasma concentration of each individual substance so that the clearance can be expressed directly, then we have:

$$\frac{UV}{P} = C_{in} \qquad \text{(inulin)} \qquad \text{(a)}$$

$$\frac{UV}{P_g} = C_{in} - \frac{Tm_G}{P_g} \qquad \text{(glucose)} \qquad \text{(b)}$$

$$\frac{UV}{P_H} = C_{in} + \frac{Tm_{(PAH)}}{P_H} \qquad \text{(PAH)} \qquad \text{(c)}$$

The two lower equations are those of a rectangular hyperbola and appear as such in Figure 9. Since the clearance of inulin is equal to the glomerular filtration rate and is constant, it appears as a straight line which does not vary with the plasma concentration.

It is apparent that the clearance of a substance reabsorbed by the tubules increases with rising plasma levels (glucose is a reminder), but that the

13

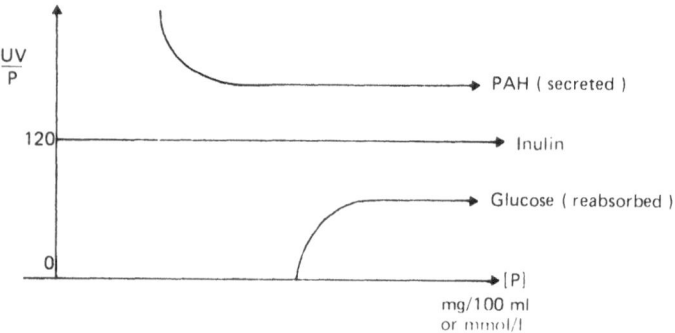

Figure 9.   The concept of clearances

clearance of a substance secreted by the tubules decreases as the plasma level rises (as in the case of PAH).

WATER REABSORPTION AND CLEARANCE

The *osmolal clearance* consists of the number of mls of plasma that are cleared of osmotically active solutes by the kidney in 1 min. The value is given by the conventional formula

$$C_{osm} = \frac{U_0 \times V}{P_0}$$ where U_0 is the urine osmolality

and P_0 is the plasma osmolality

If the urine osmolality is equal to that of plasma, then $C_{osm} = V$, the urine volume.

Free-water clearance, C_{H2O}, is the solute-free water that can be removed from the final urine and yet leave the urinary solutes iso-osmotic to plasma. If the urine is very dilute (hypo-osmolar), then the free-water clearance is positive. In fact when the kidney is excreting a maximally dilute urine, representative values for the equation might be

$$C_{osm} = \frac{45 \times 20}{300} = 3.0 \, ml/min \qquad C_{H2O} = 17 \, ml/min$$

where $U_0 = 45$, $P_0 = 300$ and $V = 20$ ml/min. The kidney is then excreting the osmoles contained in 3 ml plasma in 20 ml urine, and so is removing pure water from the body at the rate of $20 - 3 = 17$ ml/min. Thus free-water clearance is expressed by the general formula $V - C_{osm}$.

14

Conversely *free-water reabsorption*, Tc_{H_2O}, is the amount of water that needs to be added to a concentrated hyperosomotic urine in order to make the solute concentration iso-osmotic to plasma. Under these circumstances the osmolar clearance might be

$$C_{osm} \quad \frac{1400 \times 0.8}{300} \quad = \quad 3.7\,\text{ml/min} \quad Tc_{H_2O} = 2.9\,\text{ml/min}$$

This means that the excretion of the osmoles from 3.7 ml plasma in 0.8 ml saves 2.9 ml/min of free water for the body. Thus free-water reabsorption is expressed as the formula $Tc_{H_2}\hat{O} = C_{osm} - \text{vol}$. So with urine hyperosmotic to plasma the free-water reabsorption is positive, and with hypo-osmotic urine it is negative.

Action of diuretics

A brief reference to pharmacological agents, in particular the diuretics, which inhibit the transport of sodium out of the ascending loop of Henle, serves to emphasize the normal function of the system. Ethacrynic acid, frusemide and the mercurials stop solute reabsorption so that there is a large delivery of solute with water to the collecting tubules. The result is that there is an increase of the amount of water reabsorbed by the collecting tubules and in turn this dilutes the medullary interstitial fluid. So not only is there a massive loss of sodium and water in the urine, but both urinary concentration and dilution are stopped. In technical terms we say that an agent which stops the ascending-loop pump lowers the clearance of free water (C_{H_2O}) at any particular urine volume; it also impairs the reabsorption of free water (Tc_{H_2O}) at any level of the osmolar clearance, C_{osm}.

Physiological influences

The following physiological factors influence the concentration/dilution mechanism:

(1) the rate of blood flow through the vasa rectae;
(2) the flow rates through the loop of Henle and collecting tubules;
(3) the degree of hydration and rate of solute excretion, which depend in turn on dietary salt and protein content;
(4) the availability of antidiuretic hormone (ADH);
(5) interference with Na transport.

Flow through the vasa rectae will clearly affect the rate at which solute is removed from the medullary interstitium. Thus in a water diuresis it is recognized that medullary blood flow is increased so that there is 'washout' of solute with a fall in the osmolality of the medulla. In a similar fashion a rise of arterial pressure (as in hypertension) will increase medullary blood flow, since unlike the cortex it is not autoregulated, and the result is a reduction in the concentrating ability of the urine. In shock also there is impairment of the concentrating ability, for the cessation of cortical flow means that there is insufficient delivery of sodium to the nephron, and therefore the medulla, and yet the maintenance of some medullary blood flow results in medullary washout.

If the rate of flow of saline down the tubules is increased, then the sodium pump mechanism will increase sodium reabsorption up to a point (the limiting gradient) but will nevertheless not be able to reduce the sodium in the effluent to the same extent as with a smaller load. Meantime, however, the increased deposition of solute in the interstitial fluid will augment the reabsorption of free water (Tc_{H2O}) from the collecting ducts. So solute loads lead to increased urine flow (osmolar clearance) and simultaneous increase of free-water reabsorption.

A mannitol diuresis will tend to lower the osmolality of the medulla. Indeed this is likely to happen with foreign molecules such as mannitol. However if sodium chloride or urea are given, medullary osmolarity is maintained.

Of course with 12–24 h of dehydration the *U/P* osmolality is maximal at 4.0. The highest values are found at low urinary flow rates. This maximum value decreases progressively with increasing urinary flow.

The highest *U/P* ratios are attained in young men who are both fasting and thirsty. A value of 4.8 can be attained when taking 100 g of glucose/day as nourishment, or a value of 5.0 when on a high protein diet!

Causes of impaired urinary concentrating ability

In a clinical setting *hypotonic polyuria* can be classified under the following causes:

(1) *Metabolic*
   (a) Osmotic diuresis;
   (b) Hypercalcaemia or hypokalaemia (which impair the concentrating mechanism);
   (c) Low protein diet or low urea excretion (as in the neonate or in malnutrition)
   (d) Sustained water drinking.
(2) *Haemodynamic*   Increase in renal blood flow or rise of blood pressure.

16

(3) *Hormonal* Lack of antidiuretic hormone—diabetes insipidus; hyperthyroidism (thyroxine) or adrenaline administration.
(4) *Pharmacological,* due to diuretics, angiotensin or pyrogens.
(5) *Medullary damage* as in sickle cell disease or post-obstructive diuresis.

The mechanisms of impairment of urine concentration might then be visualized as in Figure 10 below.

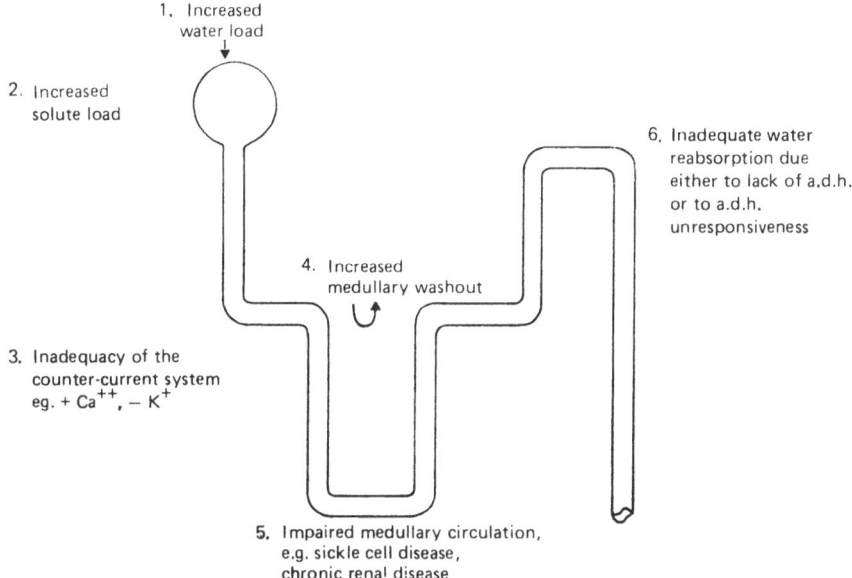

Figure 10. Mechanisms of impaired urine concentration

Impaired diluting ability

The conditions in which there is an inability to dilute the urine are:

(1) decreased glomerular filtration, i.e. chronic renal disease;
(2) hypothyroidism, hypoadrenalism, hypopituitarism;
(3) excess or inappropriate ADH administration or secretion (for example, with bronchial cancer);
(4) dilutional failure leading to hyponatraemia in sodium-retaining states such as cirrhosis, nephrosis and advanced congestive heart failure.

TESTS OF RENAL FUNCTION

The physiological tests of renal function can now be described logically in terms of the above considerations.

Glomerular filtration rate (GFR)

Under ideal experimental conditions this is done by the excretion of *inulin*, whose rate of excretion is equal to the GFR. After an inulin infusion to achieve steady plasma concentrations, the GFR is given by the standard formula:

$$GFR = \frac{[U]_{in} \times volume}{[P]_{in}}$$

A modern alternative is to use the rate of excretion of the isotope [^{51}Cr] EDTA following a single intravenous injection (Figure 11). A urine collection is not essential but instead serial plasma samples are counted so as to be able to plot the biphasic clearance of [^{51}Cr] EDTA from the plasma.

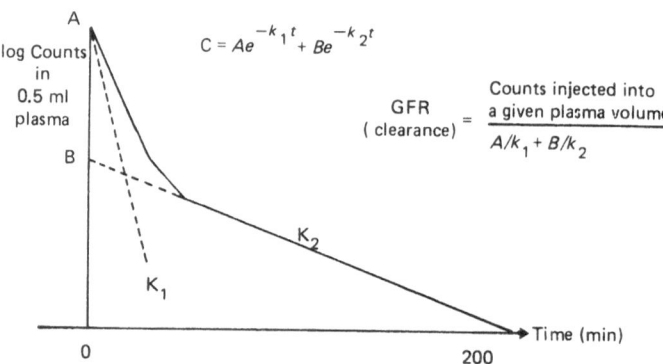

Figure 11.   GFR by single shot clearance of [^{51}Cr] EDTA

This formula arises quite simply from the fact that if there is a constant leakage (clearance) from a given volume of fluid (the plasma compartment) then:

$$clearance\ rate = volume\ of\ distribution \times k$$

where k is the decay constant or clearance constant. Measurements have to be made on a logarithmic scale since the decay values are exponential.

18

Use is made of the normal relationship:

Half-life $T\frac{1}{2} = \dfrac{2.303 \log 2}{k} = \dfrac{0.693}{k}$ so that $k = \dfrac{0.693}{T\frac{1}{2}}$

As Figure 11 indicates the clearance can be calculated from the slope (k_2) or half-life of the second prolonged part of the decay curve.

In routine clinical practice it is usual to settle for the *endogenous creatinine clearance.* Creatinine, the end-product of creatine metabolism in muscle, is excreted mainly by glomerular filtration and only slightly by tubular secretion. The technique is to obtain a blood sample and a 24 h urine collection so that the basic parameters are easily measured by the formula:

$$\text{GFR (ml/min)} = \dfrac{\text{urine creatinine conc.} \times \text{volume/min}}{\text{plasma creatinine conc.}}$$

Renal plasma flow

This is given by the rate of excretion of PAH in urine as compared with the plasma concentration. It actually measures the effective renal plasma flow (ERPF):

$$\text{ERPF} = \dfrac{\text{rate of urinary PAH excretion}}{\text{plasma PAH}} = \dfrac{U\text{PAH}}{P\text{ PAH}} = \dfrac{\text{(mg/min)}}{\text{(mg/ml)}}$$

$$= 650 \text{ ml/min}$$

Perhaps a simpler approach is to measure the clearance of radioiodinated hippurate. Although this underestimates the renal plasma flow by some 20% on account of plasma binding, it is more suitable for serial studies, for instance, after renal transplantation. The calculation is as in Figure 11.

Urinary concentration and dilution

Urine specific gravity is 1015 to 1025, and if concentrated may be 1035. If the urine loses its concentrating power (as in chronic pyelonephritis), then it becomes isotonic with plasma and has a fixed specific gravity of 1010. Moreover after a water load it will fall to 1005 since it approaches the specific gravity of distilled water. The early morning urine is examined when looking for concentration defects. In two particular situations, suspected acute renal failure and suspected diabetes insipidus, use is made of the measurement of urine and plasma osmolalities. A 1.0 molal (or 1 gmol per kg) solution of an ideal solute depresses the freezing point by 1.86 °C. The normal plasma osmolality in mosmol/kg is 300. Since it is determined by the solute particles it can be calculated roughly from the formula:

$$\text{plasma osmolality} \; = \; 2\,(Na^+ + K^+) \; + \; \frac{\text{glucose mg\%}}{18} \; + \; \frac{\text{urea mg\%}}{6}$$

and in SI units the sum in mmol/l is:

$$\text{plasma osmolality} = 2\,(140 + 5) + 5.0 + 5.0 = 300$$

An early morning urine will have an osmolality of 800–900 mosmol/kg, and after water deprivation for 16 h will be 1060 ± 200. In theory the dehydration value might be 1400; conversely, in diabetes insipidus values of 100–200 mosmol/kg are to be expected. Dehydration in fact raises the urine osmolality greater than the administration of vasopressin. In practice, it is often simplest to give five units of vasopressin tannate by injection and collect the urine samples serially over 6 h. The urine osmolality achieved will be at least 750 mosmol/kg; standard figures are 980 mosmol + 250.

Clinical note In acute renal failure (acute tubular necrosis) a urine/plasma osmolality ratio of less than 1.1 confirms the diagnosis. This situation often has to be distinguished from prerenal uraemia (dehydration), from the 'hepatorenal' syndrome when there is concurrent jaundice, or from urinary tract obstruction. The following table summarizes some distinguishing features.

Table 1

	Urine volume per day	Osmolality U	Osmolality P	Sodium concentration U	Sodium concentration P
Prerenal	800 ml	500	320	<10 mmol/l	raised
ATN	500 ml	310 – equal – 300		>20 mmol/l	any value
Urinary obstruction	variable	same as in ATN			
'Hepatorenal'	80 ml	400	260	<10 mmol/l	lowered

Urine testing and examination

The art of routine urine testing has been debased by the arrival of the 'dipsticks', which nevertheless give a quick reliable assessment of the urine content of glucose, protein, bile, blood and ketones, together with the pH.

This is fortunate because the chemical tests should no longer detract from the importance of careful microscopy of the urinary sediment. One may remember that Addis collected a 12 h urine and took the deposit from 10 ml for counting in a special counting chamber. The upper limit of normal for a 12 h urine was 1000 hyaline casts, 70 000 red cells and 300 000 white cells. How red and white cells enter normal urine is not known but their excretion is increased by fever or by exercise. Examination of an unspun urine sample is now used; 24 h collections can be preserved by the addition of thymol, formalin or phenol. Normally there are no red cells or casts but one sees one leukocyte per h.p. field in the male and one to five in women or children. Some tubular epithelial cells may be seen and always squamous epithelium from the female genital tract (Figure 12).

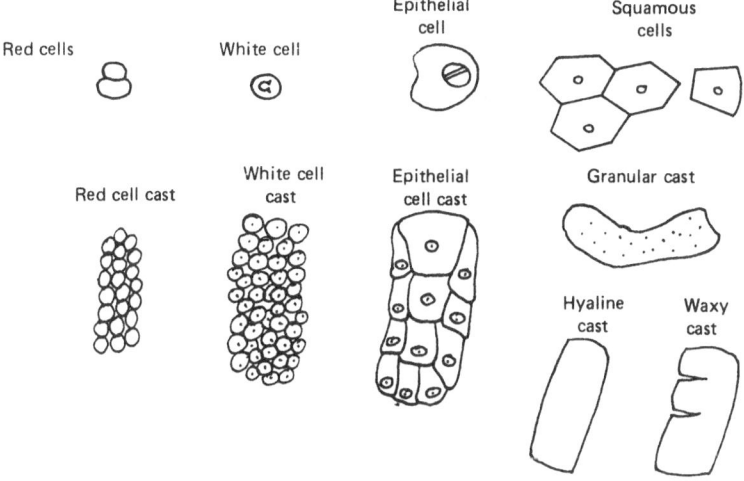

Figure 12. Types of cast in the urine

Casts are cylindrical bodies formed by conglomeration of cells and debris in the Tamm–Horsfall mucoprotein of the distal tubules. Hyaline casts have little significance, but red cell casts indicate a glomerulitis, and white cell casts indicate acute or chronic pyelonephritis. Degeneration then leads to granular change and possibly to the formation of waxy casts. When there is heavy proteinuria, as in the nephrotics, there are fat globules in the urine and fatty casts appear. In hypertension there is trace proteinuria and the sediment may show a few red cells and an occasional granular or hyaline cast, until the accelerated phase when red cells and casts all increase. The 'telescoped sediment', in which there are all types of cast, is seen typically in polyarteritis nodosa but also in systemic lupus erythematosus (SLE) nephritis.

21

In urine infections pus cells are present; nevertheless bacteruria can occur without pyuria. If there are more than 100 000 organisms (colonies) per ml of urine when plated in appropriate serial dilution, then there is a definite urinary tract infection.

Causes of cast formation

Table 2

Vascular damage	Glomerular damage	Tubular damage
Non-specific	proteinuria	epithelial cells and casts
	lipiduria	pus cell casts
	red cells	granular casts
	red cell casts	waxy casts

THE FUNCTIONS OF THE KIDNEY

This is a convenient point to summarize the functions of the kidney, many of which will now seem obvious.

(1) To excrete waste products of metabolism (urea, uric acid and creatinine) and also toxic substances (such as the phenol glucuronides and sulphates) and drugs such as salicylate.

(2) To retain those substances vital to the body; these are reabsorbed in the proximal renal tubule, as is the case for glucose and the amino acids. Likewise insulin, renin, and a whole variety of small polypeptides are reabsorbed or catabolized in the renal tubules.

(3) To maintain the constancy of the *milieu intérieur*:

(a) by regulating the water content of the body;

(b) by regulating the sodium and electrolyte content of extracellular fluid;

(c) by regulating the acid–base equilibrium of the blood. The kidney can excrete alkali directly as bicarbonate or as alkaline sodium phosphate ($Na_2H\,PO_4$); alternatively, it can excrete acid as acid sodium phosphate ($NaH_2\,PO_4$) or by the formation of ammonium ($NH_3 + H^+ = NH_4^+$).

Regulation of salt and water balance

Knowledge of how the body regulates extracellular fluid volume is still incomplete. One has to consider the role of:

(1)   glomerular filtration rate and peritubular capillary oncotic pressure;
(2)   antidiuretic hormone;
(3)   aldosterone;
(4)   the hypothetical 'natriuretic hormone';
(5)   the intrarenal prostaglandins.

Glomerular filtration and peritubular oncotic pressure
Expansion of the extracellular fluid volume will cause a rise of GFR, especially if there is a reduction of the colloid osmotic pressure of the blood so that net filtration pressure rises (see Figure 3). An increased extracellular fluid volume also causes a rise in blood pressure accompanied by a reduction of the renal vascular resistance. The overall result is a reduction in the reabsorption of salt and water, as shown in Figure 13 below.

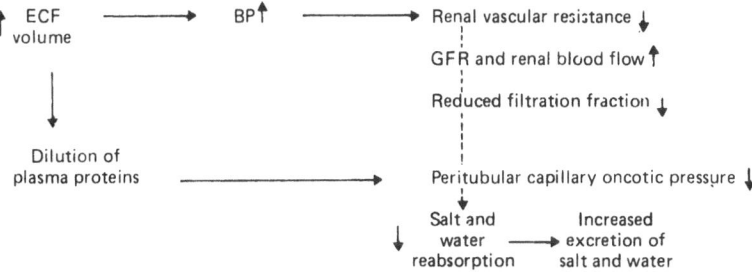

Figure 13.   Mechanism of loss of excess salt and water

There are two points to note:
(1)   The rate at which fluid is reabsorbed from the proximal tubule depends on the osmotic pressure of the blood in the peritubular capillaries.
(2)   The result of a considerable increase in renal blood flow coupled to a smaller increase in GFR is that there is a reduced filtration fraction and therefore a lowering of osmotic pressure in the peritubular capillaries. Fluid reabsorption is therefore reduced.

The converse applies in haemorrhage: there is profound vasoconstriction due to the sympathetic nervous activity and additional release of humoral catecholamines. The result is a reduction in both GFR and salt and water excretion.

In renal disease there is a fundamental difference between conditions that result in salt retention and hypertension due to glomerular damage and reduced filtration, and those conditions resulting in medullary (Henle) damage and thereby salt-wasting (Table 3).

23

Table 3

	Salt-retaining nephritis	*Salt wasting nephritis*
Features		
	Hypertension	Normal or hypotension
	Raised venous pressure	Postural hypotension
	Oedema	Possible dehydration
Causes		
	Cortical diseases	Medullary diseases
	Glomerulitis	Pyelonephritis and stone

Antidiuretic hormone
ADH is produced by the osmoreceptors of the supraoptic nuclei of the hypothalamus whenever they sense a rise in osmotic pressure of the blood. Neural impulses to the posterior pituitary then cause ADH release, and in turn this causes water reabsorption by increasing the permeability to water of the distal tubules and collecting ducts. This is possible because the ADH octapeptide which is synthesized in the supraoptic nuclei passes down the axons to the posterior pituitary whence it is released. The ring structure, as depicted below, is essential for its action. In the collecting ducts ADH activates adenylate cyclase to produce intracellular cyclic AMP, which is the 'second messenger' mediating the increase in permeability of the tubular epithelium to water.

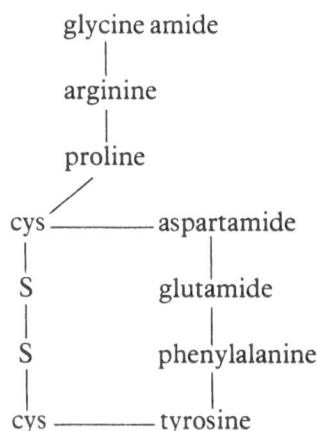

The renin–angiotensin–aldosterone mechanism
The juxtaglomerular apparatus (Figure 6) consists of baroreceptors in the wall of the afferent arteriole, which monitor the blood flow through the renal cortex, together with cells of the macula densa that are receptive to changes in

the chloride (or sodium) content of the fluid in the distal tubules of the nephron.

Thus, either renal ischaemia and/or a lowered sodium content of the distal tubule cause the release of the enzyme renin from the JGA cells. Renin is an enzyme which acts on alpha-2-globulin renin substrate, produced by the liver, and gives rise to the decapeptide angiotensin I. While passing through the lungs this is changed by the 'converting enzyme' to the octapeptide angiotensin II.

renin

$$\text{alpha-2-globulin} \xrightarrow{} \text{angiotensin I} \xrightarrow{\text{converting enzyme}} \text{angiotensin II}$$

substrate

$$(\text{angiotensinogen})(NH_2\text{---}..\text{phe-his-leu-COOH}) \longrightarrow (NH_2\text{---}..\text{phe})COOH$$
$$+ NH_2\text{-his-leu-COOH})$$

Angiotensin II is not only a powerful vasoconstrictor but it also stimulates the zona glomerulosa of the adrenal cortex to release aldosterone, and this directly stimulates the reabsorption of sodium by an action on the first part of the collecting tubule. Thus by adjustment of renin release aldosterone can be used to monitor the body's need for sodium. In effect, however, this mechanism only accounts for some 2% of the sodium that is reabsorbed (Figure 14).

Natriuretic hormone (the 'third factor')
When the extracellular fluid volume is expanded there is a reduction in salt reabsorption by the proximal tubules. Hence it has been postulated that there must be a salt-losing hormone. However, the above-mentioned changes in peritubular oncotic pressure can explain this. Furthermore, in advanced renal disease where the remaining nephrons retain a remarkable capacity for salt and water excretion, some natriuretic products of metabolism such as the hippurates and guanidines are likely to be responsible.

The prostaglandins and distribution of renal blood flow
The short nephrons of the outer renal cortex have a smaller capacity for sodium reabsorption than the longer juxtamedullary nephrons. Thus corticomedullary diversion of blood tends to cause fluid retention. This occurs when the extracellular fluid volume decreases.

For a long time it had been realized that the renal medulla produces some lipid vasodilator material, whose release in hypertension offsets the action of

25

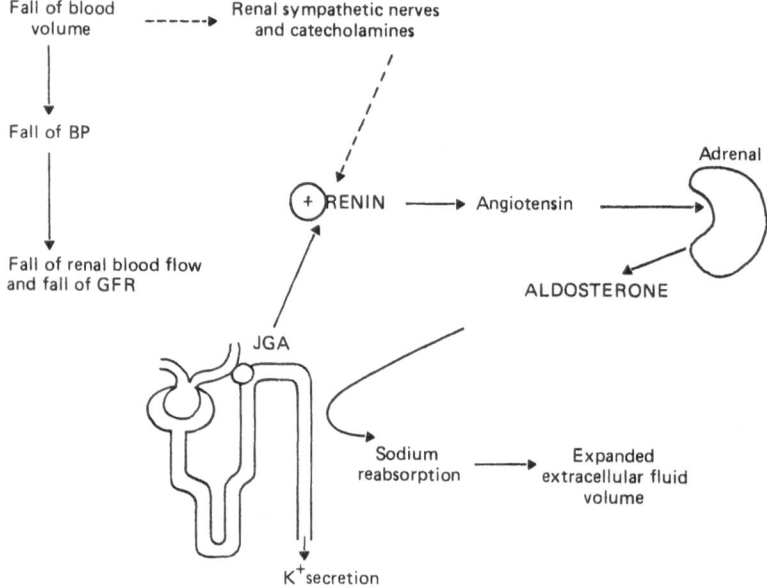

Figure 14.   Renin and aldosterone control

angiotensin. This material has been identified as prostaglandins, which are synthesized in the walls of blood vessels and also in the renomedullary interstitial cells.

The prostaglandins are 20-carbon unsaturated fatty acids with a five-membered cyclopentane ring. Synthesis is from arachidonic acid, an essential fatty acid, which becomes the substrate for prostaglandin synthetase. If there is a ketone at position 9 they are E-type, and F-type when there is an hydroxyl.

The prostaglandins

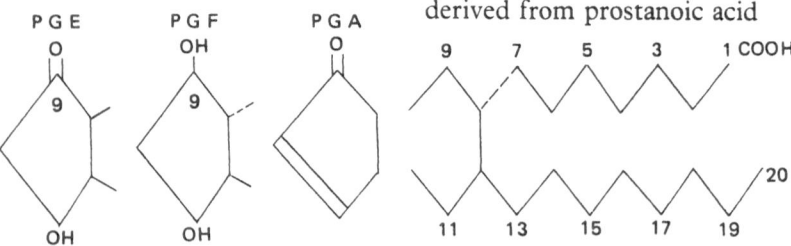

PGE_2 is the major product of the interstitial cells of the kidney. It regulates excretion of water in the collecting ducts (in opposition to ADH) but is inactivated by conversion to $PGF_2\alpha$. Kallikrein and bradykinin effects work through PGE_2.

26

It was soon found that when angiotensin II was injected into a renal artery its vasoconstrictor response was offset by the release of prostaglandin PGE. PGE causes vasodilation of the arterioles of the inner renal cortex. Thus its infusion leads to an increase in renal blood flow and to an osmotic diuresis accompanied by increased sodium and potassium excretion. Indeed the actions of acetylcholine, saline infusion, and of frusemide and ethacrynic acid could all be partly mediated by prostaglandins. Conversely when indomethacin is given to inhibit prostaglandin synthetase, there is a reduction in renal cortical blood flow. Hence there is fluid retention.

Thus E-type prostaglandins ensure adequate blood flow to the inner cortex and renal medulla, especially when circulating angiotensin is increased. It is now realised that additionally there is *a powerful hormone named prostacyclin that is produced by vascular endothelium*. In the renal cortex it, also, offsets the action of any pressor hormones, and it prevents the deposition of platelets and products of coagulation.

It is postulated that a relative deficiency of prostaglandins is relevant to hypertension. Thus in prostaglandin deficiency (as produced by indomethacin) there is inner cortical vasoconstriction with hypertension. It is reasonable to think that prostacyclin formation causes redistribution of flow within the kidneys so as to produce sodium and water loss giving protection against hypertension. However during PGF infusion renal function is hardly affected, yet there will be a pressor response related to an increased cardiac output consequent upon an enhanced vasomotor tone.

Kallikrein

There is a kallikrein in the renal tubules whose excretion seems to correlate with sodium excretion. Its urinary loss is increased in chronic renal failure, primary aldosteronism, or when there is a phaeochromocytoma. Additionally when patients are showing the 'escape phenomenon' from mineralocorticoid administration, urinary kallikrein is again increased. In about half of the patients with essential hypertension excretion is diminished; on the other hand it is increased in pregnancy hypertension.

Acid–base balance and the kidneys

The kidneys play an important role in the excretion of acids and conservation of bases:

(1) by excreting hydrogen ions;
(2) by the controlled reabsorption of bicarbonate;
(3) by producing ammonia which crosses from the cells into the tubules and there combines with hydrogen ion to form unabsorbable ammonium ions that are excreted.

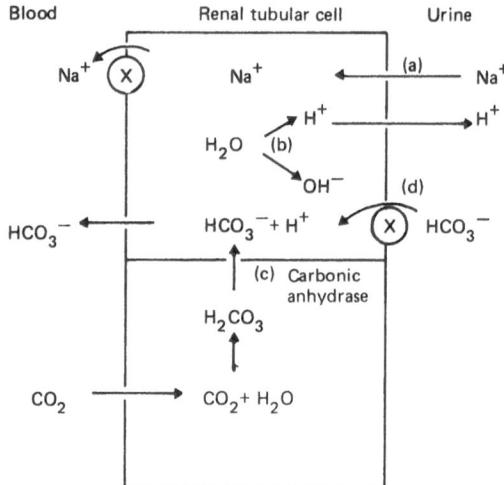

Figure 15.   Secretion of hydrogen ions and bicarbonate reabsorption

Hydrogen ion secretion/bicarbonate reabsorption
Figure 15 shows how by an active transport process hydrogen ions are secreted into the renal tubules in exchange for the reabsorption of sodium (*a*). The hydrogen ions are created from carbonic acid (*b*), (*c*). Reabsorption of bicarbonate thus occurs (*d*).

Carbonic anhydrase plays a major role in hydrogen ion secretion in the proximal tubules and luminal acidification in the distal tubules.

Bicarbonate is the most important buffer in the urine. Much is reabsorbed in the proximal tubules and the amount is in inverse proportion to the excretion of hydrogen ion. There is increased bicarbonate reabsorption and an elevation of the threshold above a serum level of 27 mmol/l:

(1)   in chronic lung disease when the pCO_2 is elevated (respiratory acidosis);
(2)   when there is chloride or potassium depletion;
(3)   when there is excessive production of adrenal hormones.

In fact, in the *proximal tubules* the urine has a pH of 6.7; in the *distal tubules* the urine has a pH of 6.4; and in the *collecting ducts* it can be as low as 4.5.

Phosphate buffering
Within the tubules the other important buffer anion is phosphate:

$$H^+ + NaHPO_4^- \quad = \quad H_2PO_4^- + Na(reabsorbed)$$

Since the phosphate carries a negative charge, it is insoluble in lipid and cannot diffuse readily into the blood. Acid is therefore excreted in the urine and sodium is reabsorbed.

Sulphate, like phosphate, is produced as part of normal protein metabolism. In the renal tubules the kidney converts the alkaline to acid salts, so bicarbonate is conserved:

$$Na_2HPO_4 \;+\; H_2CO_3 \longrightarrow NaH_2PO_4 \;+\; NaHCO_3 \text{ (reabsorbed)}$$

$$Na_2SO_4 \;+\; 2H_2CO_3 \;+\; 2NH_3 \longrightarrow (NH_4)_2SO_4 \;+\; 2NaHCO_3$$

Ammonia formation
The main source of ammonia is glutamine, which contributes both its amide and aminonitrogen to the formation of ammonium:

$$\text{glutamine} + H_2O \xrightarrow{\text{glutaminase I}} NH_4^+ + \text{glutamate}$$

$$\text{glutamate} + H_2O \xrightarrow[\text{NAD/NADH}]{\text{deaminase}} NH_4^+ + a\text{-ketoglutarate}$$
$$\text{bicarbonate}$$

Further ammonium can also be produced by the process of transamination. The overall effect, therefore, is for acids arising from protein metabolism to be excreted as *titratable acid plus ammonium.*

$$NH_3 \;+\; H^+ \longrightarrow NH_4^+ \longrightarrow \text{excreted}$$

The classical explanation is that ammonia diffuses into the lumen of the tubules and combines there with hydrogen ion to form ammonium which is excreted in the urine.

Yet with its pK of 9.1 only some 5% of the total ammonium is free ammonia, that is able to diffuse across cell membranes. However it could be that ammonium is transported by an ion pump. What is clear is that the production of α-ketoglutarate (oxoglutarate), which is a Kreb's cycle intermediate, will lead to the production of bicarbonate that is then available for intracellular buffering.

When a normal diet is consumed, protein metabolism produces 50 mmoles/day of hydrion(H^+). They arise as sulphate from sulphur containing amino acids and as phosphate and organic acids. Some 10–30 mmoles H /day can be excreted by the kidneys bound to phosphate and another 30—50 mmoles H^+ excreted bound to ammonia. The ability to excrete the anions of the organic acids depends on the glomerular filtration rate. In fact acid excretion can be represented by the formula:

urine sulphate + organic acids + 1.8 x (moles of phosphorus fed).

Patients with chronic renal disease are unable to excrete the normal acid load, a restriction largely due to an impaired ability of the kidneys to form ammonia. Additionally those patients who have a *renal tubular acidosis* are unable to reabsorb bicarbonate. Thus in chronic renal patients the plasma bicarbonate is reduced but it does nevertheless remain stable for a long period of time. Although there is retention of almost 20 mmoles/H^+ ions each day, plasma bicarbonate is steady. It is thought that this acid is buffered by the slow dissolution of the calcium salts of the skeleton and thus in the long term contributes (perhaps significantly) to renal bone disease, which appears to be worse in children and adolescents who have slowly progressive renal disease with marked acidosis. There are however alternative explanations (see page 51).

REFERENCES

Urine concentration and dilution

Berliner, R.W. (1971). Outline of renal physiology. In M.B. Strauss and L.G. Welt (eds.). *Diseases of the Kidney.* (Boston: Little Brown and Co.)

Black, D.A.K. (1965). Renal rete mirabile. *Lancet,* **ii,** 1141

Brenner, B.M. and Berliner, R.W. (1969). Peritubular protein and fluid reabsorption. *J. Clin. Invest.,* **48,** 1519

Dosseter, J.B. and Gault, M.H. (1971). *In Nephron Failure.* (Springfield, Ill: C.C. Thomas) The urinary concentrating mechanism

Giebisch, G. (1969). Effect of peritubular oncotic pressure changes on proximal tubular fluid reabsorption. *Nephron,* **6,** 260

Giebisch, G. (1972). Organisation of proximal and distal tubular electrolyte transport. *N. Engl. J. Med.,* **287,** 913

Gottschalk, C.W. (1964). Maximum urine concentration. *Am. J. Med.,* **36,** 670

Green, R., Windhager, E. and Giebisch, G. (1974). Action of anti-diuretic hormone. *Am. J. Physiol.,* **226,** 265

Jamison, R. L. and Maffly, R.H. (1976). Osmotic concentration and dilution of the urine. *N. Engl. J. Med.,* **295,** 1059

Miles, B.F., Paton, A. and de Wardener, H.E. (1954). The counter-current system (role of the loop of Henle). *Br. Med. J.,* **2,** 901

Orloff, J. and Handler, S. (1964). *Amer. J. Med.,* **36,** 686

de Rouffinac, C. (1972). Coupled ion and fluid transport in the kidney. *Kidney Int.,* **2,** 297

Smith, H.W. (1956). *Principles of Renal Physiology*. (Oxford: Oxford University Press)
Spitzer, A. and Windhager, E.E. (1970). Intra-renal control of proximal tubule reabsorption of sodium and water. *Am. J. Physiol.*, **218**, 1188
de Wardener, H.E. (1976). *The Kidney*. (Boston: Little Brown and Co.)
Windhager, E.E., Lewy, J.E. and Spitzer, A. (1969). Relation of peritubular albumin to sodium reabsorption. *Nephron*, **6**, 247

Sodium metabolism

Bricker, N.S. (1967). Effect of spironolactone on urinary kallikrein. *Am. J. Med.*, **43**, 313
Bricker, N.S. (1967). Control of sodium excretion with normal and reduced nephrons: role of third factor. *Am. J. Med.*, **43**, 313
Earley, L.E. and Daugharty, T.M. (1969). Sodium metabolism. *N. Engl. J. Med.*, **281**, 72
Editorial. (1978). Salt and hypertension. *Lancet*, **i,** 1136
Mills, I. (1970). Renal regulation of sodium excretion. *Ann. Rev. Med.*, **21,** 75
Seino, M. (1977). Effect of spironolactone on urinary kallikrein. *Tokohu J. Exp. Med.*, **121**, 111
Smith, H.W. (1957). Salt and water volume receptors. *Am. J. Med.*, **23,** 623

Acid–base balance

Garello, S., Chang, B.S. and Kahn, S.I. (1975). Dilution acidosis and contraction alkalosis. *Kidney Int.*, **8**, 279
Gennari, F.J. and Cohen, J.L. (1975). Potassium homeostasis and acid–base balance. *Kidney Int.*, **8**, 1
Lemann, J. and Relman, A.S. (1965). Net balance of acid in subjects given large loads of acid and alkali. *J. Clin. Invest.*, **44**, 507
Krebs, H.A. and Vinay, P. (1975). Regulation of renal ammonia production. *Med. Clin. N. Am.*, **59**, 3, 595
Pitts, R.F. (1964). Renal production and excretion of ammonia. *Am. J. Med.*, **36**, 720
Pitts, R.F. (1971). Ammonia and acid-base balance. *N. Engl. J. Med.*, **284,** 32
Relman, A.S. (1968). The acidosis of renal disease. *Am. J. Med.*, **44**, 706
Welbourne, T.C. (1975). Renal ammonia production in chronic acidosis. *Med. Clin. N. Am.*, **59** 3, 629
Wrong, O. and Davies, H. (1969). Excretion of acid in renal disease. *Qt. J. Med.*, **28**, 259

Renal tubular acidosis

Buckalew, V.M. (1974). *Medicine (Baltimore)*, **53**, 229

Feest, T.G., Wrong, O.M. (1975). *Ann. Intern. Med.*, **82**, 584

Gennary, F., Cohen, J.J. (1978). *Ann. Rev. Med.*, **29**, 521

Symposia on renal pathophysiology

Kurtzman, N.A. (1973). *Arch. Intern. Med.*, **131**, 779

Thurau, K. (1976). *Kidney and Urinary Tract Physiology. MTP Int. Rev. Science and Physiology.* Series One. Vol. 6. (Lancaster: MTP)

Renal circulation

Barger, A.C. and Herd, J.A. (1971). *N. Engl. J. Med.*, **284**, 482

Pomeranz, B.H., Birtch, A.G., Barger, A.C. (1968). Neural control of intrarenal blood flow. *Am. J. Physiol.*, **215**, 1067

Thurau, K. (1964). Renal haemodynamics. *Am. J. Med.*, **36**, 698

Renal function tests

Braude, H., Forfar, J.O., Gould, J.C. and McLeod, J.W. (1967). Cell and bacterial counts in urine of children. *Br. Med. J.*, **4**, 697

Britton, K.E. and Brown, N.J.G. (1971). Clinical renography. (London: Lloyd-Luke)

Brody, L.H., Salladay, J.R. and Armbruster, K. (1971). Urinalysis and sediment. *Med. Clin. N. Am.*, **55**, 243

Chantler, C., Garnett, E.S., Parsons, V. and Veall, N. (1969). Measurement of G.F.R. by single injection of E.D.T.A. *Clin. Sci.*, **37**, 169

Kassirer, J.P. (1971). Evaluation of glomerular function. *N. Engl. J. Med.*, **285**, 385

Kassirer, J.P. (1971b). Evaluation of tubular function. *N. Engl. J. Med.*, **285**, 499

Ram, M., Evans, K. and Chisholm, G.D. (1967). Measurement of effective renal plasma flow by clearance of 125-hippuran. *Lancet*, **ii**, 645

Urine analysis

Free, A.H. and Free, H.M. (1975). C.R.C. Press.

2
Diuretics and renal metabolism

Most clinicians use a wide range of diuretic agents. The following is a standard classification, and indicates their principal site of action.

(1) *Osmotic diuretics*—mannitol (5%)
(2) *Inorganic and organic mercurials* (20%)
(3) *Sulphonamide derivatives*—acetazolamide—proximal tubule (5%); thiazides—proximal tubule and distal cortical diluting segment inhibitors (10%)
(4) *High-ceiling diuretics*—basically loop inhibitors; bumetanide, frusemide and ethacrynic acid (25%)
(5) *Potassium-sparing diuretics* (distal tubule inhibitors)—triamterene and amiloride, 2–3% each); tienelic acid (also uricosuric)
(6) *Aldosterone antagonist*—acting at the distal tubule; spironolactone (2%)

The figure in parentheses gives the % filtered sodium loss caused by the diuretic. It is advisable at this point to refer again to the physiology of the reabsorption of sodium and chloride, which is shown in Figure 7

There are really only three points that need be emphasized.

33

(1) As much as 70% of the filtered sodium and water is reabsorbed iso-osmotically in the proximal tubules. At this level bicarbonate reabsorption and in turn the action of the enzyme carbonic anhydrase are vital (see Figure 15).

$$CO_2 + H_2O \longrightarrow HCO_3^- \quad + \quad H^+ \longrightarrow H^+ \text{ secreted}$$

$$Na^+ \longleftarrow Na^+ \text{ reabsorbed}$$

(2) Active reabsorption of chloride ions is now known to be the primary process in the ascending thick loop of Henle. Reabsorption of chloride causes the voltage to be positive within the lumina of the Henle loops and thus sodium transport becomes a passive process driven by that voltage.

(3) There are several functional levels in the distal tubule that should be carefully distinguished:

   (a) the cortical diluting segment where NaCl is reabsorbed leaving water in the lumen;
   (b) the distal tubule exchange segment where Na^+ is reabsorbed and K^+ secreted;
   (c) the aldosterone-sensitive segment, which is the early part of the collecting duct.

Osmotic diuretics

Mannitol is the standard example. Its several actions are as follows:

(1) Infusion causes a diminution in the osmotic pressure of proteins in the afferent arterioles and peritubular capillaries and therefore diminished reabsorption of sodium.

(2) It causes an increase in renal plasma flow and glomerular hydrostatic pressure secondary to vasodilation of the afferent arteriole.

(3) There is an osmotic effect in the proximal tubule withdrawing water into the lumen.

(4) Reduction in the osmolality of the renal medulla, in part due to increased flow in the vasá rectae, means less sodium chloride reabsorption in the ascending loop of Henle and less water reabsorption in the descending loop of Henle and collecting ducts.

Mercurials

Mercury is well known as an inhibitor of the sulphydryl groups of enzymes and proteins. It binds non-specifically to many proteins, including the binding protein metallothionein of the renal tubules, and also to mitochondria. Indeed it is quite likely that mercury stops proton transport across the inner mitochondrial membrane. Additionally it inhibits glycolysis and sodium–potassium ATPase.

The main action of the mercurials, in fact, is to inhibit active chloride transport in the ascending loop of Henle.

Sulphonamide derivatives

In 1949 it was realized that patients with congestive heart failure who were receiving sulphanilamide showed an increased excretion of sodium and water. This was found to be due to inhibition of the enzyme *carbonic anhydrase*. From this observation came the development of acetazolamide (Diamox).

The feature common to these molecules is the *sulphamoyl group*, as is evident from the following structural formulae:

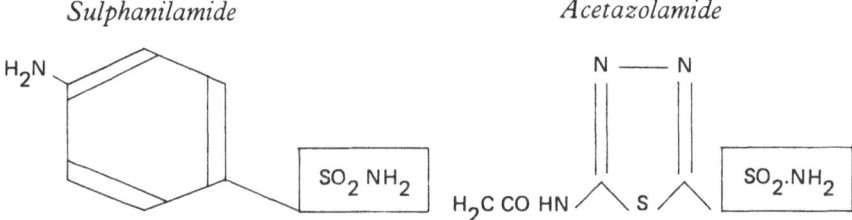

In time this led to the synthesis of the *thiazides*, as can be seen from the sequential formulae:

The thiazides form a whole series of diuretics of widely varying potency. Many are carbonic anhydrase inhibitors but this is not vital to their action. They all tend to inhibit Na–K ATPase, glycolysis, uptake of free fatty acids and energy metabolism in mitochondria.

Their major action is distal to the ascending loop of Henle. Indeed any proximal tubule effects are probably due to inhibition of carbonic anhydrase so that bicarbonate is flushed down the tubules. Since it is not absorbable distally, it acts as an osmotic diuretic. The chloride loss which they cause is due to inhibition of metabolism in the distal tubules. Thiazides are also known to be inhibitors of the aerobic glycolysis that is a feature of the renal medulla and of fatty acid metabolism in the distal tubules.

Chlorthalidone (Hygroton) has an action that can last 72h. It does not undergo metabolic degradation in the body, but shows preferential and prolonged binding to the renal tubules.

Chlorthalidone

High-ceiling diuretics

The most powerful diuretics are those which inhibit chloride transport in the ascending loop of Henle. They are derived from the thiazides.

Frusemide

Bumetanide

On the other hand ethacrynic acid is derived from aryloxy-acetic acid. The aryloxy-group has an active sulphydryl binding propensity and, in fact, ethacrynic-cysteine is the active diuretic within the tubule.

Aryloxy-acetic acid

Ethacrynic acid

36

The following points about high-ceiling diuretics should be noted:

(1)   Since these agents decrease the clearance of free water (CH_2O) during water diuresis, that is, they cause the addition of solute, and stop the reabsorption of free water (TcH_2O) during hydropenia, their action must be on the ascending limb of the loop of Henle.

(2)   As they also cause loss of phosphate and bicarbonate in the urine, both frusemide and bumetanide must have proximal tubular inhibitory actions.

(3)   Additionally they cause a redistribution of renal blood flow so that washout of medullary solute occurs.

(4)   The potassium loss notable with these agents is consequent on the delivery of increased sodium to the distal tubule, so that there is increased sodium–potassium exchange. (Figure 20.)

The exact mode of action of high-ceiling diuretics is contentious. Three basic processes have to be considered:

(1)   inhibition of Na–K ATPase;
(2)   inhibition of glycolysis;
(3)   inhibition of mitochondrial oxidative phosphorylation.

Sodium–potassium ATPase has certainly a high activity *distally* in the renal tubules and this suggests an important role in sodium reabsorption. One will recall that the sodium pump mechanism works according to the scheme as shown:

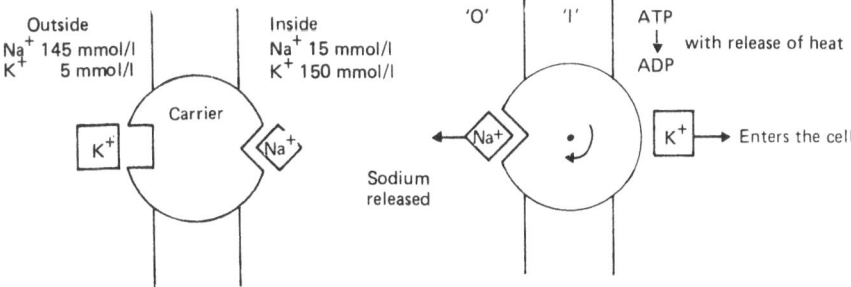

Figure 16.   The sodium pump

The object is to pump sodium ions out of the cell and concurrently to move potassium inwards. This is done by means of a carrier which is the actual ATPase enzyme, driven by the energy of ATP. Since energy conservation is limited, some heat is liberated. The important point is that the Na–K ATPase is located in the distal tubules. Indeed its synthesis (but not its activity) is regulated by aldosterone. Normally it only accounts for a small fraction (2%) of sodium reabsorption.

When one kidney is removed the other has to take on increased sodium reabsorption. The remaining kidney then shows an adaptive increase of its Na–K ATPase by some 55%. Adrenaelectomy prevents this adaptive response.

Na–K ATPase is easily inhibited by frusemide and ethacrynic acid, as well as by the mercurials. On the other hand the thiazides have little effect. Spironolactone has no direct action but it does prevent synthesis of the enzyme. At all levels of the renal tubule sodium reabsorption is an energy-dependent process proportional to the utilization of oxygen; cyanide and other metabolic inhibitors are known to cause diuresis. In the kidney the proximal tubules and loops of Henle, but not the distal tubules, are rich in mitochondria. Thus in the proximal tubules it is mitochondrial oxidative phosphorylation that provides the energy. Studies of inhibition of oxidative phosphorylation by mitochondria, using the oxygen consumption rate as measured in a Warburg manometer or the Gilson oxygraph, show that the diuretic dosages required to produce 50% inhibition can be arranged in the order—chloromeradrin<ethacrynate<frusemide<thiazide<acetazolamide. Thus these diuretics act by reducing ATP production.

Potassium-sparing diuretics

Amiloride and triamterene are alike in structure. They each act on the distal exchange segment, where normally three ions of sodium are reabsorbed for each of two ions of potassium and one of hydrogen that are excreted. In this part of the distal tubule the negative potential of the lumen is independent of mineralocorticoid.

Amiloride   *Triamterene*

Amiloride is a guanidine, which is known to inhibit oxidative phosphorylation and may, in fact, function as a 'third factor' natriuretic substance in patients with renal failure.

Tienilic acid (an ethacrynate derivative) also acts as a diuretic at the diluting segment of the distal tubule. It is particularly noted for its uricosuric property since it inhibits urate reabsorption in the proximal and distal tubules.

The aldosterone antagonist: spironolactone

The early part of the collecting duct is the aldosterone-dependent segment, and here some 1% of the filtered sodium can be reabsorbed. Spironolactone is an antagonist which acts by competition with aldosterone for its cytoplasmic receptors. Normally aldosterone would be translocated thence onto the DNA of the nuclei, where it can then affect the rate of transcription of enzymes such as ATPase. Since the affinity of spironolactone for the receptor is only 1/1000 that of aldosterone, Aldactone has to be given in large doses (100 mg b.d. SR or 50 mg q.i.d. of Aldactone 25) and there is a characteristic delay of 3–4 days before it is effective.

Summary of diuretic action

The above information on diuretics shows that there has been a phase of uncertainty as to how the diuretics actually work. In reality much of the confusion has stemmed from a lack of appreciation of the fact that sodium reabsorption in the proximal tubules must differ from that in the distal tubules.

These differences can be summarized as follows:

(1) *Proximal tubule reabsorption and the ascending loop of Henle.* Chloride reabsorption occurs with that of sodium and water. Here it is not inhibited by ouabain, but it is inhibited by ethacrynic acid, which inhibits mitochondria.

(2) *The distal tubule.* Sodium reabsorption occurs in exchange for potassium by the pump mechanism, which depends on the activity of Na–K ATPase, and this is directly inhibited by ouabain.

Thus when considering proximal tubule inhibition one has to take account of mitochondrial oxidative phosphorylation and its inhibition by most diuretics. Such agents act by reducing ATP production. Those diuretics which also inhibit Na–K ATPase have a distal tubule diuretic action. Since aldosterone controls the synthesis rate of Na–K ATPase, its antagonist, spironolactone, also acts at the distal site.

At a fundamental level, then, there is still controversy as to how each diuretic functions, but the knowledge to date can be summarized as in Table 4.

Table 4 Mode of action of the diuretics

	Ethacrynate	Frusemide	Thiazides	Mercurials	Aldactone
Inhibition of glycolysis	+	+	+	+	
free fatty acid uptake		+	+	+	
Oxidation by mitochondria	++	++	+	+++	
Vital enzymes SH enzymes	+			+++	
carbonic anhydrase ATPase	+	+	+/o	++	synthesis
Effect R Na/Q_{O_2}	↓	↓	O_2 ↓	O_2 ↓	

Each reduces sodium reabsorption (RNa) for a given oxygen consumption (Q_{O2}).

MODE OF ACTION OF DIURETICS

Sodium reabsorption from the mucosal to the serosal side of the *toad bladder* can be measured by the short-circuit current needed to reduce the potential difference across the membrane to zero. Either oxygen consumption or anaerobic glycolysis can be measured. It can be shown that the transport depends on the action of Na–K ATPase which is inhibited by ouabain. Indeed aldosterone promotes sodium reabsorption after a delay of some 4 h, which is the time required to stimulate RNA and enzyme-protein synthesis.

Vasopressin (ADH) enhances the permeability of the mucosa to water, by means of cyclic AMP stimulation. At the same time there is an increased flux of sodium by 'solvent drag' together with an increase in oxygen consumption.

Studies with erythrocytes

There are probably three types of sodium pump in the red cell but the principal one determines outflux of sodium and is coupled to the inward movement of potassium. It is inhibited by ouabain. There is a second pump which is inhibited by ethacrynic acid. It is therefore possible to examine some diuretics by their ability to inhibit the efflux of ^{24}Na from erythrocytes. If N_0 are the counts inside at time zero, and N_t the remaining counts at time t, then a plot of log $1-\dfrac{N_t}{N_0}$ against time expresses the rate of

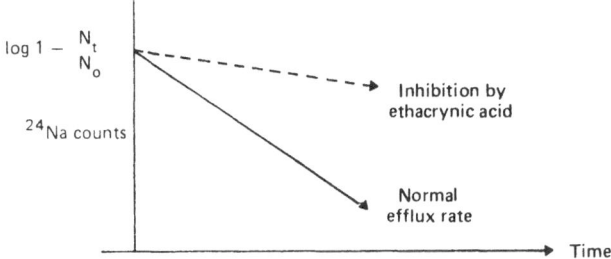

Figure 17.   Efflux of sodium from erythrocytes

extrusion of sodium from the red cells. The slope is reduced by an ATPase inhibitor, such as ethacrynic acid.

Stop–flow analysis

This has been used in the intact animal. A mannitol diuresis is started and when there is a high urine flow, the ureters are clamped for 15 min. The various portions of the tubule then equilibrate at their own levels so that when the clamp is released the tubular fractions can be collected sequentially for analysis.

Micropuncture studies

These give a better idea of what is happening in the tubules, but results have differed in the hands of various workers and certainly local drug action cannot be differentiated from changes due to an altered body composition or to changes in renal haemodynamics. There are various approaches.

Stop–flow micropuncture
It is clear that the glomerular hydrostatic pressure is equal to the sum of the stop–flow pressure and the colloid osmotic pressure of the blood.

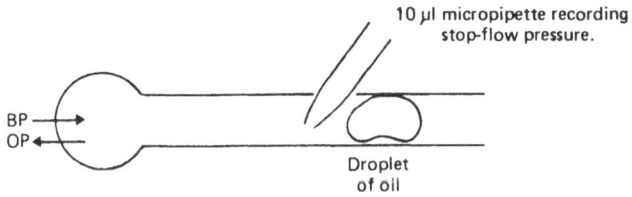

Figure 18   Stop–flow micropuncture

Free-flow micropuncture
This is performed in a similar manner by placing a pipette in the proximal tubule which is identified by intravenous injection of lissamine green. Osmolarity, inulin concentration and electrolytes are measured. At any point along the tubule the inulin concentration is a measure of the amount of sodium that has been absorbed (Figure 19a).

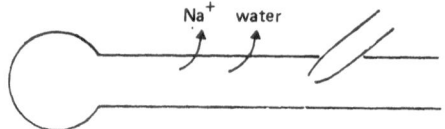

Figure 19. (a) Free–flow micropuncture

The split oil droplet technique
Two droplets of oil are placed in the tubule and fluid is injected between them. One can then measure the rate at which saline is reabsorbed by means of rapid-sequence photography over a period of some 10 sec. (Figure 19b).

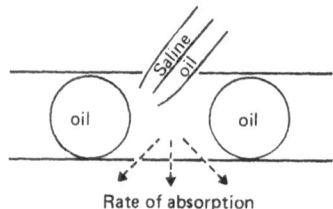

Figure 19. (b) Split oil droplet technique

Clearance studies in man

First it is necessary to establish a water diuresis by giving 1½ l of fluid at 7 am and a further litre at 8 am. Inulin is then infused in normal saline so as to calculate GFR under steady state conditions. The urine is collected in quarter hourly aliquots for analysis and at the same time an equivalent replacement quality is given by mouth. After 2 h the influence of a particular diuretic might be examined. Typical results are as shown below:

	U_{osmol} (mosmol/kg)	U_{Na} (nmol/min)	C_{H_2O} (ml/min)
Control period	55	150	11.5
Diuretic period	150	2000	12.2

METABOLIC COMPLICATIONS OF DIURETIC THERAPY

Metabolic alkalosis with potassium depletion

It is now realized that metabolic alkalosis and potassium depletion are the result of chloride deficiency caused by long-term diuretic administration.

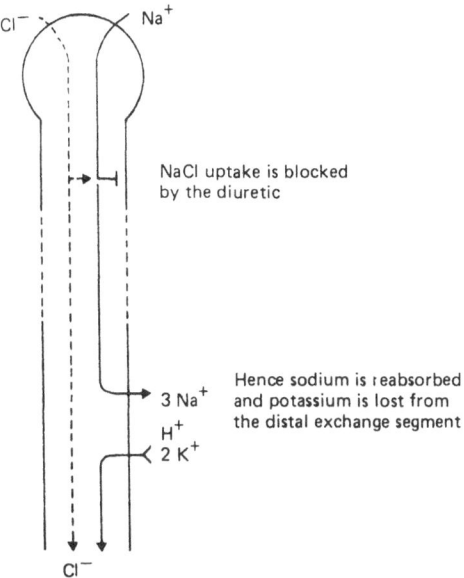

Figure 20. **Diuretic induced metabolic alkalosis with hypokalaemia**

It has been found by experience that administration of sodium or potassium without chloride does not restore either the potassium or the bicarbonate levels to normal. Chloride is essential for correction of the alkalosis. In a post-diuretic alkalosis the urinary chloride is less than 20 mEq/l, so chloride administration (usually as potassium chloride tablets) re-establishes the normal acid–base balance.

Potassium depletion may present with muscle weakness or ileus, though this is uncommon. Certainly digitalis intoxication is a greater risk. In patients with chronic bronchitis and respiratory insufficiency the metabolic alkalosis of diuretic therapy raises the plasma bicarbonate even further and is thus dangerous. For each rise of bicarbonate of 1 mEq/l the pCO$_2$ will rise by 0.9 mmHg.

Potassium chloride supplements have to be administered carefully in chronic renal failure patients or diabetics as the serum potassium may rise rapidly. The alternative (which can also be dangerous in the risk groups) is to use one of the potassium-sparing diuretics.

Hyperuricaemia

Uric acid is freely filtered at the glomeruli, reabsorbed in the proximal tubules and then secreted again in the distal tubules.

Since most diuretics are organic acids and are secreted by the proximal tubules they exert competitive effects on the tubular absorption/secretion processes. As the thiazides compete for secretory sites they cause hyperuricaemia by inhibition of uric acid secretion. Contraction of the blood volume also plays a part because, although ethacrynic acid and frusemide reduce uric acid clearance, this is not so if the plasma volume is maintained by saline infusion. Occasionally gout may be precipitated by diuretics.

Hyponatraemia

This occurs because of the inability of the tubule to excrete free water because of the inhibition of sodium reabsorption at the dilution site. As it is a dilutional hyponatraemia it responds to water restriction. More rarely there may be true salt depletion and signs of dehydration.

Hyperglycaemia

Thiazides and frusemide may either aggravate pre-existing diabetes or cause it in individuals so predisposed. Not only do they decrease insulin secretion, but they also inhibit the utilization of glucose by adipose tissue.

Effects on calcium metabolism

Most of the reabsorption of calcium and magnesium occurs in the proximal tubules. Calcium, however, is also reabsorbed in the loop of Henle, and magnesium in the distal convoluted tubules. Hence many diuretics produce a significant increase in calcium excretion. In fact, frusemide infusion can be used to correct hypercalcaemia.

On the other hand, as the thiazides are known to reduce urinary calcium excretion, they have been used to treat idiopathic hypercalcuria with calculus formation. They are also used for prophylaxis of immobilization osteoporosis.

Water intoxication

Since chlorothiazide reduces the excretion of free water by stimulating adenylcyclase in the collecting ductules and facilitating the action of vasopressin, it has been applied to the treatment of partial diabetes insipidus. Occasionally its use in other situations will lead to the development of water intoxication as is evident from hyponatraemia. Chlorpropamide and carbamazepine have a similar effect.

DIURETIC USAGE

Some 200 l of extracellular fluid are filtered each day by the kidneys, yet the normal urine volume is only 1–1½ litres. An increase flow of urine may be produced by the following means:

(1) by a diuretic;
(2) by an increase of the cardiac output and renal blood flow, as when digitalis is given for heart failure or dopamine is infused in cirrhosis;
(3) by maintaining the colloid osmotic pressure of the blood and raising the blood volume by protein infusion in patients with nephrotic syndrome;
(4) by inhibition of release of antidiuretic hormone by means of intravenous ethanol.

In oedema

Diuretics are used for congestive heart failure, nephrotic syndrome or hepatic ascites. Each of these conditions may be complicated by secondary aldosteronism. Of all the diuretics frusemide is most valuable to the nephrologist since its low toxicity permits dosages as high as 2 g/day for long periods. In addition to its powerful action on the loop of Henle it tends to redistribute renal blood flow from the inner to the outer cortex so that there is better nephron perfusion and an increase of the glomerular filtration rate. Clearly a greater response with less risk of potassium depletion can be obtained if frusemide is combined with spironolactone (Aldactone 25 mg q.i.d. or 100 mg b.d.).

Water diuresis is often impaired in advanced nephrosis, cirrhosis and congestive failure. This is due to (a) reduced glomerular filtration, (b) depression of osmolar clearance (C_{osm}) or rate of sodium excretion, and (c) persistence of high levels of vasopressin (ADH). In fact, impaired water output seems to correlate closely with the severity of the illness. Apart from frusemide, both ethanol and mannitol are known for their ability to clear water from the body. Thus in cirrhotics, in whom the urine is known to remain hypertonic even after water loading, a mannitol infusion will increase the C_{osm} and the water clearance.

In nephrotic syndrome

For many years the standard treatment has been a low salt, high protein diet (in so far as this is not a paradox). At times of plasma volume depletion associated with severe hypoproteinaemia, salt-free albumin infusions are used (20–40 g albumin). Today the patient's diuretic response is titrated, whilst gradually increasing doses of frusemide and spironolactone are added. In the 'minimal change' types, and often in focal or proliferative disease, steroid therapy is used. There is no doubt that this helps by increasing the GFR and it may reduce the permeability of the basement membrane to protein. Prednisone, however, has many undesirable side-effects. Thus it adds to the potassium loss and must therefore be prescribed with care.

In hepatic ascites

The avid retention of sodium at GFR levels of 20–90 ml/min can be explained by a combination of hyperaldosteronism and reduced renal perfusion. It is presumed that a raised intrahepatic pressure is the cause of the renal cortical hypoperfusion and that this causes renin release and so hyperaldosteronism. Pressure on the inferior vena cava by the liver also leads to sodium retention. The problem is further complicated by the fact that patients do not 'escape' from the sodium-retaining effects of aldosterone, and this could result from impaired production of a natriuretic hormone. More likely it is related to a failure to expand the effective blood volume, which in cirrhosis is always lower than anticipated owing to pooling in the splanchnic area and as a result of fluid leakage into the peritoneum in the formation of ascites.

The treatment is akin to that of the nephrotic syndrome. A low salt diet is given together with a high protein intake, if that is not contraindicated by the risk of hepatic failure. The dosage of frusemide is adjusted while the patient also receives spironolactone. As far as possible removal of ascites is to be avoided since it depletes the body of protein, but ascitic fluid reinfusion into a vein by means of the Rhône–Poulenc apparatus is being advocated since it certainly produces a diuresis. There is a risk of bacteraemia and intravascular coagulation. Better alternatives are the use of ultrafiltration (p. 352) or the insertion of a LeVeen shunt (p. 281).

In chronic renal failure

When the patient with chronic renal failure has a GFR of less than 10 ml/min he has little freedom with his fluid intake, which usually has to be strictly controlled. However, the use of frusemide increases the urinary flow and gives slightly greater flexibility. The possible side-effects are nausea and loss of hearing.

In hypertension

Salt plays an integral role in the hypertensive process as is shown by the increased sodium content of the smooth muscle of the arterial walls. Even so, subjects with hypertension excrete salt readily. This is explained by a decrease in the reabsorption of fluid by the proximal tubules due to an alteration of renal haemodynamics. However, once renal failure develops, the blood pressure increases in proportion to the degree of salt retention and therefore correlates with the body weight.

Diuretics are used in hypertension (a) because a reduction of blood volume reduces the cardiac output and so lowers the blood pressure, and (b) because the associated sodium depletion reduces the vascular reactivity and lowers the pressor responses. Thus, although the use of powerful diuretics causes renin release and angiotensin generation, there is no practical problem in treatment.

A thiazide diuretic or chlorthalidone is generally used. Frusemide is chosen either when rapid sodium depletion is needed for severe hypertension, or when there is complicating chronic renal insufficiency and a need to increase the GFR.

RENAL METABOLISM

The above section on diuretic action serves to emphasize how interest in the details of renal metabolism is developing. An overall scheme of energy production and utilization has to be envisaged. The basic foods are glucose, fatty acids and amino acids and the aim is the production of energy at ATP, as shown in Figure 21.

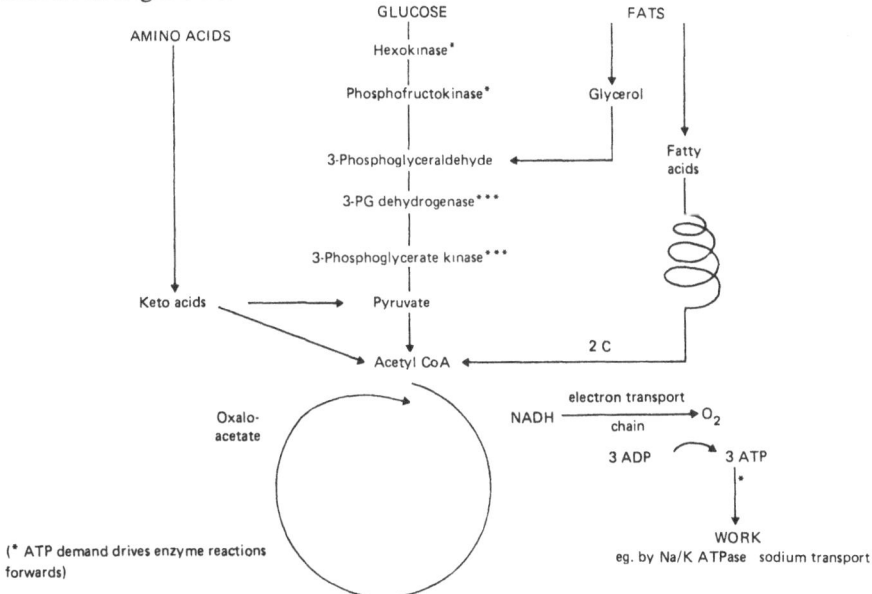

Figure 21. Production and utilization of ATP

The crucial question is how is the utilization of ATP geared to demand and so to the flux in the glycolytic pathway and the Kreb's cycle? In fact, ATP accumulation by feedback inhibition (for example, on hexokinase) and by allosteric regulation (for example, on phosphofructokinase) can exert restraint on glucose utilization. Such points are marked (*). However, the main regulatory step is where ATP demand is pulling the glyceraldehyde dehydrogenase and the phosphoglycerate kinase step forwards (***).

It becomes apparent, therefore, that the use of ATP for sodium pumping by Na–K ATPase in turn promotes further ATP formation (a) by promotion of glycolysis, and (b) by increased oxidative metabolism.

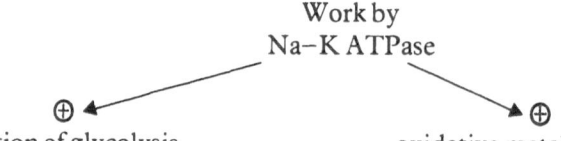

Work by
Na–K ATPase

promotion of glycolysis $\oplus$ oxidative metabolism is stimulated
via glyceraldehyde-P-dehydrogenase   because ADP release stimulates
and phosphoglycerate kinase   mitochondrial respiration $\oplus$

1:3 diP-glycerate + ADP = 3.P.glycerate + ATP

As already explained, mitochondrial metabolism and energy production is of prime importance for sodium reabsorption in the proximal tubules and loop of Henle. The actual substrates utilized by the kidneys are shown in Table 5.

Table 5 Production of energy by the renal cortex

From:				
glucose			20–25%	
FFA	(palmitate) (ketones)		20%	
citrate			10%	
lactate	(alkalosis) 40%			(acidosis) 10%
glutamine (alkalosis) 10%				(acidosis) 40%

It is a remarkable fact that the kidneys appear to abstract no glucose from the blood, but of course they have an amazing capacity for gluconeogenesis. In fact, in starvation they produce as much as 40g/day of glucose, which represents 45% of whole body gluconeogenesis. Naturally glucose is a suitable substrate for providing the kidneys with energy. Although they only form 0.5% of the body weight, they account for 10% of the basal oxygen consumption and this is expended on the 99% reabsorption of filtered sodium that they have to maintain. Some thirty moles of sodium are reabsorbed per mol of oxygen utilized. With a P/O ratio of 3, this means that 6 mmol ATP are produced for each molecule of oxygen consumed and in turn this energy reabsorbs 30 mmol of sodium. Thus the kidneys can reabsorb 5 mmol of sodium for every 1 mmol of ATP formed. This is high efficiency for only 3 mmol of sodium are transported per 1 mmol ATP in muscles, erythrocytes and the skin.

As Table 5 above shows free fatty acids, particularly palmitate, are used up avidly by the kidneys. Palmitate is, in fact, used preferentially to glucose by the renal cortex; 1 mole of palmitate does provide 130 moles ATP! On the other hand the renal medulla prefers aerobic or anaerobic glycolysis, but in this way 1 mol of glucose only produces 38 mol ATP.

Both lactate and glutamine are abstracted by the kidneys. Lactate utilization is greatest in alkalosis when the glycolytic rate is normally highest. Conversely glutamine utilization is greatest in acidosis when the need is to produce ammonia.

It appears that blood flow to the renal cortex, and glucose and oxygen consumption are all closely correlated with the reabsorption of sodium. The kidney is the only organ in the body in which oxygen consumption is related to blood flow. Moreover, when sodium reabsorption is inhibited the partial pressure of oxygen in the urine actually rises. Glucose will support sodium reabsorption to the extent of at least 95% of the filtered load, since oxidative phosphorylation is particularly high in the renal cortex and there is aerobic or anaerobic metabolism in the medulla. It has long been recognized, however, that the respiratory quotient of the renal cortex is 0.75 and this must mean that fatty acids and acetoacetate are normally being used as a fuel. Indeed fatty acid oxidation is known to be great in the ascending loops of Henle.

When the kidneys are deprived of glucose as in starvation or with the insulin lack of uncontrolled diabetes, then there is a switch to gluconeogenesis using lactate as a basic fuel. The renal cortex and medulla oxidize fatty acids during starvation. So there is an elevation of citrate which by its feedback inhibition of phosphofructokinase lowers glucose utilization. At the same time the oxidation of fatty acids gives rise to acetyl-CoA, there is an inhibition of pyruvate dehydrogenase, and pyruvate is then reconverted back to glucose. Additionally the alanine abstraction of the kidneys rises markedly when it is being mobilized from the muscles in starvation, and it is used as substrate for gluconeogenesis.

Naturally studies have been made of the distribution of enzymes in the various parts of the nephron. As already mentioned, Na–K ATPase is found mainly in the distal tubules where its activity can be promoted by aldosterone. Hexokinase shows a low activity in the proximal and a high capacity in the distal tubules, as also do the other enzymes of glycolysis such as glyceraldehyde-phosphate dehydrogenase and pyruvate kinase. The Kreb's cycle enzymes and marker enzymes for gluconeogenesis, namely glucose-6-phosphatase and phosphoenolpyruvate carboxykinase, are found mainly in the proximal tubules. The key enzyme of ammoniogenesis, glutamic dehydrogenase, is also found in the proximal tubules.

Ammonia formation

The ability of the kidney to increase ammonia formation so as to facilitate hydrogen ion excretion is enhanced in the metabolic acidosis that accompanies chronic renal failure or renal tubular acidosis, and also in starvation. As explained above (page 29) ammonia is derived from glutamine, some two-thirds coming from the amide nitrogen and the other third from the amine-N of glutamine. Whatever the intimate cause of this adaptive change it is slow, taking several days to become established.

Bourke emphasizes that acidosis influences the urea cycle so that nitrogen is diverted to ammonium formation. Acidosis stops the utilization of bicarbonate (which is the first step in the urea cycle), so that this is then available for buffering. The ammonium in the liver becomes attached as glutamine, which is then carried by the blood to the kidneys.

Parathormone and the renal tubules

Parathormone (PTH) causes phosphate reabsorption in the proximal tubules, which is a cyclic AMP-mediated process. In fact PTH acts in the peritubular capillaries on the base of the renal tubular cells, and the cAMP that is formed within the cell stimulates the formation of a protein kinase which then induces phosphate reabsorption at the brush border.

In hyperparathyroid disease the serum chloride is raised so causing a hyperchloraemic acidosis, which correlates with a reduced ability of the tubules to reabsorb bicarbonate. Moreover, even in the anephric patient parathormone can influence the body acid–base balance; this probably results from its ability to affect the intake of phosphate by other tissues.

Renal tubular acidosis

Renal tubular acidosis (RTA) is when the kidney is unable to acidify the urine normally. In the *distal tubule* type this is because of an inability to maintain the necessary hydrogen ion gradient for secretion. It is thus called 'gradient-limitation RTA'. Patients cannot acidify their urine and may lack carbonic anhydrase in their distal tubules.

In the *proximal tubule* form there is a failure to reabsorb bicarbonate, so more than 15% of the filtered bicarbonate is lost. This proximal type is accompanied, as might be expected, by loss of phosphate, glucose and amino acids. There can also be urinary loss of potassium giving rise to severe hypokalaemic weakness. Osteomalacia occurs in some cases because of calcium

50

loss and acidosis. Bicarbonate-wasting RTA is sometimes due to hyper-parathyroidism.

By definition the 'titratable acidity' is subnormal and, in fact, ammonia excretion may account for an increased percentage of the hydrogen ion that can be excreted. The *definitive test* is to give a load of 7g of encapsulated ammonium chloride and to monitor the urinary pH over 3–5h. Normally urinary pH should fall to less than 5.3; the urine remains alkaline in RTA cases.

A variety of causative factors have now been identified.

Causes of renal tubular acidosis

Congenital
(1)   Sporadic or familial;
(2)   associated with diseases such as galactosaemia or fructose in-tolerance;
(3)   medullary sponge kidney.

Acquired
(1)   Toxins: lithium, toluene, amphotericin B, acetazolamide, old tetracycline;
(2)   with interstitial nephritis (cf. rabbits immunized with renal antigens);
(3)   as part of pyelonephritis, after renal transplantation, and with stones;
(4)   due to hypokalaemic tubular nephropathy caused by excess use of diuretics;
(5)   due to hyperparathyroidism or vitamin D damage.

Hypergammaglobulinaemic states and immune disorders
(1)   As a result of myeloma;
(2)   in Sjögren's syndrome;
(3)   in active chronic hepatitis or primary biliary cirrhosis.

Since carbonic anhydrase plays a major role in renal tubular acidification in the distal tubules as well as hydrogen ion secretion in the proximal tubules, it would make sound sense if a defect in this enzyme were to account for renal tubular acidosis. In fact there are sporadic case reports of an inactive carbonic anhydrase in the red cells of some families with primary renal tubular acidosis.

Damage to renal tubular epithelium in various subtle ways, as well as interference with ATP production in the cells, would appear to explain other cases. Thus it is now known that the complete Fanconi syndrome, with loss of glucose, phosphate and amino acids can be produced by infusing rats with maleate, which is the *cis*-isomer of the Kreb's cycle intermediate fumaric acid; it complexes with thioles.

$$O$$
$$\|$$
Maleic $H—C—C—OH$ $H_2—C—COOH$
acid $\|$ $|$
            $H—C—C—OH$ $\boxed{Pr\sim S}—C—COOH$
                   $\|$ $|$
                 O H

In this way maleate inhibits the tricarboxylic acid cycle of the kidney mitochondria. Substrate level phosphorylation is blocked so that ATP formation is stopped. Lack of energy alone does not explain the bicarbonate diuresis, for this is not caused by poisons like arsenite. It is therefore possible that maleate also interferes with a bicarbonate-stimulated ATPase.

Gradient-limiting RTA is treated by giving bicarbonate (1 mmol/kg per day) to correct the acidosis. Potassium repletion is often required. However in the case of bicarbonate-wasting RTA alkali administration simply results in bicarbonate loss in the urine and a marked hypokalaemia. Sometimes it can be treated by the daily use of hydrochlorothiazide to produce mild volume depletion; large potassium supplements are needed.

Hyperchloraemic acidosis of renal insufficiency

Hyperchloraemic acidosis is a common feature of mild renal insufficiency, especially when caused by tubulointerstitial disease. These patients can still acidify their urine and bicarbonate wasting is thus suspected. This might be due (a) to direct tubular damage, (b) elevated parathormone levels, or (c) enhanced chloride reabsorption.

Hypokalaemia and the renal tubules

Depletion of potassium within the renal tubular cells impairs mitochondrial oxidative metabolism, and this correlates with an inability to concentrate the urine. Vacuoles appear within the tubular cells. Both a polyuria and a tubular proteinuria are evident.

There are many causes of potassium depletion that might lead to a renal defect:

(1)   malnutrition or gastrointestinal loss, for example, vomiting and diarrhoea;

(2)   drug-induced losses of potassium due to diuretics; laxatives; liquorice or carbenoxalone; amphotericin B therapy;

(3)   adrenocorticoid-induced potassium depletion as in primary or secondary aldosteronism, or other cause of corticosteroid excess;

(4)   renal potassium loss, as in renal tubular acidosis.

Bartter's syndrome

This is a rare autosomal recessive condition that may present in childhood or adult life as persistent hypokalaemia. The features are:

(1)   juxtaglomerular hyperplasia; and thus
(2)   hyper-reninaemia and hyperaldosteronism; leading to
(3)   hypokalaemic alkalosis due to renal potassium wasting
(4)   elevated plasma noradrenaline levels and resistance to both noradrenaline and angiotensin II.

It is now thought that the whole syndrome is due to excessive activity of prostaglandin synthetase leading to excess renal prostaglandin production. Indeed hyperplasia of the interstitiorenal medullary cells can be shown. Excess of renal prostaglandins decreases proximal tubular sodium reabsorption, and thus leads to increased sodium delivery to the distal nephron and increasing urinary potassium loss.

Normalization of the low serum potassium does not correct the hyper-reninaemia *per se*. The treatment is to administer indomethacin to inhibit the prostaglandin synthetase and to curtail urinary potassium loss by spironolactone.

REFERENCES

Physiological action of diuretics

Beyer, K.H. and Baer, J.W. (1961). *Pharmacol. Rev.*, **13,** 517
Ford, R.V. (1961a). *N. Engl. J. Med.*, **264,** 1204
Ford, R.V. (1961b). *Med. Clin. N. Am.*, **45,** 961
Seldin, D.W. (1966). *Ann. N.Y. Acad. Sci.*, **139,** 273

Tubular action

Imai, M. and Kokko, J.P. (1974). *J. Clin. Invest.*, **53,** 393
Jacobson, H.R. and Kokko, J.P. (1976). *Ann. Rev. Pharmacol.*, **16,** 201
Suki, W.N., Eknoyan, G., Martinez-Maldonado, M. (1973). *Ann. Rev. Pharmacol.*, **13,** 91-106

Loop of Henle

Burg, M. (1973). *Am. J. Physiol.*, **225,** 119
Khuri, R.N., Agulian, S.K., Bogharian, K. (1974). *Am. J. Physiol.*, **227,** 1352

Diuretics and renal haemodynamics

Hook, J.B., Blatt, A.H., Brady, M.J. and Williamson, H.E. (1966). *J. Pharmacol. Exp. Ther.*, **154,** 667

Moyer, J.H., Onesti, G. (1971). *Am. J. Cardiol.*, **27,** 407

Osmotic diuresis

Gennari, F.J., Kassirer, J.P. (1974). *N. Engl., J. Med.*, **291,** 714

Mersalyl

Burg, M.B. and Green, N. (1973). Effect of mersalyl on the ascending loop. *Kidney Int.*, **4,** 245

Evanson, R.L. (1972). Mercurial diuretics and tubular sodium and potassium transport. *Am. J. Physiol.*, **222,** 282

Vogh, A. (1950). Discovery of the organic mercurials. *Am. Heart J.*, **39,** 881

Carbonic anhydrase

Maren, T.H. (1967). *Physiol. Rev.*, **47,** 597

Bicarbonate reabsorption

Gyory, A., Brendel, U. and Kinne, R. (1972). *Pflügers Arch.*, **335,** 287

Ross, B., Leaf, A., Silva, P. and Epstein, F.H. (1974). *Am. J. Physiol.*, **226,** 642

Thiazides

Beyer, K.H. (1958). *Ann. N.Y. Acad. Sci.*, **71,** 363

Weller, J.M. and Malvin, R.L. (1969). *Med. Clin. N. Am.*, **53,** 1321

Frusemide

Allison, M. and Kennedy, A.C. (1971). Diuretics in chronic renal disease: high dose frusemide. *Clin. Sci.*, **41,** 171

Burg, M. (1973). *Am. J. Physiol.*, **225,** 119

Ethacrynic acid

Cannon, P.J., Heinemann, H.O., Stason, W.B., Laragh, J.H. (1965). *Circulation*, **31,** 5

Diuretics and renal metabolism

Bumetanide

Symposium (1975). *Postgrad. Med. J.*, **51,** suppl. 5

Potassium-sparing agents

McKenna, T.J., Donohoe, J.F., Brien, T.G., Muldowney, F.P. (1971). *Br. Med. J.*, **2,** 739

Amiloride

Bentley, J. (1968). Inhibitor of sodium transport across the toad bladder. *J. Physiol. (Lond.).*, **195,** 317

Spironolactone

Fanestil, D.D. (1968). Binding to kidney mineralocorticoid receptors. *Biochem. Pharmacol.*, **17,** 2240

Complications of diuretic therapy

DeRubertis, D., Michaelis, M.F., Beck, N. and Davis, B.B. (1970). *Metabolism*, **19,** 709
Van Ypersele de Strihou, C. (1972). *Adv. Nephrol.*, **2,** 241

Prostaglandins

Lee, J.B. (1971). Prostaglandin Ai: antihypertensive and renal effects. *Ann. Intern. Med.*, **74,** 703

Renal metabolism

Cahill, G.F. and Aoki, T.T. (1975). Renal gluconeogenesis and amino acid metabolism in man. *Med. Clin. N. Am.*, **59** 3, 751
Cohen, J.J. (1975). Metabolic support for renal sodium reabsorption. *Med. Clin. N. Am.*, **59,** 523
Costello, J. Scott, J.M., Wilson, P. and Bourke, E. (1973). Glucose utilization and production by the dog kidney *in vivo* in metabolic acidosis and alkalosis. *J. Clin. Invest.*, **52,** 608
Kamm, D.E. and Fuise, R.E. (1967). Acid–base alterations and renal gluconeogenesis. *J. Clin. Invest.*, **46,** 1172
Weidemann, M.J., Krebs, H.A. (1969). The fuel of respiration of rat kidney cortex. *Biochem. J.*, **112,** 149

3
The kidney and hypertension

It is difficult, considering the volume of literature available on the subject, to present a brief synopsis of the kidney and hypertension. The crux of the matter, however, is that the juxtaglomerular apparatus (Figure 22) consists of stretch receptors in the wall of the afferent arteriole working in conjunction with the sodium-sensitive cells of the macula densa, so that either ($\div$) diminished renal blood flow or ($\div$) a decrease in the sodium being delivered to the distal tubule will cause the release of renin (see Figures 6 and 23). This structure, described by Goormaghtigh in 1932, can be pictured as shown.

The JGA occupies the vascular pole of the glomerulus. Immunofluorescence confirms that its granules contain renin. There is a rich sympathetic nerve supply, and when there is increased sympathetic drive there is constriction of the afferent arteriole, so the pressure of the JGA is lowered and renin release enhanced. This happens in hypertension, cirrhosis, or shock, when there is raised intracranial pressure, or diminished flow due to obstruction to the circulation as in renal artery stenosis. It might also happen under the influence of ganglion-blocking drugs, for although the renal arterioles are dilated, the pressure at the JGA is low. On the other hand, if there is postural hypotension due to autonomic dysfunction (as in diabetic neuropathy), there is a failure to release catecholamines on standing. In this situation there is no

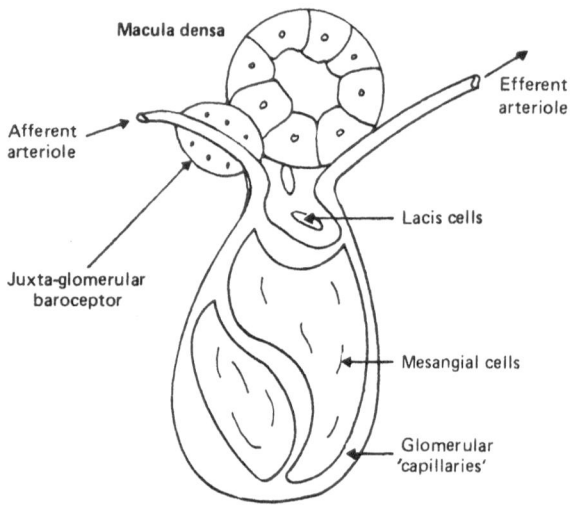

Figure 22. The juxtaglomerular apparatus

compensatory renin release, as occurs in the normal person in an upright posture. The JGA is therefore part of the baroreceptor system which includes the carotid body, aortic and atrial stretch receptors.

As the sodium flux down the tubules increases there is increased reabsorption by the ascending loop of Henle up to a limit, but inevitably the sodium concentration in the distal tubule must rise and this switches off renin release. Conversely in sodium depletion, renin–angiotensin–aldosterone generation will be activated, for it is the physiological sodium-conserving mechanism. Figure 23 summarizes renin and aldosterone control.

In normal persons and those with essential hypertension it is the sympathetic drive to the JGA which determines renin release. Yet the baroceptor is relatively insensitive as the renal artery pressure has to drop by 50% before renin release is increased!

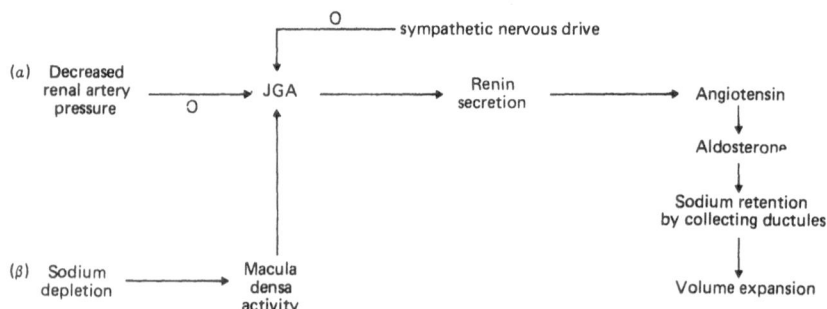

Figure 23. Renin and aldosterone control

HYPERTENSION AND ITS CAUSES

The pressure within arterioles is determined by:

(1) the cardiac output;
(2) the volume of fluid in the arterial system and its viscosity;
(3) the vasomotor tone of the peripheral arterioles, for this determines resistance to flow.

Peripheral vascular resistance (PVR) can thus be raised on account of:

(a) sympathetic nervous activity;
(b) the myogenic response of the muscle of the arterioles;
(c) vascular damage as in arteriosclerosis.

The known vasoconstrictor factors include noradrenaline and angiotensin II. Angiotensin II interacts with hormonal receptors on the vascular smooth muscle cells. The opposing vasodilators include the prostaglandins and the kallikrein-kinins.

In the United States the incidence of hypertension is as high as 10%, and constitutes a major health problem. Primary essential hypertension accounts for the high incidence, to which smoking and obesity are additive; secondary causes such as renal or adrenal disorders account for less than 3% of the total cases. It is important to see this in perspective.

The classification of hypertension

This follows traditional lines as listed below.

(1) Primary essential hypertension
(2) Endocrine and like causes
    (a) Coarctation of the aorta
    (b) Cushing's syndrome; oral contraceptive administration
    (c) Conn's syndrome—primary aldosteronism
    (d) Liddle's syndrome (BP is normal in Bartter's syndrome)
    (e) Phaeochromocytoma, with adrenaline or noradrenaline production.
(3) (a) Disease of the renal vasculature:
        (i) atheromatous renal artery stenosis
        (ii) fibromuscular hyperplasia
        (iii) obliterative endarteritis of arcuate and interlobular vessels
        (iv) renal infarction
        (v) rarely a renin-secreting tumour (JG cell or Wilms).
    (b) Parenchymal disease:
        (i) acute and chronic glomerulonephritis
        (ii) chronic pyelonephritis

(iii)   polycystic disease

(iv)   post-toxaemia of pregnancy

Other diseases include diabetes, amyloid, gout, polyarteritis, scleroderma.

ESSENTIAL HYPERTENSION

This is a family trait whose inheritance depends on the interaction of several genes. More recently it has been realized that an individual's diastolic or systolic blood pressure is closely related to his plasma or urinary output of noradrenaline—indeed the person with essential hypertension seems to be readily geared for 'fear, flight or fight', so his blood pressure rises more in response to stress or the cold pressor test. It is well known that there is an increased vascular responsiveness in the skin and muscle vascular beds of patients with essential hypertension. Additionally one has to be aware that autonomic activation in essential hypertension can be regional rather than generalized. A selective increase in renal vascular resistance does seem to occur. This may be either because of an enhanced intrinsic responsiveness of the vascular smooth muscle, or on account of an enhanced mechanical advantage of that muscle. The latter results from an increase in the muscle wall thickness-to-lumen ratio, so resulting in a large reduction in radius with even small degrees of muscle shortening. Yet in fact this phase of muscular hypertrophy may be a later consequential phase.

In accordance with their increased adrenergic responsiveness young persons with essential hypertension may show evidence of tachycardia, palpitation and increased cardiac output. At this stage their circulation is hyperdynamic, the hypertension is labile and the systolic blood pressure recordings are relatively high, although they may only complain of sweating or flushing, cardiac awareness or tightness in the chest.

Mechanisms of and treatment for essential hypertension

Renal haemodynamics differ from normal in essential hypertension. Thus when saline is infused those patients with an elevated renal vascular resistance show a natriuresis. They also have an increased filtration fraction which must reflect an increased pressure in their glomeruli, and this means that they will have an increased peritubular oncotic pressure. Yet natriuresis must occur because there is also an increased pressure in the peritubular capillaries. Usually the patients have a suppressed plasma renin, although there is no evidence that they have an expanded plasma volume. In fact they are in sodium balance. (Of course, there is an increased sodium content of arteriolar walls).

It has been shown further that patients with essential hypertension can be subdivided into those with low, normal or elevated plasma renin levels.

60

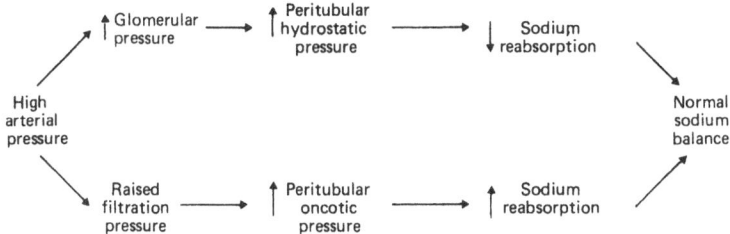

Figure 24. Sodium reabsorption in essential hypertension

High renin levels are said to predispose to vascular complications, such as stroke or coronary thrombosis. Few people agree with this—patients with essential hypertension and high renin levels may already have intrinsic disease of the renal arterioles and therefore renal ischaemia. They do tend to be younger. In fact renin levels in patients with essential hypertension fall off with age and this may reflect senescence, that is nephrosclerosis, and hence diminished baroceptor responsiveness. It remains to be seen whether patients who initially have high renin levels develop lower values as they get older.

There are other possible explanations for low renin hypertension (LRH). Such patients might be producing an excessive amount of an unidentified adrenal steroid, which could be deoxycorticosterone, 18 hydroxydeoxy-corticosterone or a potentiator of aldosterone 16a, 18 dihydroxydeoxy-corticosterone. These patients have low plasma renins and a low plasma aldo-sterone.

Older hypertensives with low plasma renins respond well to mild diuretics. Conversely, those who have a high plasma noradrenaline output and thus an elevated plasma renin, or those who have a high renin due to renal ischaemia, are ideally suited for either beta- or combined alpha/beta blockade. Indeed since the beta-blocking drugs prevent the action of catecholamines, it is logical to treat anxiety symptoms or the early hyperkinetic heart syndrome of hypertension with a regime such as propanalol 20–80 mg three times daily. Smoking should be forbidden, as it is a potent stimulus to catecholamine release. In practice many of the clients in a hypertension clinic fall into this category!

It has been emphasized that essential hypertension is a reflection of the setting of the sympathetic nervous system. In turn this may depend on central and peripheral nerve neurotransmitter activity. In fact those who have a high output of adrenaline and noradrenaline when under stress, show a better performance in a variety of tests and often a higher IQ.

Concurrently there may be a decrease of hypothalamic dopamine, for prolactin levels are raised in patients with essential hypertension. Release of prolactin from the pituitary is under constant inhibition by 'prolactin-inhibitory factor' (PIF), whose own control is determined by the dopamine in the hypothalamus. Administration of the dopamine agonist bromocriptine or of L-dopa can be shown to lower the blood pressure in persons with essential hypertension.

Effects of essential hypertension

Essential hypertension means that the blood pressure at the time of diagnosis exceeds 140/90 and that no cause other than anxiety, a positive family history and middle age are evident. Indeed the condition usually begins between the ages 20–50 and becomes worse with age. Females are affected more than males but seem to suffer less from the long-term effects, such as left ventricular hypertrophy and congestive heart failure, cerebral haemorrhage or stroke. Fewer than 5% suffer such severe nephrosclerosis that they die of uraemia (Figure 25). The hypertension may precipitate other conditions such as subarachnoid haemorrhage from a berry aneurysm, dissecting aneurysm of the aorta or a mesenteric thrombosis.

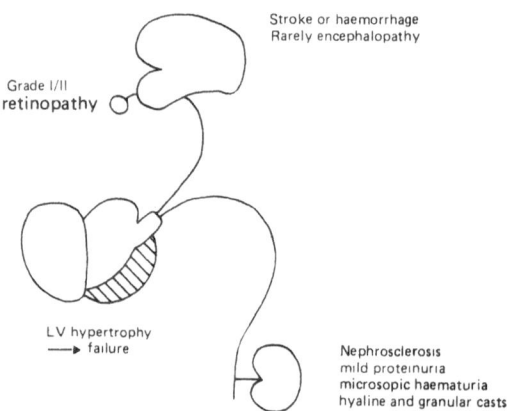

Stroke or haemorrhage
Rarely encephalopathy

Grade I/II retinopathy

LV hypertrophy
⟶ failure

Nephrosclerosis
mild proteinuria
microsopic haematuria
hyaline and granular casts

Figure 25. Anticipated sequelae of essential hypertension

The nephrosclerosis is part of the generalized *arteriosclerosis*, which shows in the renal arterioles as onion-skin lamellation of the endothelium, splitting of the internal elastic lamella and smooth muscle hypertrophy of the media. The lesions can look complicated because of additional atherosclerosis. This is determined by other factors such as the level of the serum cholesterol, obesity, diabetes mellitus and genetic tendencies.

Advanced arteriolar disease of the kidneys leads to *glomerular collapse and sclerosis* with hyalinization, atrophy of the renal tubules and, in all, some loss of renal mass and progression to a smaller kidney (11 cm) with a granular pitted surface (Figure 26). There is also an increase of the renal interstitial connective tissue.

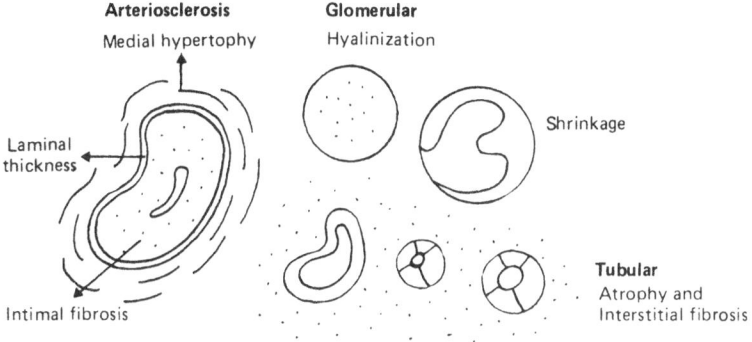

Figure 26.   The kidney of essential hypertension ... nephrosclerosis

RENAL HYPERTENSION

Renin was discovered in 1898 when Tigerstedt and Bergman found that a crude saline extract of rabbit kidneys would raise the blood pressure of other rabbits. Then in 1934 Goldblatt described the production of hypertension following the application of a clip to one renal artery of an animal. He had been impressed by the frequency with which persons with hypertension are found to have disease of their renal arteries at autopsy, and he found that a clip constricting one renal artery led to an elevation of blood pressure, which could later be cured by removing either the clip or the whole kidney.

In recent years similar experiments have been performed in rats who either have a clip on one artery and a normal contralateral kidney in position (the so-called two-kidney rat), or in which the opposite kidney is removed (the one-kidney model). In the two-kidney rat enhanced renin secretion from the clipped kidney is the stimulus to the elevation of blood pressure, as can be shown by the fall produced by the infusion of an angiotensin II inhibitor. On the other hand fluid retention and expansion of the blood volume is the cause of the raised blood pressure in the one-kidney animal. In this latter case the blood pressure does not fall when an angiotensin antagonist (saralasin) is infused (Figure 27).

Volume expanded (low renin) hypertension—as in the one-kidney animal

It is usual for a phase of increased cardiac output to precede the increase of peripheral resistance that signifies established hypertension.

Three possibilities should be considered.

(1)   *Auto-regulation.* The natural myogenic response of the renal arterioles means that the vessels respond by vasoconstriction so as to maintain a stable blood flow when they are faced with an increase of the cardiac output. In this way the process of blood volume expansion will result in hypertension.

(2)   *Vascular restructuring* will also occur, although more gradually, so that the walls of the arterioles become hypertrophied.

(3)   *The electrogenic Na–K pump* of the arteriolar walls might be decreased in the volume-expanded type of hypertension. This could result in an increased intracellular sodium and an increased contractility of the heart, arteries and veins. There is little evidence of this at the present time. Yet often leucocytes show decreased ATPase.

The two-kidney model and human disease

The animal models which have been outlined above can be contrasted as in Figure 27.

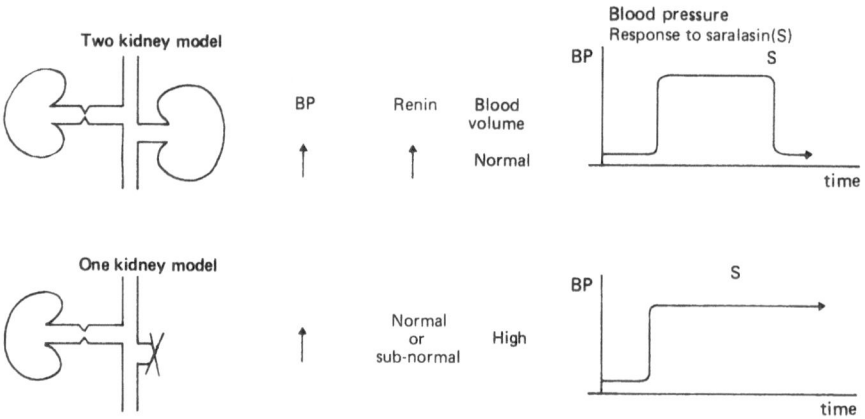

Figure 27.   The two-kidney and the one-kidney rat models

In the one-kidney model, in which there is overexpansion of the blood volume and a suppressed renin, there can be no response to saralasin. There is a clearcut response when renin secretion is high as in the two-kidney model. The interest in these models really relates to their human counterparts.

Classical renal artery stenosis is the equivalent of the two-kidney, one-clip model. The stenosed kidney suffers from ischaemia and so produces excess renin. In theory the hypertension can be cured by repair of the stenosis with reanastomosis of the artery, or by nephrectomy. The critical test is clearly to measure the renin produced from each renal vein. It will be high from the stenosed kidney and low from the contralateral kidney, which in fact should show suppressed renin production. One normally expects the renal vein renin of the stenosed kidney to be at least twice that of the opposite kidney (values of 1.5–2.0x are regarded as diagnostic). The situation becomes complicated by the fact that renin is already present in the renal artery and an ischaemic kidney is merely adding extra renin. One therefore has to allow for renal plasma flow through the affected kidney:

renin secretion = renal plasma flow x renal vein renin increment

= PAH clearance x (vein renin–artery renin)

In practice the peripheral vein renin can be assumed to be equal to the arterial renin concentration, so that

renin secretion = PAH clearance x (renal vein renin–peripheral vein renin)

The details are discussed below as part of the investigation scheme; typical results are shown in Figure 28.

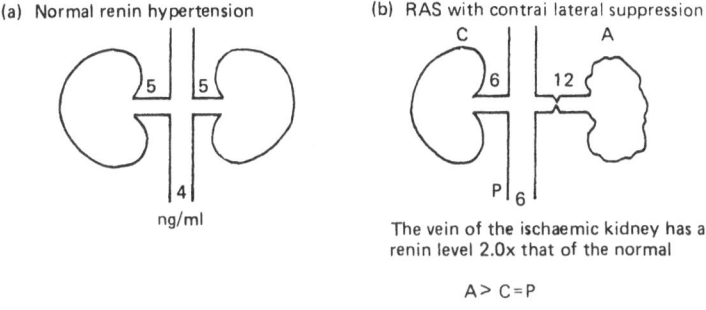

(a) Normal renin hypertension

5   5

4

ng/ml

(b) RAS with contrai lateral suppression

C   A

6   12

P 6

The vein of the ischaemic kidney has a renin level 2.0x that of the normal

A> C = P

Figure 28.   Typical renin values in renal artery stenosis

In reality the human RAS often resembles the one-kidney model because the hypertension has usually caused vascular damage in the contralateral unprotected kidney so that this other kidney is unable to excrete sodium normally. There is therefore fluid retention and a suppression of the plasma renin which obscures the underlying problems. Likewise patients with bilateral chronic renal disease resemble the one-kidney rat model, as they are fluid-overloaded and their hypertension can only be cured by haemodialysis.

The renin-angiotensin sequence is so important that it should be considered again (Figure 29).

In the case of hypertension caused by the oestrogen contraceptive pill, oestrogen causes the release of excess renin substrate from the liver so that it is suspected that there is then increased generation of angiotensin II and

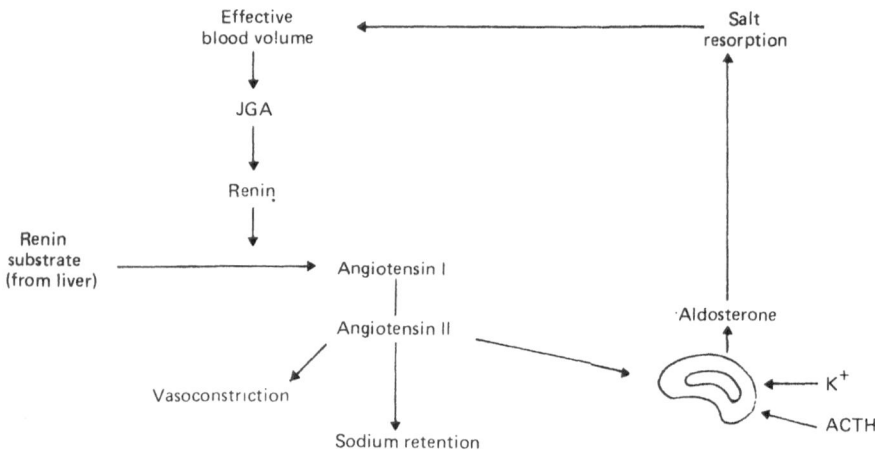

Figure 29.   Hormonal effects of excess renin release by a kidney

aldosterone; some of these patients, therefore, may show a slightly lowered serum magnesium as in primary aldosteronism.

The differential diagnosis of renal hypertension

The standard screening tests consist of:

(1)   urine analysis and microscopy for evidence of nephritis or pyelonephritis, even though there is no urinary sediment in renovascular disease;

(2)   an intravenous pyelogram (preferably a rapid sequence urogram);

(3)   blood urea and electrolytes;

(4)   peripheral renin and 24h aldosterone in relation to 24h urine sodium.

The way in which the types are recognized are discussed briefly below.

Essential hypertension
By definition this is hypertension for which no renal cause has been found. It may be familial, often the patient is a smoker, and the symptoms are those of adrenergic responsiveness. Headache is not so prominent as has been thought in the past. Apart from tachycardia and sweating, patients may have faintness or giddiness. Female patients should be questioned as to whether they are taking the contraceptive pill.

The IVP is normal, renin may be normal or slightly elevated or lowered, exchangeable sodium and fluid volumes are normal and there is no evidence for production of a salt-retaining steroid.

Coarctation of the aorta
The diagnostic feature is the delay and weakness of the femoral pulses when compared with the radial pulsation. Since there is a constriction in the aorta the renal blood flow is reduced (and is presumably the cause of the hypertension) although the glomerular filtration rate is normal.

Phaeochromocytoma
When the tumour is in the adrenal gland the product is mainly adrenaline, but it is noradrenaline when in an extraneous site. Although the tumour accounts for less than 0.5% cases of hypertension one should be vigilant for the triad of headache, sweating and palpitations. Since the blood pressure fluctuates it may be recorded as normal. However, raised blood levels of catecholamines are found between attacks and this must mean continuous active synthesis, since there is virtually no storage within a phaeochromocytoma. Moreover, catecholamines in the plasma are rapidly inactivated by catecholomethyltransferase together with monoamineoxidase. In fact the diagnosis is usually made by a 24h urine estimation of HMMA (vanillylmandelic acid—or more correctly 4-hydroxy-3-methoxy-mandelic acid— normal value 0.7–7.0 mg/day) or of urinary metanephrine and normetanephrine (normal less than 1 mg/day). In each case the substance is extracted and is oxidized by periodate to vanillin which can be assayed spectrophotometrically.

Provocation tests are now used less than formerly. The phaeochromocytoma can be made to secrete by the intravenous injection of 0.025 mg histamine, 300 mg tetraethylammonium bromide, 1 mg glucagon or 0.5–1.0 mg tyramine.

The alternative is to monitor the blood pressure response to 5 mg phentolamine (Rogitine) given intravenously. In the case of phaeochromocytoma the blood pressure falls more than 35/25 mmHg within 5 min. After this the drug should be continued orally 20 mg q.i.d. for alpha-blockade and be combined with propranolol as a beta-blocker. Patients in hypertensive crisis due to phaeochromocytoma can be treated very adequately with the new combined alpha and beta-blocking drug labetolol. It is rather less active on the alpha than the beta-receptors so that the heart is protected by beta-blockade, while there is not too much arteriolar dilatation. The dose of labetolol is 1.5 mg/kg given intravenously as a bolus dose or as an infusion.

Renal parenchymal disease
Whereas renovascular disease produces no urinary abnormalities, in glomerulonephritis there is a proteinuria with red cell casts, and in pyelonephritis the urine shows numerous white cells. Renal biopsy is essential in glomerulonephritis, since the histology may have prognostic significance

and may also determine the treatment. Pyelonephritis is usually evident from the pyelogram which shows a cortical scar opposite a clubbed calyx (page 200).

Endocrine hypertension
The hypertension of Cushing's or Conn's syndrome may present its own unique diagnostic problems. However, quite often the Cushing's appearance is typical with a moon face, fat body and thin weak limbs which may be bruised, a buffalo hump on the back and striae on the abdomen and thighs. As well as hypertension there is glucose intolerance, and the urinary-free cortisol level is greater than 300 μg/day (over 380 nmol/l). The plasma ACTH is raised in cases of pituitary origin.

To the nephrologist the common practical problem is posed by a hypertensive patient with hypokalaemia. In this case the use of diuretics, enemas or the consumption of liquorice has to be ascertained but ultimately it must be discovered whether there is renal potassium wasting. That means that the urinary potassium is greater than 20 mmoles per day, when the serum potassium concentration is less than 3.0 mmol/l per day. This might simply be a result of chronic pyelonephritis, but usually the next step is to search for the steroid-dependent causes of renal potassium loss.

Table 6   Causes of mineralocorticoid-induced renal potassium wasting

Raised urinary cortisol	Normal urinary 17-OH-corticoids	Decreased urinary 17-OH-corticoids
Cushings (3)	Primary aldosteronism (1)*	11-Hydroxylase deficit
Ectopic ACTH	Secondary aldosteronism (5)	17-Hydroxylase deficit (4)
	Mineralocorticoid excess (2)	
	Increased renin	*Increased aldosterone*
	2 Aldosteronism (5)	Primary aldosteronism (1)
		Idiopathic aldosteronism
	or	Dexamethasone responsive
	Decreased renin	
	Primary aldosteronism (1)	*Decreased aldosterone*
	Mineralocorticoid excess (2)	Mineralocorticoid excess (2)

* The numerals refer to the summary below

Causes of hypertension with steroid-dependent renal potassium wasting

(1)   Primary aldosteronism (adenoma) (Conn. 1954)
       Idiopathic aldosteronism (hyperplasia)   increased aldosterone
                                                              and
       Dexamethasone responsive aldosteronism   decreased renin

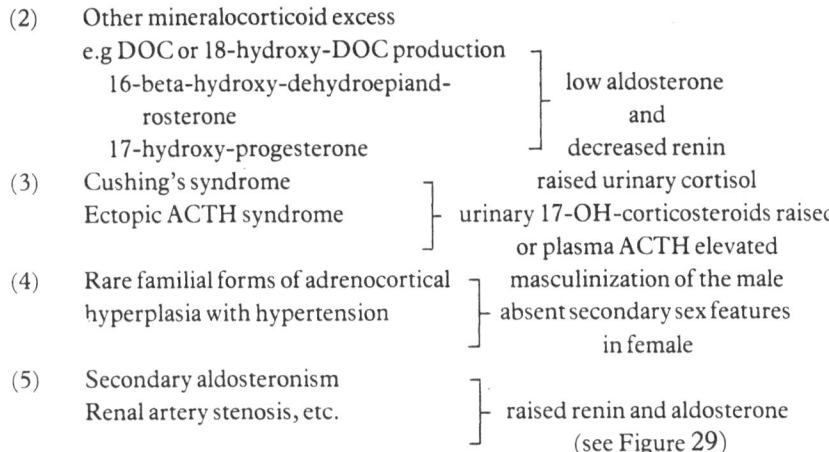

(2) Other mineralocorticoid excess
e.g DOC or 18-hydroxy-DOC production
16-beta-hydroxy-dehydroepiand-
rosterone
17-hydroxy-progesterone
⎤
⎦ low aldosterone
and
decreased renin

(3) Cushing's syndrome
Ectopic ACTH syndrome
⎤
⎦ raised urinary cortisol
urinary 17-OH-corticosteroids raised
or plasma ACTH elevated

(4) Rare familial forms of adrenocortical
hyperplasia with hypertension
⎤
⎦ masculinization of the male
absent secondary sex features
in female

(5) Secondary aldosteronism
Renal artery stenosis, etc.
⎤
⎦ raised renin and aldosterone
(see Figure 29)

In order to establish steroid-dependent potassium wasting the patient is placed on a high sodium intake of 200 mmoles sodium together with 100 mmoles potassium for 7–10 days, so that in this way the distal tubule exchange segment will be overworked at sodium reabsorption with the consequent development of urinary potassium loss and hypokalaemia. By way of subsequent confirmation it can then be shown that urinary potassium loss is reduced when the patient takes spironolactone (Aldactone-A), 50 mg q.i.d.

The approach to the differential diagnosis is as follows:

(1) Measure the plasma and urinary-free cortisol to exclude Cushing's.
(2) Take 24 h urine aldosterone and the aldosterone secretion rate. Note that in order to do this it is necessary first to replete the body potassium, since low body potassium reduces aldosterone secretion. Having done this, the patient who is found to excrete more than 18 μg per day of aldosterone metabolites while on a high salt diet is suspect.
(3) Measure any other steroids such as DOC or 18-DOC as a guide to steroid-suppressible hypertension.
(4) Estimate plasma renin using augmentatory procedures such as sodium deprivation, upright posture, infusion of sodium nitroprusside, or blood pressure reduction by hydrallazine.
(5) Observe for dexamethasone-responsive aldosteronism (or other adrenal excess) by the administration of dexamethasone, 2.0 mg/day orally. There is remission of both hypertension and hypokalaemia within 7–14 days.
(6) Attempt to localize the tumour by catheterization of the adrenal veins and determination of the aldosterone concentration from each side, or by [131I] 19-iodocholesterol scanning.

Note that Liddle's syndrome is another form of hypertension with hypokalaemia which is not steroid dependent. In this case there is no response to spironolactone, but triamterene corrects both the hypokalaemia and the hypertension.

Procedure for the collection of renal vein renin samples
(1)   Fasting patient who is recumbent at all times;
(2)   30 min before test give 2 g *p*-amino-hippurate (PAH) into drip;
(3)   next 500 ml dextrose-saline with 2 g PAH over 4 h;
(4)   in this time perform bilateral femoral vein catheterization by Seldinger;
(5)   take 10 ml blood samples in EDTA anticoagulant and keep in icebath:

   (a) from the IVC;
   (b) simultaneous renal vein samples whilst lying;
   (c) renal vein samples 2, 4, 6, 8 min after 300 mg diazoxide i/v;
   (d) on withdrawal of catheters, another IVC sample below renal veins.

Classical renal artery stenosis (RAS)

This has two main causes:

(1)   Due to *fibromuscular hyperplasia*. The patient is often a young woman with hypertension; the condition is frequently found in pregnancy. One or both renal arteries are narrowed by intimal and muscular hyperplasia, which on an arteriogram presents the 'sausage string' appearance. It has been proposed that this condition develops when there is excessive mobility of the kidneys. Certainly the pseudo-stenoses may cause functional stenosis in the erect position but not when prone.

(2)   Due to *atherosclerosis*. The patient is usually a male over the age of 40 who is a smoker, or who has some other cause for hyperlipidaemia of type II, IIb or IV, and who has stenosis of one or both renal arteries by atheromatous plaque. This either surrounds the artery orifice or is just beyond the origin. The presentation is as hypertension, often of accelerated type, together with polyuria and potassium loss due to the associated hyperaldosteronism. Rarely there is an episode of haematuria or loin pain which points to a renal infarct. On clinical examination some 50% patients have a loud bruit either posteriorly in the appropriate loin or in the epigastrium laterally over a renal artery.

It is important to have a precise approach in establishing a diagnosis. For this purpose one must remember that the kidney with the stenosed artery will be a smaller kidney, which forms a small volume of glomerular filtrate from which a higher proportion of sodium and chloride will be reabsorbed, so that the concentration of the urine on that side is high. Of course the clearance by that kidney of inulin, creatinine or PAH will be low.

Thus the features of renal artery stenosis are as follows. Beyond the stenosis is a small kidney/with reduced renal blood flow (PAH)/reduced GFR (inulin or creatinine clearance)/and the increased secretion of aldosterone causes sodium reabsorption.

The intravenous pyelogram (IVP) or 'rapid sequence urogram'
The IVP is really done to exclude pyelonephritis. At the same time one is looking for a 1.5 cm shrinkage in size of the affected kidney (although in fact some 10% of a group of patients with hypertension may show this). Additionally some 5% of those patients who do have renal artery stenosis will be found to have a non-functioning kidney.

A rapid-sequence urogram in which the films are taken at 1 min intervals for the first 5 min is of great value. The following points are to be noted with care:

(1)   delayed appearance of the nephrogram at 30 sec or 1 min on the abnormal side;
(2)   delayed appearance of the dye in the minor calyces;
(3)   spastic appearance of the calyces;
(4)   any notching of the renal pelvis and ureters due to a collateral circulation;
(5)   an increase in the concentration of dye on the affected side at 10 min; this can be brought out particularly well when the patient has been given a water load to drink, so that the dye contrast is much less dense in the unaffected kidney.

This sounds simple and is, if the appearances are classical. However only in 70% cases of RAS is there a dense nephrogram. In a large series by Maxwell some 40% of genuine cases showed a difference in the size of the kidneys, and of these 40% showed increased concentration on the affected side, as is expected, but all the others showed a decreased concentration. False negative results, that is, lack of a specific abnormality on the pyelogram, occur in at least 25% of cases of RAS diagnosed by means of a renal arteriogram. Bilateral renal artery stenosis is also common, and then of course there will be little difference in the appearance of the two kidneys.

Renal angiograms
Selective renal angiography is performed by the Seldinger technique in which

a flexible catheter is passed up the aorta through a needle and guide wire inserted into the femoral artery. Clearly in a patient with atheroma there is a calculated risk of femoral, iliac or renal embolism.

The following types of abnormality may be shown:

(1)   fibromuscular hyperplasia in the young female;
(2)   proximal atheromatous stenosis with post-stenotic dilatation;
(3)   multiple stenoses or malformative aneurysmal dilatation;
(4)   narrowing of interlobar or arcuate arteries.

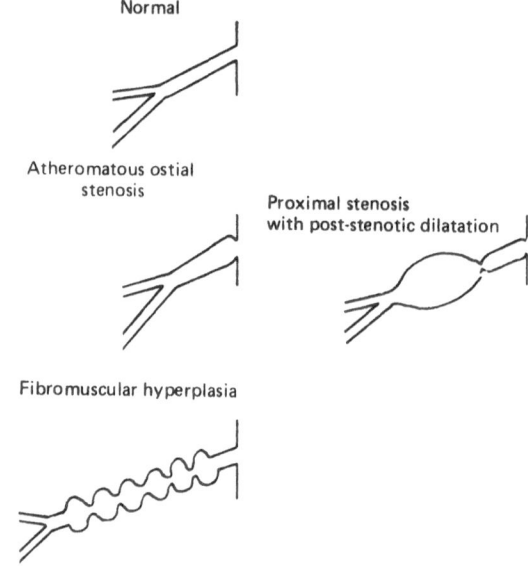

Figure 30.   Illustrative renal angiograms

Since atheroma is so common in middle age, it comes as no great surprise to find that one-third of renal arteriograms will show some abnormality regardless of the level of the blood pressure. Therefore if a stenosis is demonstrated, it is obligatory to prove its *functional* nature. In other words it must be shown that a stenosed kidney is producing excess renin. Demonstration of a lesion is not proof that it is the cause of the hypertension.

Isotope renography
This is a very useful screening test, but unfortunately it may be accompanied by a number of false-positive results. Sodium iodohippurate-I[131] is given intravenously and a scintillation crystal over each kidney plots the time-course of the gamma counts as they pass through the renal circulation into the urine. Normally there is a rapid rise of counts within 30 sec and then an

attenuated rise to a peak at 3–4 min, after which there is a steep fall-off. In renal artery stenosis there is a delayed and reduced peak, whose difference from the normal can be accentuated by a water load.

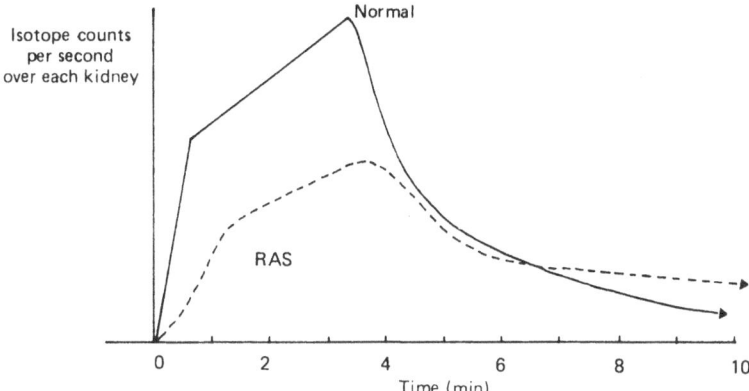

Figure 31.   Isotope renogram in renal artery stenosis

When looking for renal infarcts or cysts, or merely in order to measure kidney size, it is also simple to scan the kidneys after the administration of isotope-labelled chloromeradrin.

Renal biopsy
In theory this should show the difference between a kidney with a stenosed artery and a contralateral kidney which may be suffering from the effects of the hypertension. In practice it is dangerous to biopsy patients with hypertension and anyway useful information is often not obtained since the changes may be patchy.

Table 7

	Side of the stenosis	*Contralateral side*
Glomeruli	Normal but crowded	Normal
Tubules	Atrophic	Normal
Arterioles	Normal	Hyalinosis or endarteritis
JGA	Hypertrophic	Normal

Divided renal function tests (the Howard or Stamey technique)
This is an involved procedure whose use is limited to special units. The idea is to look for:

(1)   a 3:1 decrease of urinary flow rate on the stenosed side; and
(2)   a 100% increase in the urinary PAH concentration on the same side.

At the same time one has to verify that the renal plasma flow in the contralateral 'normal' kidney is at least 200 ml/min (normal 350 ml/min) and that this kidney has a creatinine clearance of at least 50 ml/min.

The patient drinks excess water, then 40 g of urea in 1 l of normal saline are infused over about 90 min so that a good urinary flow is obtained. Using a low spinal anaesthetic that will not affect renal blood flow, ureteric catheters are passed up to a level of 15 cm and are wedged so that there is no leak. Then PAH is infused to measure renal plasma flow, and urine collections are made for successive periods. The urinary sodium, PAH and creatinine are assayed. Table 8 illustrates the type of result. Naturally there are technical problems. Some 80% of patients only show the expected differences, and of course the test is of limited value when the disease is bilateral. Worse still, false-positive results occur when there is bilateral nephrosclerosis with asymmetrical disease.

Table 8

	Urine flow rate ml/min	Urine PAH mg/100 ml	PAH clearance ml/min	Urine creatinine mg/100 ml	Creatinine clearance ml/min
Normal	20	30	270	5	90
RAS	0.5	180	20	40	5

Renin assays

As discussed above it is hoped to establish that the stenosed kidney's renal vein renin has a value of 1.5–2.0 times that of the unaffected side. Moreover, it is important to demonstrate that there is suppressed renin production on the normal unaffected side. If A signifies the renal vein renin on the affected side, C on the contralateral side and P is the peripheral venous or arterial renin, then we hope to find (see Figure 28) that

$$A > C = P$$

The sensitivity of the procedure can be increased by the use of controlled hypotension. As already explained one should derive the 'renin-secretion rate' by estimation of the renal plasma flow and the $V-A$ differences for renin (page 65). Results indicating that $A = C > P$ or $A = C = P$ show that removal of one kidney is not to be considered.

In addition, increased prostaglandins can be detected in the renal venous blood of an ischaemic kidney.

Treating renal hypertension

Finally of course a decision must be reached as to whether treatment should be by surgery or medical management of hypertension. The hope is to reconstruct the artery or to remove an offending kidney. Sometimes one can do an autotransplantation by implanting the kidney in the patient's iliac fossa by attachment to an iliac artery. The real successes are obtained in patients with fibromuscular hyperplasia. However, in view of the nature of atheroma, it is not too surprising that even in patients under 40 who have the operation for renal artery stenosis the 1 year follow-up figures are broadly 50% cure, 25% improvement and 25% failure. This result has to be judged against an initial perioperative mortality of around 5%. Moreover although the blood pressure may fall at first, it often rises again by 4 years and only some 25% of subjects are still normotensive after 6 years.

It is therefore now regarded as more rational and simpler to deal with the patient's hypertension using conventional medical treatment. In this respect the beta-blocking drugs have proved to be excellent, since they work in the supine and standing position and avoid postural hypotension. They reduce both the cardiac output and the secretion of renin. One of their particular advantages is that they reduce blood pressure swings due to mental or physical stress. Those agents which have a cardioselective beta-blockade, namely the beta-1 blocker drugs such as acetbutalol, are just as effective as beta-1 and beta-2 blockers and they have the advantage that they cannot precipitate asthma. Additionally of course one may make use of the varied choices of ganglion-blocking drugs and diuretics. When there is secondary aldosteronism, spironolactone is invaluable.

Many of these patients present with accelerated hypertension and deterioration of renal function. Improvement may only occur after 2 to 3 months of effective antihypertensive therapy. There may be some dilemma as to how to deal with the malignant phase. The current availability, however, of diazoxide, trimethapan (Arfonad) and minoxidil or sodium nitroprusside should eliminate the need for urgent unilateral or bilateral nephrectomy.

Renin and the evaluation of therapy in patients with hypertension

It is useful to be aware of all of the conditions in which there may be *unilateral elevation of a renal vein renin:*
(1)   renal artery stenosis;
(2)   asymmetrical interlobar nephrosclerosis;
(3)   vascular malformations;
(4)   pyelonephritis;
(5)   segmental renal infarction;
(6)   unilateral hydronephrosis

These are important since investigation might falsely suggest a main artery stenosis.

It has already been stressed that selective renal vein renin determinations aim to detect a 1.5:1 ratio of the involved to non-involved sides. Indeed experience has shown that a normal peripheral vein renin does not exclude renal vascular disease since 40% of such patients may have a normal baseline renin. As in the experimental situation the use of the angiotensin II antagonist saralasin (1-sar-8-ala-angiotensin II) has shown that those patients who exhibit a fall of blood pressure have an elevated plasma renin activity. However, as might be expected, the evidence is that the occurrence of sodium overload may prevent the decrease in blood pressure that should occur with saralasin infusion in angiotensinogenic hypertension. It is therefore important to use a potent diuretic before the test. Volume expansion is also the explanation for the fact that although propranolol is highly effective in high renin hypertension, it can be without hypotensive action in low renin hypertension.

Rare causes of a raised plasma renin
Two rare causes of hypertension and high plasma renin activity occur—there can be a renin-producing tumour of the JGA or a renin-producing Wilm's tumour in children. They cause an accelerated hypertension and secondary aldosteronism with hypokalaemic alkalosis. This will be corrected by excision of the tumour. Likewise obstruction of the urinary tract by a hydronephrosis has been known to increase renin secretion leading to severe hypertension, which is cured by relief of the obstruction.

A low plasma renin activity
This clearly indicates that hypertension is due to excessive amounts of mineralocorticoids. Primary aldosteronism, as described by Conn in 1954, is characterized by mild hypertension but marked hypokalaemia and alkalosis, and normal or elevated serum concentrations of sodium and chloride. It accounts for some 0.5% of hypertensive patients. In the case of adenoma the aldosterone secretion is not influenced by the upright posture with stimulation of renin secretion, but does show a circadian rhythm so that there are high plasma aldosterone levels in the morning and a decline during the day. Conversely in idiopathic bilateral adrenal hyperplasia there is no circadian rhythm but the aldosterone levels do increase with upright posture. Surgery is not generally successful in the idiopathic hyperplasia syndrome and therefore preoperative differentiation is advisable. In *idiopathic hyperplasia as compared to adrenal* adenoma one should note that (a) the hypokalaemia and the alkalosis are milder because (b) the aldosterone secretion rate is less, and so (c) the plasma renin levels are not so low and can be stimulated to a greater extent by sodium depletion.

A response to spironolactone or to conventional diuretics is to be anticipated. Since the dose of Aldactone may be as high as 400 mg/day (a dosage that will often induce side-effects), a standard diuretic such as amiloride is often preferred. Beta-blockade often does not help low renin hypertension and may leave a-adrenergic constriction unopposed.

MALIGNANT (ACCELERATED) HYPERTENSION

Malignant or accelerated hypertension is often seen in renal hypertension but is uncommon in essential hypertension. There is necrotization or hyalinization of arterioles in many tissues including the kidneys. Thus the media of the vessels is swollen and anuclear and stains a deep red. The intimal endothelium is separated from the elastica by hyaline material which is due to an insudation of plasma protein (*plasmatic vasculosis*). It is now realized that angiotensin II causes contraction of the endothelial cells of the arterioles and a widening of the intraendothelial junctions. The high intravascular pressure has this same effect and drives proteins, even those of high molecular weight such as fibrinogen, into the arterial walls. This may lead on to *endarteritis fibrosa* in which there is a proliferative thickening of the intima at the expense of the vessel lumen (see Figure 32).

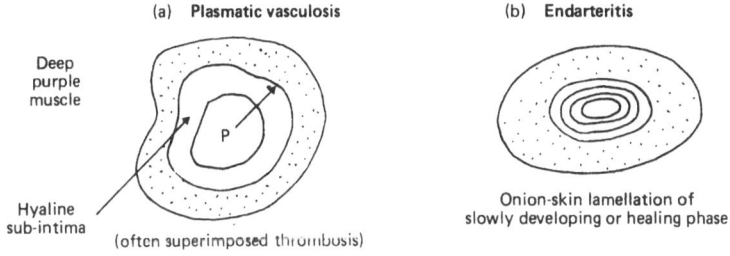

Figure 32. Vascular changes of malignant hypertension

In malignant hypertension symptoms are directly related to the level of the blood pressure. As described by Volhard, arterial spasm plays a large part. There is retinopathy with haemorrhages, exudates, papilloedema, encephalopathy and a progressive deterioration of renal function. A vicious cycle is initiated in which renal damage causes sodium retention due to renin and aldosterone output. The normal feedback inhibition of sodium is defective so that *inappropriately high renin secretion persists* and perpetuates vascular damage.

Further studies using angiotensin II infusions have shown that it produces *constriction of arterioles that alternate with areas of segmental dilatation,* and that these latter zones are the sites of increased vessel wall permeability. In reality hypertension in the animal first causes a diffuse peripheral vasoconstriction, yet the blood supply to tissues remains normal. Thereafter there is superimposed focal pathological spasm which, although it is transient, leaves damage due to arteriolar necrosis in the dilated segments and an increase of capillary permeability with oedema. In the brain this results in focal arterial necrosis and infarcts, and capillary and large haemorrhages. In the flea-bitten kidneys one will see focal necroses and capillary aneurysms. The hypertensive disease becomes irreversible at the stage when there is necrosis of the arterioles of the kidneys.

At this phase of acute vascular damage exposure of subendothelial arteriolar tissue leads to the onset of platelet aggregation and focal but widespread intravascular coagulation due to the formation of fibrin thrombi in the arteriolar system. The result of this is that red cells become torn on fibrin strands, and also by being wedged in between endothelial cells, and a *microangiopathic haemolytic anaemia* with characteristic *fragmented red* cells is seen.

If the kidney is not severely damaged by malignant hypertension, the condition is likely to be reversible with therapy, but there is usually a dramatic fall in urea and creatinine clearances. Damage also shows as proteinuria, sporadic haematuria and oliguria. Left ventricular failure and encephalopathy are to be expected (cf. Figure 25).

The genesis of vascular damage

It is useful to form a conceptual diagram of the interacting mechanisms which lead to damage to the vessel walls in uncontrolled hypertension (Figure 33).

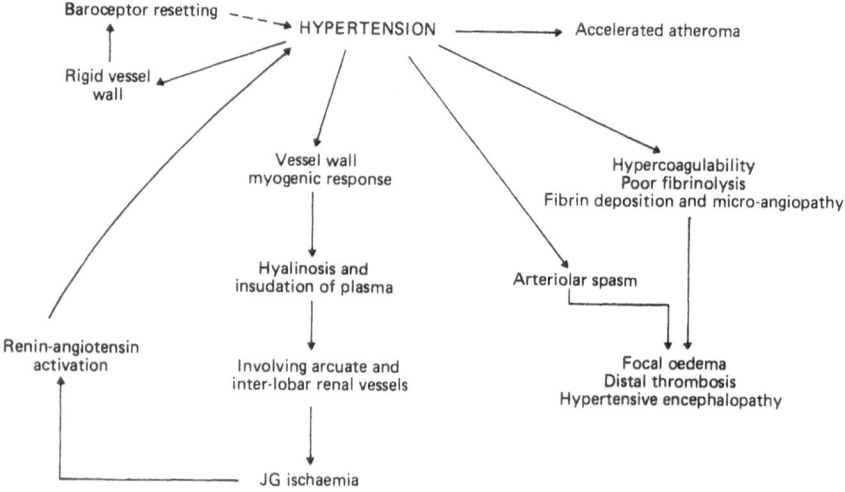

Figure 33. The vicious circle of vascular damage in hypertension

Briefly the interacting mechanisms are as follows:

(1) *The primary problem* is hypertensive arteriolar vasoconstriction which raises the blood pressure and, by its involvement of the kidneys, causes renin–angiotensin activation. Once established the persistent hypertension leads on to:

    (a) accelerated atherosclerosis, since the high pressure will drive lipoproteins into the arterial walls;

    (b) rheological changes due to hypercoagulability and poor fibrinolysis.

(2) As vessel walls harden with ageing, or with arteriosclerosis due to hypertension, one would anticipate a decreased arterial distensibility and a diminished sensitivity or even a degeneration of carotid sinus and aortic arch baroceptors. Such a poorly compliant arterial system could blunt baroreceptor reflexes.

In fact carotid baroreceptor activity is retained in most hypertensive subjects and thus will act to oppose either hypotension or hypertension. It turns out however that the reflex is not as active as in normotensive subjects, who with decrease of baroceptor activity show a greater increase in blood pressure than hypertensive persons.

RENAL INFARCTION

This occurs as a result of:

(1) renal artery emboli (75% cases) including atheromatous embolization;

(2) atherosclerosis;

(3) trauma to the flank;

(4) renal vein thrombosis.

It is appropriate to consider renal infarction at this stage as it might also complicate those vasculitides, such as polyarteritis nodosa and scleroderma, which can give rise to malignant hypertension. Indeed renal infarction *per se* can give rise to a sudden and perhaps transient hypertension.

The diagnostic features are often clear cut: flank pain and tenderness, with fever and haematuria, and the development of hypertension, accompanied by elevation of the SGOT and alkaline phosphatase (which arise from the renal tubules). Urinary tract infection or obstruction is to be considered, but in the case of renal infarction the IVP will be normal.

Sources of emboli such as bacterial endocarditis are always sought but emboli of atheromatous material from the aorta are much more common and are difficult to recognize clinically. Only the pathology is distinctive since the embolus will contain cholesterol clefts and there is a wedged-shaped infarct.

If the whole renal artery is obstructed and the diagnosis can be made early by aortography, then a surgical endarterectomy or embolectomy may be performed. Otherwise the decision is whether anticoagulation is justified.

HYPOTENSIVE THERAPY

Hypertension causes premature ageing of the arteries of the brain, causing a marked liability to cerebral thrombosis and haemorrhage, with an increased prevalence of coronary thrombosis and myocardial disease. Thus in men aged 35–45 years a diastolic pressure of 95 mmHg increases the mortality 5 fold. Smirk found in New Zealand the following five-year mortality rates in mild hypertension:

	Untreated	*Treated*
Men	44%	24%
Women	25%	15%

The actual principles of hypotensive therapy are presented here only in outline as the various categories of drug and their dosages will be familiar to the practising physician. It is important to recognize, however, the site of action of the various agents and these are detailed in Figure 34.

The diuretics

These produce relaxation of arteriolar walls by depleting the extracellular fluid and the arterial walls of salt. In moderate and severe hypertension the powerful diuretics are used, such as *frusemide* 40 mg–0.5 g/day; or *bumetanide* 1–mg, in combination with low salt diet (0.5 g). Long-term thiazide therapy is particularly suited for the middle-aged patient with mild hypertension, but in the elderly it should not be used owing to the risk of potassium loss, precipitation of diabetes, hyperuricaemia and even salt depletion.

Thiazide dosages should be built up gradually. Thus one might use hydrochlorothiazide 50 mg/day for one week, 75 mg/day in the second week and 100 mg/day thereafter. In this way an adaptation keeps the extracellular fluid volume near to normal. The maximum daily dose of bendrofluazide is 20 mg and for chlorothalidone 200 mg.

Spironolactone is often used for its potassium-conserving effect and its specific antialdosterone action; daily dosages are 50–100 mg. Particularly suited for this form of therapy are either patients with mineralocorticoid hypertension or those with low renin hypertension.

Centrally acting agents

Reserpine from rauwolfia
This has been used for many years: so it is well known that it may cause nasal

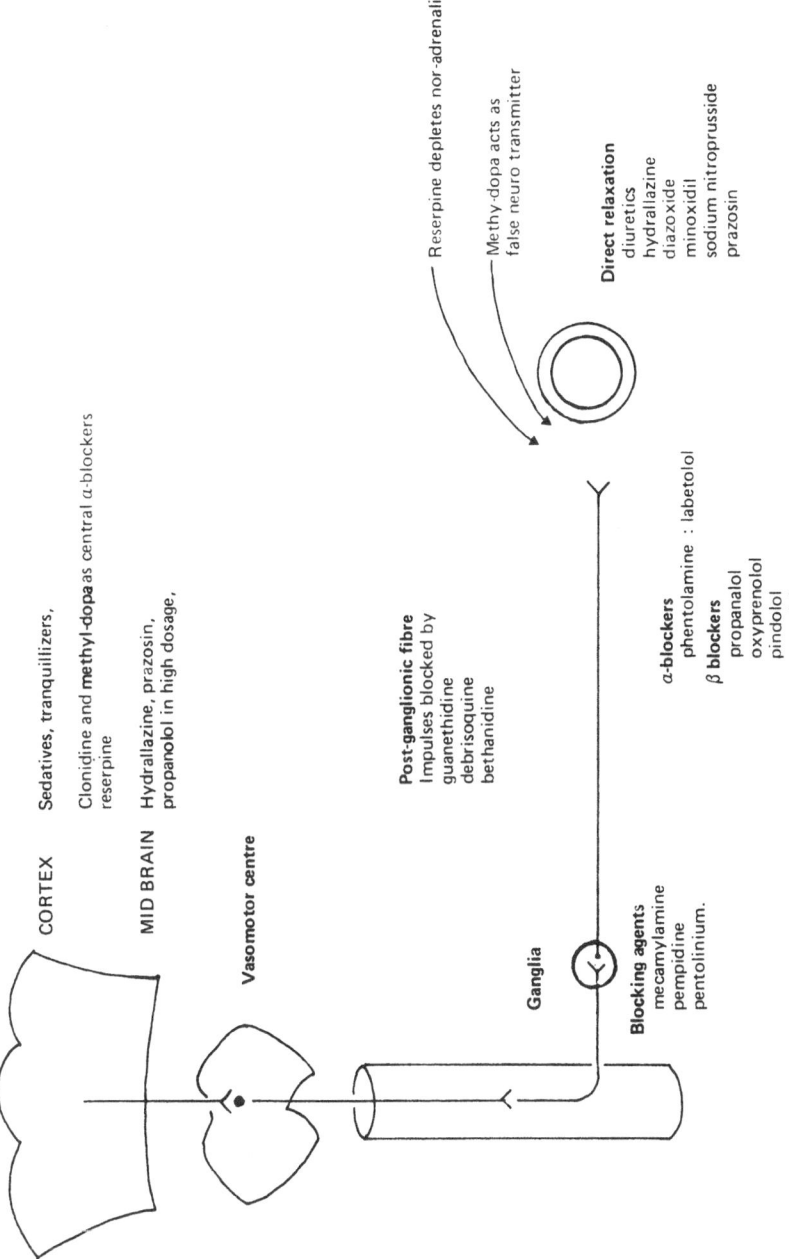

Figure 34. Sites of action of the hypotensive drugs

81

stuffiness, lethargy and depression. An advantage is that it works in the recumbent as well as the upright posture. A dose of 2.5 mg i/m is useful in a hypertensive crisis.

Methyl-dopa

This acts by causing alpha-methyl-noradrenaline (false transmitter) formation in the sympathetic nerve endings, and thereby reduces sympathetic outflow from the brain. Since plasma renin is lowered it is particularly good for patients with a degree of renal failure. It may cause drowsiness, confusion or depression, and if used in high dosage a Coomb's positive haemolytic anemia.

At the standard dosages of 250–500 mg q.i.d. there is good control with little tendency to postural hypotension; renal blood flow actually increases.

Clonidine

This has an alpha-blocking action within the brain that results in decreased sympathetic drive. It does cause sedation and it is perhaps best to start therapy with 0.1 mg at bedtime.

Prazosin

This has some central action but mainly it acts by causing peripheral dilatation of both arteries and veins; it is particularly good if the patient has heart failure. A small test dose of 0.5 mg must be given first and thereafter 0.5–1.0 mg t.i.d.

Ganglion-blocking drugs

These drugs which block both the sympathetic and parasympathetic nerves are currently out of favour because of their side-effects. They include hexamethonium, mecamylamine (2.5–15 mg three times daily) and pempidine.

In an emergency Arfonad can be used to good effect. The initial dose is 10 mg given in 10 min and this is followed by the intermittent infusion of 30 mg every 30 min.

Adrenergic neurone blocking drugs

These sympatholytic drugs are more commonly employed. Unfortunately guanethidine (Ismelin), bethanidine (Esbatal), debrisequine (Declinax) and guanoxan (Envacar) all carry the risk of postural hypotension, exertional hypotension and impotence. Diarrhoea and rectal urgency can also occur.

Guanethidine, however, is very useful as an adjunct to hypotensive therapy in refractory cases, or indeed for any case of severe hypertension. Like prazosin it dilates the veins (the capacity vessels); a drop in cardiac output is the major cause of the fall of the blood pressure; later the peripheral resistance is reduced.

Beta-receptor blocking drugs

These produce a reduction of cardiac output (which is very dangerous if there is any tendency to failure) and they cause peripheral arteriolar dilatation and a reduction in renin release by the kidneys. They are currently in vogue, but they are dangerous in the elderly, and they must never be used in chronic bronchitis because of the increase in airways resistance.

Propranolol is the prototype. A dose under 80 mg per day is only weakly hypotensive, unless combined with a diuretic. As dosages increase the cardiac output is reduced. Although the peripheral vascular resistance tends to go up at first, it falls later, and circulating renin is lowered. These effects are generally beneficial and seem only to cause trouble in patients who also have peripheral vascular disease.

The dose of propranolol (Inderal) can be 120–480 mg/day; oxyprenolol (Trasicor) 160–320 mg/day; and pindolol (Visken) 10–45 mg/day. Tenormin (atenolol) can be given as a single dose (100 or 200 mg/day); not only is it long-acting but it is also cardioselective (beta-1 blocking), and should not cause bronchoconstriction. Metoprolol is a similar drug, given at a dose of 100 g.t.d.

Alpha-receptor blocking drugs

These have their application in refractory hypertension or in the treatment of phaeochromocytoma. Even in essential hypertension alpha-blockade will contribute to lowering of the blood pressure. Generally phentolamine and phenoxybenzamine (Dibenyline) are used only for phaeochromocytoma.

Combined alpha- and beta-blockade

This combination as *labetolol* at a dosage of 200 mg t.i.d. is the current fashion for the treatment of phaeochromocytoma or for severe hypertension. Blockade of the alpha-receptors lowers the peripheral resistance, and concurrent beta-blockade protects the heart from reflex sympathetic drive. The baroreceptor reflexes, however, remain sufficiently active to avoid postural hypotension.

Direct arteriolar relaxants

These are available as follows.

Hydrallazine (Apresoline)

This is a peripheral vasodilator, which at 25 mg three times daily is a useful adjunct to hypotensive therapy. In an emergency repeated doses can be given intramuscularly. It is known to increase renal blood flow. The drug must be treated with respect as large doses cause headache, joint symptoms and tachycardia, and even a drug-induced lupus syndrome with a positive antinuclear factor reaction.

Diazoxide (Eudemine)

This is given as 300 mg i/v or 100–200 mg t.i.d. It is very useful at the onset of treatment for malignant hypertension. When diazoxide is used it should be injected rapidly as a bolus so that it can be bound to the arterioles before it becomes fully bound to the plasma proteins. It has a slight salt and water-retaining effect, and it reduces secretion of insulin, thereby impairing glucose tolerance.

Sodium nitroprusside (Nipride)

This is given as a 0.01% solution in dextrose at a rate of 0.5–8μg/kg body weight, so as to produce a controllable peripheral vasodilatation.

Minoxidil

This is a piperidine–pyrimidine derivative which is a potent relaxant of vascular smooth muscle. It is useful for patients who are refractory to hydrallazine, propranlol, a-methyldopa or guanethidine. The starting dose is 2.5 mg orally and control may be achieved at 5–40 mg/day.

Each of the above drugs is particularly useful for accelerated hypertension or encephalopathy. The diastolic should not be lowered more than 100 mmHg for fear of oliguria.

Table 9   Recommended regimes for hypertensive emergencies

Drug	*Administration*	*Dosage*	*Onset*
Diazoxide	i/v	300 mg rapid bolus	immediate
Labetolol	i/v	50 mg stat, then	
		2 mg/min	30 min
Sodium nitroprusside	i/v	60 μg/ml	immediate
Trimethaphan (Arfonad)	i/v	1 mg/ml	immediate
Reserpine	i/m	2.5 mg	1–2 hours
Hydrallazine	i/v or i/m	10–20 mg	1–2 hours
Methyldopa	i/v	250–500 mg q.i.d.	1–4 hours
Guanethidine	oral	(individual)	days

Labetolol

This has combined beta- and alpha-blocking action so that it lowers the cardiac output and also reduces the peripheral resistance. The starting dosage is 100 mg three times daily orally but the final dose in severe hypertension may well be 1200 mg/day. For hypertensive encephalopathy it can be given intravenously at an initial dose of 50 mg or used as an infusion of 200 mg in 200 ml of dextrose given at a rate of 2 ml/min. If this drug causes troublesome hypotension, then the beta-blockade can be offset by increasing the heart rate with intravenous atropine.

Combination therapies

These are useful in hypertension but can lead to therapeutic muddles. Typical regimes are:

(1)   diuretic with beta-blocker/clonidine/sympatholytic drug;
(2)   diuretic/hydrallazine/beta-blocker;
(3)   diuretic/minoxidil/beta-blocker.

In choosing such regimes one has to be aware of the side-effects and the particular contraindications for various drugs. A knowledge of beta-blockers is important (see Table 10).

Table 10   Comparison of beta-blocking drugs

Relative potency		Beta-1 heart	Beta-2 arterioles bronchi	Membrane depressant
1. Oxyprenolol	2.0	++	+	+
2. Propranolol	1.0	++	+++	+
3. Pindolol	0.04	++	+	0
4. Sotalol	0.1	++	+	0
5. Practalol acetbutolol metoprolol	0.5	++	0	0

Table 11 shows a synopsis of drug contraindications. Some particular positive indications should also be stressed. If there is a liability to hypokalaemia with oedema then spironolactone, triamterene or amiloride should be part of the diuretic combination. Beta-blocking agents are advisable for hypertensive heart disease complicated by angina or ventricular ectopic beats. In the presence of severe renal impairment frusemide and methyldopa, hydrallazine, and prazosin or minoxidil are more effective than adrenergic neurone blocking drugs.

Table 11   Synopsis of drug contraindications

Heart failure	Beta-adrenergic receptor blocking drugs
Atrioventricular conduction defects	Beta-adrenergic receptor blocking drugs
Raynaud's disease	Beta-adrenergic receptor blocking drugs
Asthma	Beta-adrenergic receptor blocking drugs
Depression	Rauwolfia, methyldopa, clonidine and propranolol
Tricyclic antidepressant therapy	Adrenergic, methyldopa, clonidine and propranolol
Elderly patients	Beta-blockers and posturally acting drugs
Diabetes or hyperuricaemia	Thiazide diuretics and frusemide; diazoxide

REFERENCES

Recent symposium

4th Meeting of the International Society of Hypertension (1976). *Clin. Sci.* vol. **51**. suppl. 3

5th Meeting of International Society of Hypertension (1978). Clin. Sci. vol. **55**. Suppl. 4

Essential hypertension

Baldwin, D.S. and Biggs, A.W. (1958). Natriuresis in essential hypertension. *Am. J. Med.,* **24,** 893

Carey, R.M. and Ayers, C.R. (1976). Labile hypertension as a precursor of essential hypertension. *Am. J. Med.,* **61,** 811

Circulatory control and mechanisms in hypertension

Guyton, A.C. (1972). *Ann. Rev. Physiol.,* **34,** 13

Hollenberg, N.K., Borucki, L.J. and Adams, D.F. (1978). *Medicine,* **57,** 167

Ledingham, J.M. (1963). *1st Symposium. Adv. Med. Roy. Coll. Phys.,* **1,** 3

Control of renin release

Davis, J.O. and Freeman, R.H. (1976). *Physiol. Rev.,* **56,** 2

Vander, A.J. (1967). *Physiol. Rev.,* **47,** 359

Angiotensin–sodium interactions

Gavras, H. (1973). *Science,* **180,** 1369
Skeggs, L.T. (1976). *Am. J. Med.,* **160,** 737

Hypertension–two different mechanisms; renal hypertension

Brunner, H.R. (1971). *Science,* **174,** 1344
Fraley, E.E. (1972). *N. Engl. J. Med.,* **287,** 550
Goodwin, F.J. (1974). *Br. J. Hosp. Med.,* **11,** 525
Laragh, J.H. (1975). *Am. J., Med.,* **58,** 4
Stamey, T.A. (1965). *Am. J. Med.,* **38,** 829

Renal blood flow and perfusion, before and after renal hypertension

Ferrario, C.M. (1973). *Am. J. Physiol.,* **224,** 102

Pathology

Giese, J. (1973). Renin–angiotensin and hypertensive vascular damage. *Am. J. Med.,* **55,** 315
Kincaid-Smith, P. (1955). Course of malignant hypertension. *Q. J. Med.,* **27,** 117
Laragh, J. (1972). Renin–angiotensin, aldosterone in hypertensive vascular disease. *Am. J. Med.,* **52,** 633
McManus, J.F. and Lupton, C.H. (1960). Ischaemia of renal glomeruli in hypertension. *Lab. Invest.,* **9,** 413
Wiener, J. (1965). Cellular pathology and experimental hypertension. *Am. J. Pathol.,* **47,** 457

Hypertension and renal failure

Coleman, T.G. (1970). *Circulation,* **42,** 509
Craswell, P.H. (1972). *Br. Med. J.,* **4,** 749
Del Greco, F. (1975). *Kidney Int.,* **7,** S 176
Smith, P.K., Maxwell, M.H. (1975). *Kidney Int.,* **7,** S 151
Vertes, V. (1969). *N. Engl. J. Med.,* **280,** 978

Renal prostaglandins

Lee, J.B. (1976). *Am. J. Med.,* **60,** 798
McGiff, J.C. (1975). Prostaglandins and regulation of blood pressure. *Kidney Int.,* **8,** S262 Prostacyclin and kidney (1979) *Fed. Proc.,* **38,** 89

Renal Medicine

Use and limitations of saralasin

Case, D.B. (1976). *Am. J. Med.*, **60,** 825

Inhibitor of angiotensin converting enzyme

Ferguson, R.K. (1977). *Lancet,* **i,** 775

Diagnosis and localization in primary aldosteronism

Horton, R. and Finck, E. (1972). *Ann. Intern. Med.,* **76,** 855

Tyramine test for phaeochromocytoma

Engelman, K. (1968). *N. Engl. J. Med.,* **278,** 705

Aspects of hypertension treatment

Br. J. Pharmacol. Use of Labetolol. (1976). Suppl. 681
Dargie, H.J. (1977). Minoxidil in resistant hypertension. *Lancet,* **ii,** 515
Dollery, C.T. (1977). Combination therapy of hypertension. *Ann. Rev. Pharmacol. Toxicol.,* **17,** 311
Lorimer, A.R. (1976). Beta-blockade in hypertension. *Am. J. Med.,* **60,** 877

4
Glomerulonephritis

There are *three immunological mechanisms* which may initiate glomerular damage:

(1)   deposition in the glomeruli of circulating antigen–antibody (immune) complexes;

(2)   formation of an antibody against the glomerular basement membrane;

(3)   localization of antigen either in the mesangial cells or on the glomerular basement membrane followed by local reaction of antibody against it.

Immune complex disease

Since each immunoglobulin molecule has two arms with an antigen-combining site on each, antibody is bivalent. Many antigens are multivalent on account of repetitive units in their structure, as is the case with bacterial polysaccharide or a viral envelope. This means that union of antigen with antibody can give rise to a variety of polymers whose structure will be determined (a) by the nature of the antigen, and (b) by the amount and affinity of the antibody: [Antigen] + [Antibody] = [Ag/Ab complex]. The spectrum of immune complex composition is shown below.

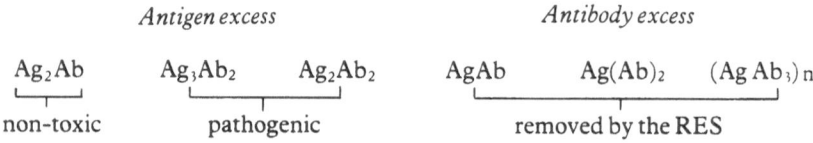

As will be seen the type of complex which produces immunopathological damage is a small unit, slightly on the side of antigen excess, with an Ag_3Ab_2 structure.

The classical model of immune complex disease is 'serum sickness nephritis' in which an animal such as a rabbit is injected with bovine serum albumin (BSA) antigen to which it will form antibodies by the 6th day. As antibody increases it will result in the rapid immune elimination of antigen and at the time formation of circulating antigen–antibody complexes. They persist in the circulation only transiently but are deposited in tissues to give rise to the classical 'serum sickness' immunopathology in the form of vasculitis with rash, arthralgia, carditis and glomerulonephritis. They can either be localized by means of isotope-labelled antigen or by the use of immunofluorescence for IgG antibody or complement components in tissues (Figure 35).

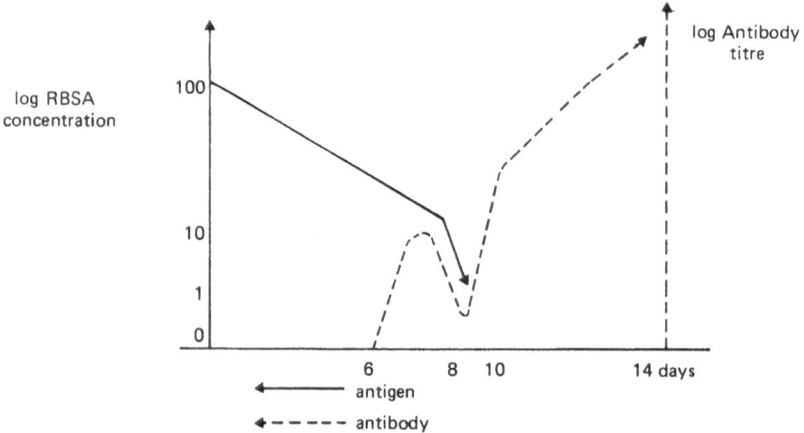

Figure 35.   The serum sickness model

As indicated the nature of the complexes depends on the valency of the antigen, and how much antibody is available and what is its 'affinity' (Figure 36).

90

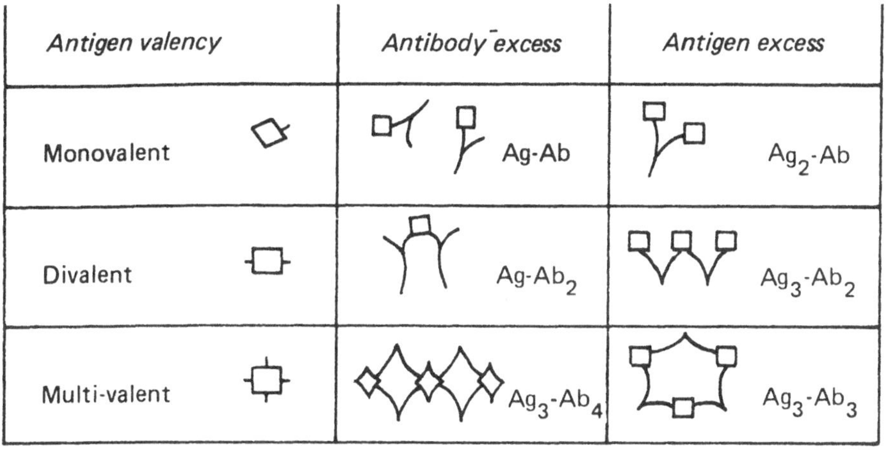

Antigen valency	Antibody excess	Antigen excess
Monovalent	Ag-Ab	Ag_2-Ab
Divalent	Ag-Ab_2	Ag_3-Ab_2
Multi-valent	Ag_3-Ab_4	Ag_3-Ab_3

Figure 36. Antigen–antibody interactions

The nature of the complexes determines their fate or their immuno-pathogenicity. Thus the large lattice structures formed by antibody excess are insoluble and are removed as foreign debris by the cells of the reticuloendo-thelial system, principally by the Kupffer cells of the liver. These are so-called *class III complexes* (Germuth).

Conversely, the soluble complexes may be so small that it is said that they produce no tissue damage at all. However one must realize that both the amount of antigen and certainly the amount of antibody is likely to fluctuate. Those complexes which in antigen excess have the structure Ag_3Ab_2 or Ag_2Ab_2 cause nephritis or vasculitis. Their activity depends on:

(1)   Their ability to fix to tissues, to react with complement, to damage platelets and leukocytes causing agglutination, and to degranulate mast cells with the liberation of vasoactive amines.

(2)   Their role in generating mediators of inflammation such as Cl-esterase, anaphylatoxin, bradykinin, fibrinolysin, and thus whether they cause an increase of vascular permeability, contraction of smooth muscle and endothelial cell proliferation.

(3)   The original nature of the antibody, as rabbit, human and guinea pig antibody form active complexes whilst bovine, chicken and horse antibodies are inactive.

As pathogenic immune complexes form the following steps take place:

(1)   In the presence of basophiles (or mast cells) which carry IgE immunoglobulin antibody, antigen interaction causes release of platelet agglutinating factor and vasoactive amines.

91

(2)   These amines cause an increased permeability of blood vessels, mainly in areas of platelet agglutination (the glomeruli, for example).

(3)   With the increase in permeability of the vessel wall complexes can permeate through to the basement membrane. The result is fixation of complement with the release of chemotactic factors and attraction of polymorphs, whose lysosomal enzymes cause digestion of the basement membrane.

(4)   Unless there is protective fibrinolysis by undamaged endothelium of the glomeruli, platelet agglutination will lead on to fibrin deposition and glomerular capillary thrombosis.

The sequence of events leading to immune complex disposition in glomeruli is as shown in Figure 37.

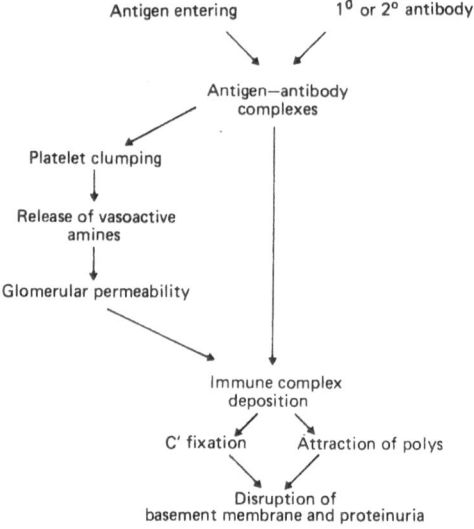

Figure 37.   Immune complex localization in glomeruli

The ultimate site of localization of complexes within the glomeruli also depends on their size. Since they are small *class I complexes* in antigen excess will traverse the basement membrane and localize as deposits on the *epithelial* side adjacent to the foot processes of the epithelial cells, which become fused. Some may remain within the membrane. Animal experiments show that complexes in these positions can be gradually removed by an excess of antigen, which presumably converts them to more soluble forms entering the urine.

Class II complexes are larger either because the antigen is bigger or because of larger antibody such as IgM. They are either taken up by the mesangial cells, which are phagocytic cells belonging to the reticuloendothelial system, or they localize on the *endothelial* side of the basement membrane.

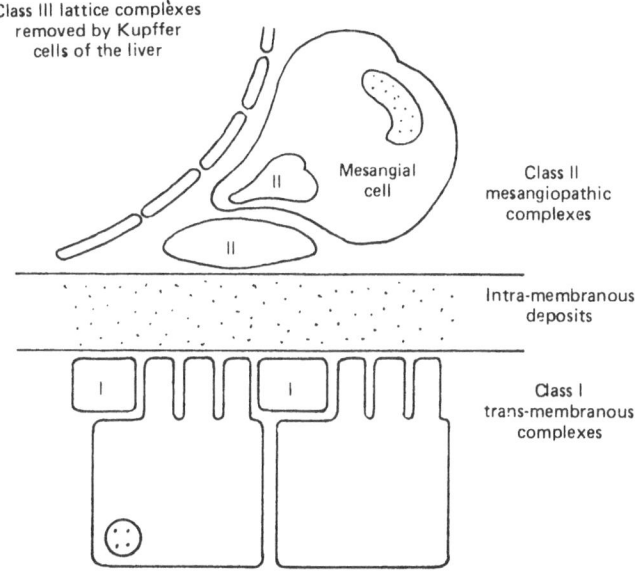

Figure 38. Complex size and glomerular localization

In the rabbit BSA model class I complexes contain IgG antibody only; their molecular weight is less than one million daltons. Class II complexes exceed 1×10^6 daltons; they often contain IgM antibody. Whereas class I cause diffuse proliferative or membranous disease, class II tend to cause focal mesangiopathic disease or mesangio-capillary lobular nephritis (Figure 38).

The nature of the antibody response is clearly of crucial importance, a point which has been developed by Germuth. Those animals which have no antibody response to an antigen are by definition 'tolerant' and although the antigen remains in the circulation, they do not develop nephritis. Those animals which develop a very good antibody response show a transient phase of antigen–antibody complex formation in antibody excess, so that there is rapid elimination of the antigen from the circulation. They develop a transient but rapidly resolving nephritis (see Figure 35 above) but most of those complexes are removed by the reticuloendothelial system. Interest focuses on those animals which have a medium or low antibody response to antigen, particularly when the experimental situation is adjusted so that small amounts of antigen are injected daily, so as to maintain circulating immune complexes in antigen excess. These animals develop a diffuse membranous type of

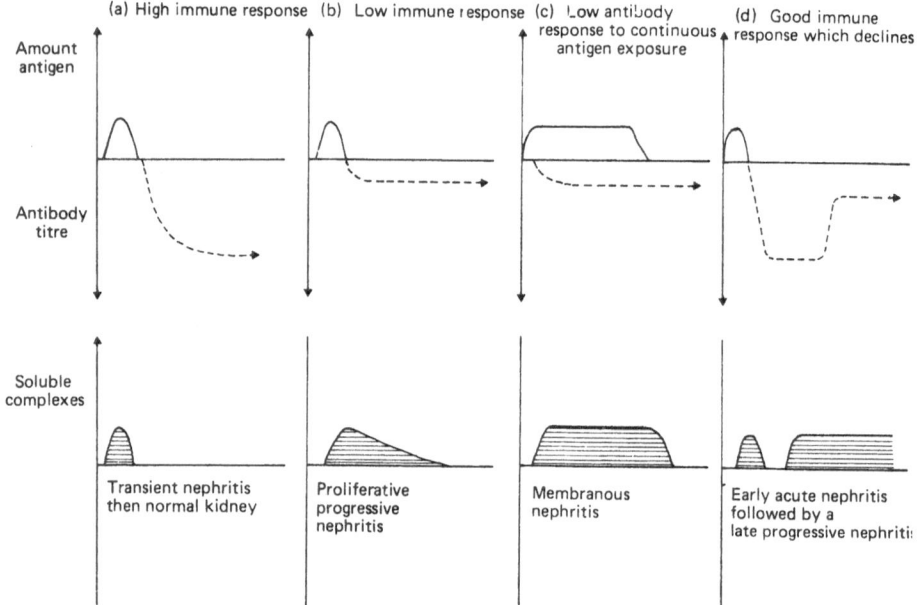

Figure 39.   **Role of antibody response (after Germuth)**

glomerulonephritis. Alternatively the nephritis will be mesangiopathic when there is rather more antibody than antigen.

Animals or individuals are genetically determined to be either good or poor antibody responders to a given antigen, and this accounts for current interest in HLA typing and in the *Ir* (immune response) genes. Situation (d) in Figure 39 is rather hypothetical. It is intended to explain the clinical observation that an early acute nephritis which apparently resolves is followed some years later by chronic nephritis. In reality it seems that this late phase may depend on slowly progressive glomerular sclerosis with the development of hypertension.

The actual amount of antibody may not be so relevant as its 'affinity'. Affinity measures the intensity of an antigen–antibody interaction and is denoted by a thermodynamic constant, k, in a reaction based on mass action principles such as:

$$[Ag] \ + \ [Ab] \ \overset{k}{\rightleftharpoons} \ [Ag.Ab]$$

Early in an immune response antibodies tend to be of lower affinity than those that appear later. It is probable that when antigen levels are high, both low and high affinity antibody is produced. Later when antigen levels are low, only those cells which produce high affinity antibodies will be stimulated. It is a crucial point because most antigen–antibody interactions operate normally in the body at low concentrations of antigen.

Low affinity antibody tends to be non-precipitating and it has a poor potential for elimination of antigen from the circulation. This may be visualized as shown in Figure 40 according to the work of Christian (1969).

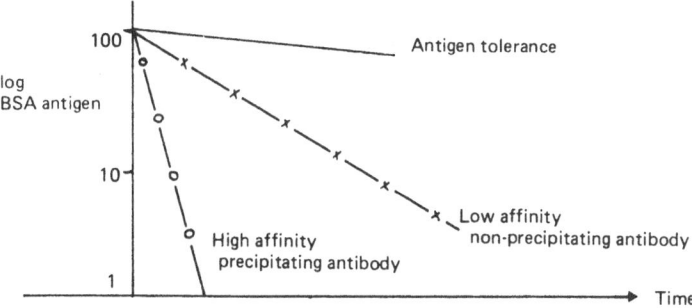

Figure 40.   Elimination of antigen by antibody

It has been claimed that those animals which develop chronic nephritis are those which produce low affinity antibodies. This is because antigen–antibody complexes persist in their circulation for long periods. Moreover Steward and Soothill have shown that strains of mice whose genetic structure and macrophage responses are such that they produce low affinity antibody to HSA (human serum albumin) are in fact those which are known to be genetically susceptible to nephritis. They found that higher affinity antibody could be produced when antigen was given in Freund's adjuvant rather than in saline.

We can see, therefore, that membranous nephritis (Figure 41) occurs when there is long-term deposition of soluble antigen–antibody complexes that are formed in antigen excess or when the antibody is of low affinity. If the deposits lodge in the membrane they give a spiky appearance which can be shown up by silver stains. Otherwise they pass through to a subepithelial position.

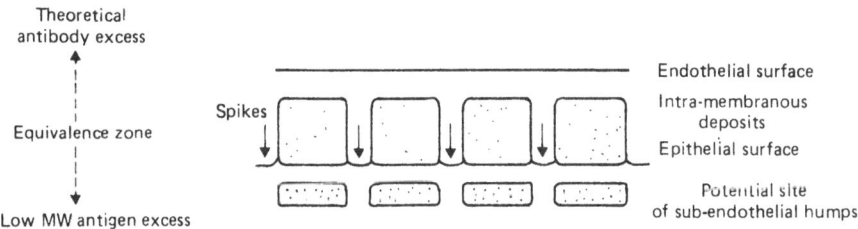

Figure 41.   Membranous nephritis

It seems that when there are immune deposits within the basement membrane, this reflects a zone of antigen–antibody equivalence. When there is a relative excess of antigen, then the complexes will pass through to the subepithelial position.

Clinical and experimental experience shows that a variety of viruses can give rise to chronic immune complex nephritis. Not only do virus antigens tend to persist but they also elicit low affinity non-neutralizing antibody. This is the case with lactic dehydrogenase virus infection in mice, and the systemic lupus erythematosus (SLE)- like syndromes of Aleutian mink disease or Gross virus infection of NZB/NZW mice.

Antiglomerular basement membrane antibody disease

This is usually produced by injecting an animal with heterologous antibody (that produced in another species) to glomerular basement membrane. In the 'heterologous phase' the foreign antibody adheres to the basement membrane and produces a transient nephritis. However this is followed after a few days by an 'autologous phase' when the host animal produces its own antibodies to the foreign gammaglobulin in the glomeruli. According to the administered dose the result can be a focal, a diffuse proliferative, or an exudative and necrotizing glomerulonephritis.

This whole process can be telescoped so as to be more dramatic, and at the same time more amenable to study, if rabbits which are presensitized to sheep IgG are injected with a sheep antirabbit GBM serum. The mechanisms are shown in Figure 42.

Thus antibody bound to its antigen (the basement membrane) causes activation of C1q and thereby both platelet agglutination and complement cascade activation; in turn there is activation of coagulation. Polymorphs are

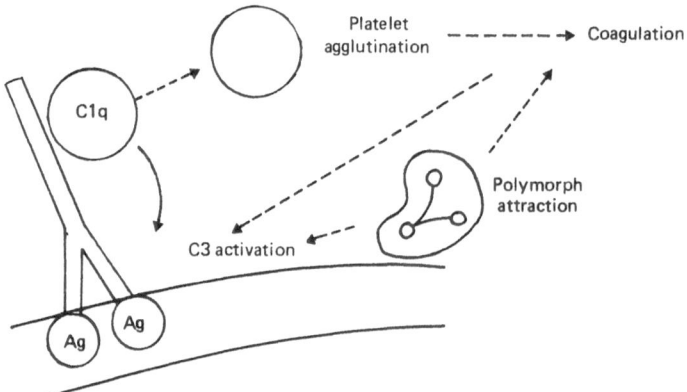

Figure 42.   Mechanisms in nephrotoxic serum nephritis

attracted to the site of damage by the complement chemotactic component C567. Release of their lysosomal enzymes is an important factor in the digestion and destruction of the basement membrane. Both reduction of plasma fibrinogen by arvinization or platelet depletion have been shown to be beneficial.

Mesangiopathic nephritis

Since the mesangial cells are part of the reticuloendothelial system, they will ingest any free particulate antigen in the circulation. It is then possible for antibody against the antigen to destroy those mesangial cells. Such a sequence has been demonstrated experimentally but its role in practice has yet to be ascertained.

Animal models of nephritis

At this stage we can summarize the animal prototypes in order to illustrate the great contribution that has been made to the understanding of the human situations.

Immune complex nephritis
This is produced in a variety of ways:

(1)   Acute serum sickness nephritis using a single large dose of BSA antigen causes a transient proliferative nephritis.
(2)   Chronic serum sickness nephritis using repeated small doses of BSA antigen causes a membranous nephritis.
(3)   Chronic serum sickness nephritis using horse serum antigen causes a mesangiopathic nephritis with a vasculitis akin to polyarteritis nodosa.
(4)   Heymann's nephritis: that is a membranous nephritis caused by the release of autologous renal tubular antigen into the circulation.

The latter model is quite important because it appears that it represents the pathogenic mechanism of idiopathic membranous disease. Thus it was originally noted that intravenous injection of an antiserum to fraction III of the renal tubules of the rat would cause a mild proteinuria, and that as a result of the tubular damage there would then be release of nephritogenic antigen so as to form immune complexes, which in their turn would give rise to a membranous autoimmune nephrosis. Further study by Barabas and Lannigan showed that the process could be telescoped by prior injection of BSA to induce an immune complex process, which itself would induce permeability of the basement membrane, so that thereafter an injection of antiserum to renal tubules would have a more profound damaging effect. In analogous fashion a previous injection of mercuric chloride, so as to damage the tubules, will magnify the amount of damage.

Antiglomerular basement membrane disease
This has two animal counterparts.

(1)   Masugi nephritis—this utilizes antiGBM antibody made in another animal (that is, heterologous antibody).

(2)   Steblay nephritis caused by using the animal's own autologous GBM as antigen. The basement membrane in Freund's complete adjuvant is injected intramuscularly and a rapidly progressive nephritis ensues.

Factors predisposing to nephritis

Clearly a paramount factor is the prevalence of bacterial or viral infection, but in addition one has to consider that often the antibody response is insufficient to result in total clearance of circulating antigen, so that immune complexes persist in the circulation. This can occur:

(1)   On account of low affinity antibodies (as discussed above).

(2)   When there is continuous release of antigen into the circulation as the result of chronic viral infection as in SLE or LCM in mice. In these situations a T lymphocyte deficiency may be acquired or inherited. Indeed it is likely that the HLA or *Ir* (immune response) genes control both macrophage and T lymphocyte potential to respond to foreign antigens.

(3)   Inherited complement deficiencies may also predispose to infection or persistence of antigen. High titre IgG-antibody is itself opsonic and will aid removal of bacteria from the circulation. Yet early in an immune response the IgM antibody that is formed in the 'primary phase' requires complement in order to effect opsonization (that is, the fixation of C3b on bacteria) so as to promote their phagocytosis.

Indeed, when there is total absence of C3, there is a marked liability to pneumonia and septicaemia. Complement is also required for the aggregation of virus particles. In fact it turns out that glomerulonephritis, SLE, polyarteritis or connective tissue diseases are relatively common when there are C1r, C2 or C4 deficiencies. However it is a curious paradox that although C3 or C5 deficiency predisposes to infection, patients need not have nephritis. Moreover in partial lipodystrophy, where there is partial C3 deficiency and often membranoproliferative nephritis, these patients are still not susceptible to recurrent or chronic infection.

Systems involved in the immunopathology of nephritis

The complement system

Union of antigen with antibodies of the IgG or IgM type results in an alteration of the Fc part of the molecule so that the complement component Clq binds and so activates the 'classical pathway'. On the other hand, bacterial polysaccharides and endotoxins, aggregated IgA and myeloma proteins, and so-called 'nephritic factor' lead to triggering of the 'alternate pathway' of complement activation. The result is that either C3 convertase from the classical pathway or C3 activator of the alternate pathway will lead to firing of the terminal complement sequence C3—C9 (Figure 43). Cell membranes to which C3b is attached are then lysed, inflammation is promoted by the influx of polymorphs which are attracted by the chemotactic unit C567, and coagulation is enhanced. There is a positive feedback whereby C3b generation promotes the activity of C3Pase of the alternate pathway. C3b is normally held in check by C3b inactivator (KAF), and other important inhibitors also serve to keep the system in check. However local activation and fixation of the hydrophobic terminal complement components on cell membranes result in cell membrane damage by a detergent-like action. Only one molecule of activated C8–C9 is required to punch a hole in the cell membrane of an erythrocyte.

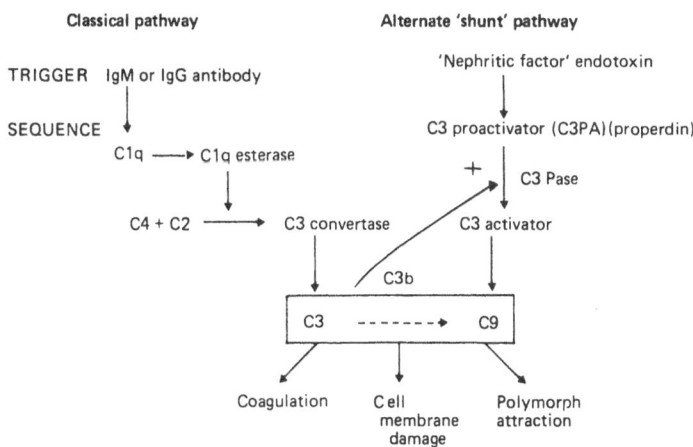

Figure 43.   Simple scheme of the complement pathway

The role of polymorphs

It is unusual to see more than an occasional polymorph in a glomerulus in nephritis, except in the condition called acute exudative nephritis in which polymorphs accumulate in the capillary lumina. All the same, polymorphs are attracted by the trimolecular complex C567, and their enzymes digest basement membrane.

They contain at least four basic proteins whose release is known to mediate vascular permeability, and their lysosomal enzymes contain cathepsins A, D and E as well as a collagenase and an elastase. These enzymes explain why GBM fragments appear in the urine, and also why new GBM (non-collagen) antigens may become exposed.

The role of platelets

As described above release of vasoactive amines from platelets seems to be essential for the localization of immune complexes. Both antihistamines and antiserotonin agents have been shown to reduce the degee of complex deposition. Once platelets are agglutinated, exposure of platelet factor III on the membrane and release of PF4 into the blood enhances the coagulation cascade. However prostacyclin of renal vascular endothelium is protective.

The role of coagulation leading to fibrin formation

Coagulation is liable to occur in the renal glomeruli in active immune complex diseases because haemoconcentration with a resultant rise of blood viscosity is a normal effect of the ultrafiltration and, of course, when platelets and immune complexes are being concentrated together coagulation is triggered by means of PF3. Additionally if basement membrane collagen is exposed, this will cause (a) direct adherence and agglutination of platelets, and (b) triggering of coagulation by activation of Hageman factor XII.

Coagulation should always be balanced by fibrinolysis. The glomeruli have some measure of protection since, unlike most arterioles, their endothelial cells release fibrinolytic activator. Additionally the mesangial phagocytic cells are known to ingest fibrin particles. The breakdown products of fibrin—

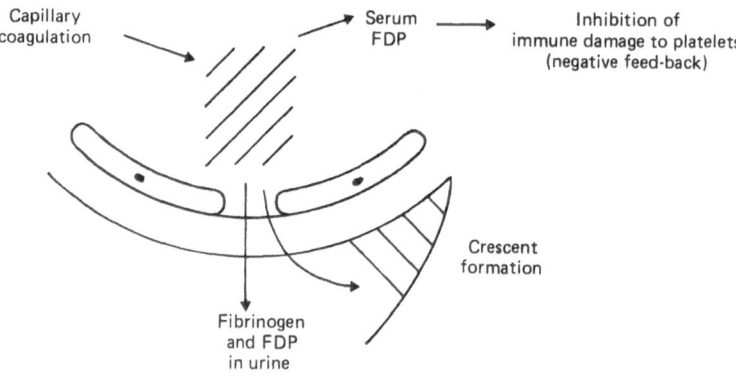

Figure 44.   Summary of the role of fibrin

FDP—are found to be elevated in the sera of patients with nephritis and they are also excreted in the urine. Although fibrinuria is mainly a measure of the degree of damage to the basement membrane, allowing a molecule as large as fibrinogen (340 000) to pass, additionally it is claimed that the amount of FDP in urine is a measure of the activity of a proliferative nephritis (Figure 44).

Leakage of fibrin into Bowman's capsule has important consequences for it stimulates the growth of epithelial crescents which eventually strangle the glomerulus. Moreover coagulation within a glomerulus is often followed by hyalinosis and collagen formation with sclerosis. In turn the impairment of renal blood flow causes renin release which leads on to hypertension.

CLASSIFICATION OF NEPHRITIS

Familiarity with the normal cell structure of the renal glomerulus is essential for understanding the classification of nephritis, since it is based on morphology (Figure 45).

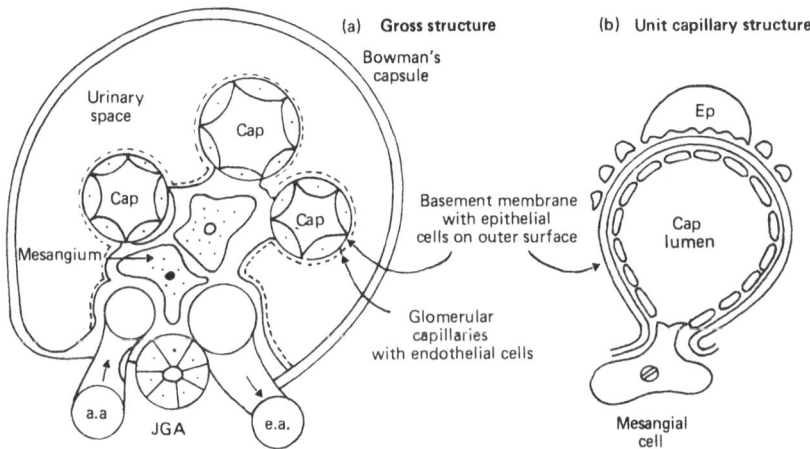

Figure 45.   Arrangement of cells in the renal glomerulus

The capillary loops are lined by endothelium between which plasma filters through the basement membrane and thence between the slit processes of the epithelial cells into Bowman's capsule. Near to the central stalk the supporting mesangial cells may insert processes beneath the endothelial cells but superficial to the basement membrane; they therefore appear as 'deep endothelial' cells. The function of the mesangial cells is phagocytic.

Morphological terms applied in nephritis classification

In the first place nephritis may be *diffuse* (involving all glomeruli), *focal*

101

(involving one or more glomeruli) or *segmental* (involving parts of glomeruli).

Secondly, when there is morphological change as seen by the light microscope, the components which are involved are:

(1)   endothelial or mesangial proliferation;
(2)   extracapillary epithelial proliferation leading to crescent formation;
(3)   basement membrane thickening as in 'membranous nephropathy';
(4)   a mixture as in mesangio-capillary disease. These changes are pictured in Figure 46.

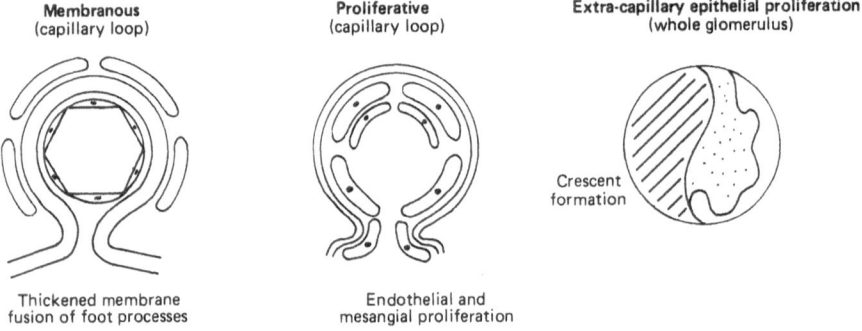

Figure 46.   **Histological types of nephritis.**
Membranous/proliferative/extracapillary

Immunofluorescent studies and classification

Immunofluorescence is used for the localization of immunoglobulins, complement components and antigens. A frozen section of a renal biopsy sample is placed on a microscope slide and is covered with antihuman IgG or antihuman complement conjugated with fluorescein isothiocyanate. After washing, viewing under ultraviolet light will show up any deposits in the glomeruli.

In the technique of 'indirect' immunofluorescence (the 'sandwich' technique) an antiserum is applied to the slide (say rabbit antiproperdin), then a second fluorescein conjugated antibody is used to reveal its localization, as is evident when a fluorescein labelled sheep antirabbit globulin is added.

Immunofluorescent patterns
Typically the deposition of immune complexes is in a '*lumpy-bumpy*' pattern in, on or beneath the basement membrane. Such a pattern with IgG immunofluorescence is quite distinctive from the *smooth linear* staining given by an antibody reacting directly with the basement membrane. There is a fundamental distinction between these types of nephritis (Figure 47).

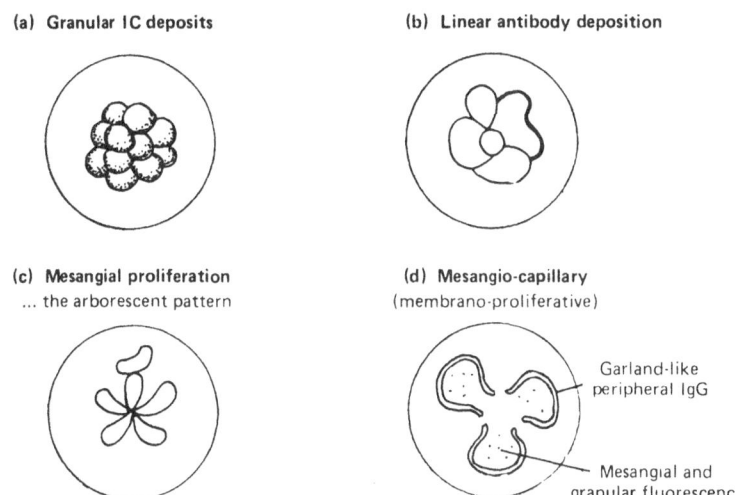

(a) Granular IC deposits

(b) Linear antibody deposition

(c) Mesangial proliferation
... the arborescent pattern

(d) Mesangio-capillary
(membrano-proliferative)

Garland-like
peripheral IgG

Mesangial and
granular fluorescence

Figure 47. Basic immunofluorescence patterns

The classification of nephritis by morphology and cause

Minimal change nephritis
No light microscope changes; specific cause ? lymphokines; occurs with pollen or milk allergy and atopy in subjects with HLA-B12.

Immune complex nephritides
(1) *Endothelial proliferation and subepithelial humps* (class I complexes); due to poststreptococcal nephritis; other bacterial infections like staphylococcus, pneumococcus; bacterial endocarditis; shunt nephritis; syphilis.
(2) *Membranous nephropathy* (class I complexes); idiopathic due to tubular antigen; infections, such as hepatitis B, malaria, syphilis; exposure to metals; neoplasms; SLE; diabetes.
(3) *Mesangiopathic proliferative nephritis* (class II complexes); SLE, DNA–anti DNA complexes; drug induced lupus; Henoch–Schönlein; polyarteritis nodosa; Wegener's granulomatosis; cryoglobulinaemia; nephrotic syndrome due to malaria.
(4) *Mesangial-nephritis*; post-streptococcal; mesangial IgA disease.

Antiglomerular basement membrane antibody
(1) The Goodpasture syndrome;
(2) in some types of rapidly progressive nephritis.

Immune-mediated tubular and interstitial damage
This is due to:

(1)   Deposition of immune complexes of IgG with C′ on the tubular basement membranes.

(2)   The formation of autoantibodies to tubular basement membrane— for example, this can be seen on rare occasions after streptococcal infection.

(3)   Lymphocyte-mediated cytotoxic damage to tubular cells. These latter mechanisms could account for those situations in which there is residual tubular damage after an interstitial nephritis.

Histopathology of nephritis

Classification is based on light microscopy supplemented when necessary by electron microscopy and by immunofluorescence, as indicated by the synopses given above.

Minimal change nephritis
The glomeruli are normal by light microscopy, but as there can be heavy proteinuria the electron microscope will reveal fusion of the foot processes of the epithelial cells; this is secondary to the proteinuria. There are no immunoglobulins to be found by immunofluorescence (Figure 48).

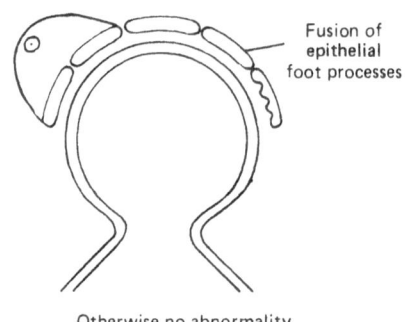

Fusion of
epithelial
foot processes

Otherwise no abnormality.
? increased permeability caused by lymphokines

Figure 48.   Minimal change nephrosis

Focal glomerulosclerosis is when there are associated focal and sclerotic lesions in those glomeruli which are in the juxtamedullary zone. Patients have microscopic haematuria and a poor response to steroids, so their overall prognosis is poor. They form part of the spectrum of disease of minimal change nephritis.

Two other entities might be confused with minimal lesions: (a) When there is some associated but slight mesangial hypertrophy, in which fluorescence will reveal IgG or IgA. These patients have haematuria and the 'mesangial-IgA' syndrome; and (b) when electron microscopy shows very early extramembranous deposits—this might be called 'minimal-membranous' and indeed it can progress to membranous disease.

Proliferative nephritis

Diffuse—Typically this occurs in poststreptococcal nephritis, in which there is proliferation of the endothelial cells of the glomerular capillaries as well as the mesangial stalk cells.

Mesangial proliferation—When the mesangial cells alone proliferate there is no narrowing of the capillary lumina, as is the case when there is endothelial proliferation. This appearance is commonly seen in resolving poststreptococcal glomerulonephritis.

Extracapillary glomerulonephritis or **'crescentic nephritis'**—This is a proliferative nephritis in which leakage of fibrin into Bowman's space has resulted in a proliferation of the epithelial cells, and the formation of 'crescents' which eventually strangle the glomeruli. It is therefore a rapidly progressive nephritis. In the typical Bacani type a virus aetiology has been suspected, since a preceding streptococcal infection is not usually found.

Membranoproliferative nephritis—In this condition there is mesangial expansion and proliferation but at the same time thickening of the capillary walls, hence the alternative name **'mesangiocapillary'** nephritis (MCGN).

Membranous nephropathy

Here there is a uniform thickening of the glomerular capillary walls. Deposits of antigen–antibody complexes actually expand the membrane (see Figure 41) so that when finger-like processes or spikes project outwards, that condition is termed 'epimembranous'. The deposits contain IgG and C3.

MONITORING THE COURSE OF A NEPHRITIS

Renal function

Following the serum creatinine, the creatinine clearance and the amount of fluid accumulated by the patient by means of daily weighing is the time-honoured and accepted means of following the course of a nephritis.

Detection of immune complexes

This is now in a stage of development, although, in contrast to the animal experiments, it is not so easy in man to relate the finding of immune complexes to an episode of deterioration. The nephrologist, however, should be aware of the following approaches.

The platelet agglutination test
As described above platelets agglutinate immune complexes. Therefore fresh washed human platelets are incubated overnight at 5 °C with heat-inactivated (50 °C) serum in appropriate serial dilution. Platelets which are agglutinated will form a dark aggregate pattern in contrast to the small white button of normally sedimented platelets.

Determination of macromolecular bound C3
If C3 (molecular weight 185 000) is separated on Sephadex G-200, it will appear in the second peak during fractionation. However, if it comes off the column together with the higher molecular weight proteins, then this is taken to mean that the C3 is bound to immune complexes. The fractions have to be measured by a sensitive microhaemagglutination inhibition assay (Figure 49).

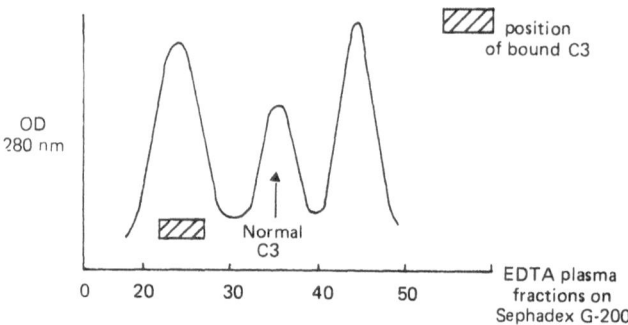

Figure 49.   Detection of macromolecular bound C3

Anticomplementary activity of sera
Immune complexes bind the complement in serum so that their presence can be detected as a depletion of haemolytic complement. A major snag is that aggregated immunoglobulins are also complement fixing and give rise to false-positive reactions.

Reactions with C1q
The first complement component C1q gives a precipitin line on a plate when there is diffusion against 19S complexes. From this observation arose a competitive binding assay. Radioiodinated C1q is allowed to bind with any immune complexes in a serum and can then be precipitated with polyethylene glycol so as to leave any free isotopic C1q in the supernatant. In this way

complexes are quantitated. Yet another approach is when the immune complexes in sera are used to inhibit the binding of radiolabelled C1q to sheep erythrocytes that have been sensitized by antibody.

Rheumatoid factor binding tests

Monoclonal IgM rheumatoid factors can be obtained from the sera of patients with lymphoproliferative diseases. These form a preciptin line on a plate when allowed to diffuse against sera which contain even small size gammaglobulin complexes. The rheumatoid factor reacts because it is an IgM antibody to an IgG molecule. On this basis it has been possible to devise a competitive binding assay in which union of rheumatoid factor with iodinated heat aggregated IgG can be competitively inhibited by preincubation with sera containing antigen–antibody complexes.

A-Protein of Staphylococcus aureus (SpA)

The A-protein of *Staphylococcus aureus* bonds to the Fc-part of IgG antibody molecules, so in order to assay immune complexes or aggregated immunoglobulins in sera the procedure is to incubate $200\,\mu l$ of serum, $200\,\mu l$ of polyethylene glycol assay buffer and $100\,\mu l$ of $[^{125}I]$ SpA. In the final event the centrifuged deposit is assayed for the amount of $[^{125}I]$ SpA that has been bound.

Uptake of immune complexes by macrophages

Denatured iodinated gammaglobulins will be taken up by macrophages. This also can be made the basis of a competitive binding assay in which the uptake of immune complexes from sera will then reduce the amount of labelled gammaglobulin that can be ingested.

Complement levels

If there are circulating immune complexes there is activation of the classical pathway of complement consumption, so that both serum C3 and serum C4 will be depressed, as also is the serum C1q. In this way the active phase of an acute proliferative nephritis or SLE nephritis can be monitored.

In the case of 'alternate pathway' complement activation, however, there will be lowering only of C3PA (properdin factor B) and of the serum C3. Many of these patients exhibit persistent hypocomplementaemia (see below, page 139). Reference to Figure 43 will clarify these statements.

Selectivity of proteinuria

When there is minimal damage to the glomerular basement membrane only small molecules such as albumin (70 000) or transferrin (molecular weight 90 000) are able to leak. This is called a 'selective proteinuria'. On the other hand when the basement membrane becomes more porous, then larger molecules such as IgG (150 000), fibrinogen (340 000) or even a-$_2$-macro-globulin (820 000) will be lost through the glomerulus and appear in the urine. This is a 'non-selective' proteinuria.

After urine concentration by a Diaflo membrane, or by means of ultrafiltration, or by absorption of water using 60% polyethylene glycol (carbowax 20M), it is only necessary to determine the urinary ratio of IgG to albumin or better still the ratio of IgG to transferrin. So, for example, an IgG/transferrin ratio of 0.2 or less signifies a 'minimal change' nephritis which will respond satisfactorily to steroid therapy. The range 0.3–0.5 is poorly selective and in these cases there is both IgA and haptoglobin in the urine. In the IgG/transferrin range 0.5–0.9 of non-selective proteinuria one will also find a-$_2$-macroglobulin present in the urine and perhaps lipoproteins (molecular weight 1×10^6).

Whereas proliferative nephritis may be selective, or at the worst poorly selective, conditions which cause non-selective proteinuria include membranous nephropathy, mesangio-capillary nephritis and focal glomerulosclerosis. It is unusual for a 'selectivity' to improve with treatment, although occasionally this occurs with the selective proteinuria of an exudative proliferative or focal proliferative nephritis.

Intrarenal coagulation

It is possible to monitor the activity of a nephritis by the daily urine output of

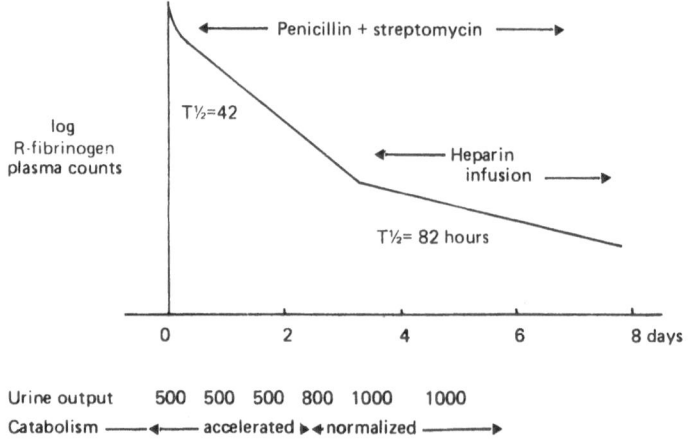

Figure 50. Radiofibrinogen catabolism in nephritis due to endocarditis

fibrin degradation products (FDP); so, for example, when indomethacin therapy is instituted a fall of urinary FDP will often be noted.

Of greater value is the radiofibrinogen catabolism study. The evaluation of these results requires a plasma protein expert for it is not really sufficient to merely compare the plasma decay of radiofibrinogen with the normal to see if there is increased fibrinogen catabolism. The breakdown rate of fibrinogen or catabolic rate has to be quantitated by the urinary excretion of free isotopic iodide as compared with the amount of radiolabelled fibrinogen within the body. In the oliguric patient this will necessitate various corrective procedures.

However, the principle of the procedure is simple, as shown in Figure 50, in which the nephritis accompanying bacterial endocarditis can be seen to improve along with the fibrinogen catabolic rate while the patient is on a heparin infusion.

Reticuloendothelial cell clearances

The main mass of the reticuloendothelial cells is formed by the Kupffer cells of the liver. If radioiodinated colloidal albumin is injected intravenously, its rate of removal is a function of the phagocytic activity of the Kupffer cells. In most immune complex diseases, inflammatory states and most nephritides there is enhanced Kupffer cell phagocytic clearance. Thus if the normal half-life of clearance is 14.0 min (Drivas, Wardle and Kerr, 1976), most cases of proliferative and membranous nephritis will show a half-life of about 10 min, whereas in IgA mesangial nephritis accelerated clearance may give a half-life of 6–8 min. This increase of RES function normally correlates with disease activity, although it will be reduced if the patient receives corticosteroid therapy.

Conversely in mesangiocapillary nephritis there can be reduced RES function, which presumably reflects saturation of the phagocytic cells by the larger immune complexes in antibody excess. Indeed this may provide an explanation why the mesangial cells are so encumbered; both the Kupffer cells and the mesangial cells might be described as suffering from 'indigestion'. In reality their Fc receptors are probably blocked.

SUMMARY OF SOME BASIC CLINICAL FEATURES OF THE NEPHRITIDES

Presentation

This may be as:

(1)   proteinuria;
(2)   haematuria—there are red cells and red cell casts in the urine;

(3)   an acute nephritic syndrome, with oliguria, oedema and hyperten-
       sion;
(4)   as a nephrotic syndrome, with massive proteinuria, oedema and
       potential hypovolaemia.

A *nephritic syndrome* can be due to:

(1)   acute exudative proliferative nephritis;
(2)   mesangial proliferative nephritis;
(3)   mesangiocapillary nephritis (membranoproliferative nephritis);
(4)   rapidly progressive extracapillary nephritis.

A *nephrotic syndome* can be a consequence of:

(1)   minimal change nephritis;
(2)   focal nephritis;
(3)   membranous nephropathy;
(4)   mesangiocapillary nephritis.

Age

It is helpful to know the age at which a particular type of nephritis is likely to
appear:

(1)   minimal change: 1–5 years (associated with allergy and HLA-B12);
(2)   acute exudative proliferative: 5–10 years (the age for streptococcal
       sore throats);
(3)   mesangiocapillary: 10–20 years;
(4)   membranous nephropathy: 20–50 years (especially associated with
       neoplasms);
(5)   rapidly progressive nephritis with crescents: 50–60 years.

Indices

A reasonable guess can be made as to the type of nephritis that will be revealed
by biopsy by taking account of the urinary sediment and differential protein
clearance, the degree of lowering of the GFR and elevation of blood pressure,
and by the level of the serum C3 (Table 13).

Haematuria is common in all those nephritides with changes on light
microscopy, as is a reduction of the glomerular filtration rate and an elevation
of the blood pressure. A low C3 complement can be found in the active stage
of an acute exudative proliferative nephritis, occasionally in rapidly
progressive crescentic nephritis, and quite commonly in mesangiocapillary
nephritis.

When considering haematuria one has, of course, to think of other

Table 13

	Haematuria	DPC	Low GFR/elevated BP	C3 Complement
Minimal change	o	Selective	—	Normal
Focal sclerosis	+	Non-selective	Common	Normal
Proliferative	+	Non-selective	Common	Normal or high but low in MCGN
Membranous	+	Non-selective	Common	Normal

possibilities (page 160) such as infection in the urinary tract, a stone or a Wilm's tumour. Patients who have overt haematuria, either after an upper respiratory tract infection or after exercise, usually have microscopic haematuria between attacks. Renal biopsy will reveal the nature of the lesion, mesangial IgA disease, for instance. This may not, however, be the case when a young woman is on the oral contraceptive 'pill' for these patients can get focal areas of renal damage due to microthrombi in intrarenal small vessels; these are only revealed by angiography.

Recurrent haematuria can be a manifestation of Alport's syndrome of hereditary nephritis with deafness. There is often a family history (page 162).

Histology

Since renal biopsy was introduced by Iversen and Brun in 1951 it has become clear that histology gives a reasonable guide to prognosis. Thus a minimal change nephritis *per se* has a good prognosis, but if there is nephrotic syndrome with it, an increase of complications such as hypertension, acute renal failure (usually precipitated by plasma volume depletion) or infections is probable. Whatever the type of nephritis the prognosis is so much the worse if there are tubular as well as glomerular lesions. Hypertension always worsens the prognosis, because, as Ellis noted in 1942, it leads to vascular damage and to a 'circulus vitiosus . Steroid therapy, also, carries the inevitable risks of peptic ulceration, liability to infection, coronary thrombosis or stroke.

As for the other nephritides the outcome simply depends on the amount of damage to the glomeruli. Focal sclerosing nephritis, proliferative nephritis, membranoproliferative nephritis and membranous nephropathy can all pursue a steady downhill course. When there are many crescents, as in the rapidly progressive glomerulonephritides, the progression to acute renal failure can occur in days, or at best within a few months.

Nephrotic syndrome

Several types of nephritis present as 'nephrosis' (Müller, 1905) in which the patient loses more than 3.0 g/day of protein in the urine so that hypoproteinaemia with oedema and also hypovolaemia develop. The pathophysiological sequence is important and can be summarized as in Figure 51.

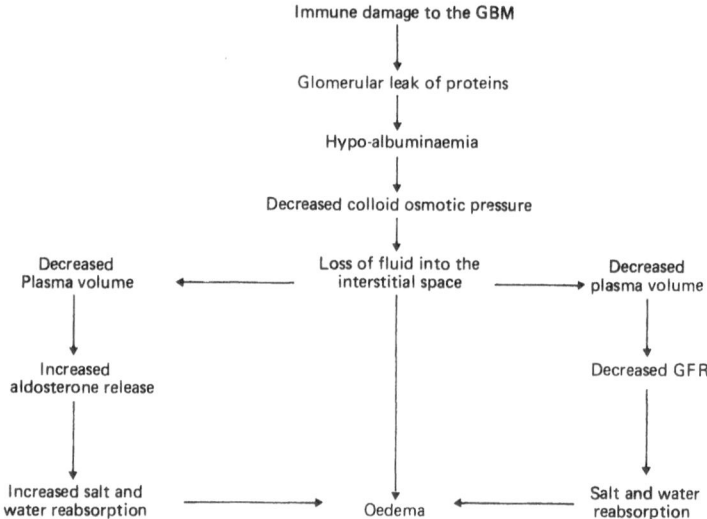

Figure 51. Operative mechanisms in nephrotic syndrome

Reduction of the plasma volume leads to oliguria, and it may be necessary to restore the serum proteins before the patient can pass sufficient urine. A low albumin due to loss through the glomeruli also gives rise to quite intense lipaemia (which will be discussed below, page 310), but in the long term there is a real risk of accelerated atherosclerosis leading to coronary thrombosis or stroke. The same patients often have a hypercoagulable state, which may be manifest as deep vein thrombosis or even superimposed renal vein thrombosis.

REFERENCES

Mechanisms of nephritis

Carpenter, C.B. (1970). Immunological aspects of renal disease. *Ann. Rev. Med.*, **21**, 1

Dixon, F.J. (1968). The pathogenesis of glomerulonephritis. *Am. J. Med.*, **44**, 493

McCluskey, R.T. and Classen, J. (1973). Immunological mechanisms in nephritis. *N. Engl. J. Med.*, **288**, 564

Merrill, J.P. (1974). Glomerulonephritis. *N. Engl. J. Med.*, **290**, 257, 313, 374

Peters, D.K. (1973). The immunological basis of nephritis. *Br. J. Hosp. Med.*, January, 63

Classification of glomerulonephritis

Berger, J. (1971). Types of immune deposit. *Adv. Nephrol.*, **1**, 11

Bohle, A., Kluthe, R., Sarne, H. and Wehner, H. (1970). Renal biopsy in the nephrotic syndrome. *German Med. Month.*, 32

Cameron, S. (1973). Glomerulonephritis. *Medicine*, **21**, 1258

Grundmann, E. and Kirsten, W.H. (1976). Glomerulonephritis classification. *Curr. Top. Pathol.*, vol. 61

Germuth, F.G. and Rodriguez, E. (1973). Immunopathology of the renal glomerulus. (Boston: Little Brown and Co.)

Kincaid-Smith, P., Mathew, T.H. and Lovell Becker (1973). *Glomerulonephritis*, Vols I and II. (New York: John Wiley and Sons.)

White, R.H.R. (1970). Glomerulonephritis in children. *Br. J. Hosp. Med.*, May, 746

Immune complexes

Bonomo, L. and Turk, J.L. (1970). *Immune complex diseases*. (Milan: Carlo Erba Foundation)

Christian, C.L. (1969). Immune complex disease. *N. Engl. J. Med.*, **280**, 878

Dixon, F.J. (1971). Immune complexes and disease (nephritis and rheumatic). *J. Exp. Med.*, **134**, no. 3, pt 2. supplement

Dixon, F.J. and Cochrane, C.G. (1970). Pathogenicity of antigen–antibody complexes. *Pathol. Ann.* 355

Pincus, T., Haberkern, R. and Christian, C.L. (1968). Experimental chronic glomerulonephritis. *J. Exp. Med.*, **127**, 819

The mesangium

Davison, A.M. (1973). The mesangial cell in nephritis. *J. Clin. Pathol.*, **26**, 198

Mauer, S.M. (1972). Acute mesangial immune injury. *Clin. Res.*, **20**, 513

Mauer, S.M. *et al.* (1972). The mesangial cell in nephritis. *J. Clin. Invest.*, **51**, 1092

Vernier, R.L. *et al.* (1971). The mesangial cell in nephritis. *Adv. Nephrol.*, **1**, 31

Polymorphs

Hersh, E.M. and Bodey, G.P. (1970). Leucocyte mechanisms in inflammation. *Ann. Rev. Med.*, **21**, 105

Janoff, A. (1972). Neutrophil proteases in inflammation. *Ann. Rev. Med.*, **23**, 177

Basement membrane

Kefalides, N.A. (1969). Chemistry and structure of basement membrane. *Arthritis Rheum.*, **12**, 427

Types of collagen

Mahieu, P. *et al.* (1972). Cell-mediated immunity to basement membranes. *Am. J. Med.*, **53**, 185

Shibata, R. *et al.* (1971). Nephritogenic glycoprotein. *J. Immunol.*, **106**, 1284

Platelets/fibrinogen/coagulation

Cameron, J.S. (1973). Glomerulonephritis. *Medicine*, **21**, 1258

McKay, D.G. *et al.* (1972). Blood coagulation and the inflammatory response. *Am. J. Pathol.*, **67**, 181

Vassalli, P. and McCluskey, R.T. (1970). The coagulation process in glomerular diseases. *Adv. Nephrol.*, **1**, 47

Wardle, E.N. (1973). Radiofibrinogen catabolism in renal disease. *Q. J. Med.*, **165**, 205

Wardle, E.N. (1974). Intravascular coagulation in renal disease: functional considerations. *Clin. Nephrol.*, **2**, 85

Wardle, E.N. (1976). The functional role of intravascular coagulation in renal disease. *Scot. Med., J.*, **21**, 83

Fibrinolysis

Myhre-Jensen, O. (1971). *Lab. Invest.*, **25**, 403

Warren, B.A. (1963). *Br. J. Exp. Pathol.*, **444**, 365

Cryoglobulins

Brouet, J.C. *et al.* (1974). Biological and clinical significance of cryoglobulins. *Am. J. Med.*, **57**, 775

Cream, J.J. (1976). Clinical and immunological aspects of cutaneous vasculitis. *Q. J. Med.*, **45**, 255

Jori, G.P. *et al.* (1977). Serum cryoglobulins in chronic liver disease. *Gut,* **18,** 245

McIntosh, R.M. (1971). Cryoglobulins in immune complex diseases. *Int. Arch. Allergy Appl. Immunol.,* **41,** 700

McIntosh, R.M. (1975). Cryoglobulins in immune complex diseases. *Q.J. Med.,* **44,** 285

Detection of immune complexes

Hallgren, R., Wide, L. (1976). IgG aggregates using protein A of *Staph. aureus. Ann. Rheum. Dis.,* **35,** 306

Johnson, A.H., Mowbray, J.F. and Porter, K.A. (1975). Detection of circulating immune complexes. *Lancet,* **i,** 762

Onyewotu, H., Holborrow, E.J. and Johnson, G.D. (1974). *Nature,* **248,** 156

Ooi, Y.M., Vallota, E.H. and West, C.D. (1977). C1q binding and sucrose gradient ultracentrifugation. *Kid. Int.,* **11,** 275

Theofilopoulos, A.N., Wilson, C.B. and Dixon, F.J. (1976). Competitive inhibition of uptake by cells. *J. Clin. Invest.,* **57,** 169

Zubler, R.H. *et al.* (1976). C1q binding and sucrose gradient ultracentrifugation. *J. Immunol.,* **116,** 232

Symposium on immune complex detection (1977). *Ann. Rheum. Dis.,* Supplement.

Complement

Alper, C.A. (1974). Infection and abnormalities of the complement system. *N. Engl. J. Med.,* **282,** 349

Cameron, J.S. *et al.* (1973). Plasma C3 and C4 in the management of glomerulonephritis. *Br. Med. J.,* **3,** 668

Hamburger, J., Crosnier, J. and Maxwell, M. (eds.) (1974). Complement in glomerulonephritis. Chapters 1–8. *Advances in Nephrology,* 4

Hunsicker, L.G. *et al.* (1972). Metabolism of the third complement component in nephritis. *N. Engl J. Med.,* **287,** 835

Peters, D.K. *et al.* (1973). Mesangiocapillary nephritis, partial lipodystrophy and hypocomplementaemia. *Lancet,* **ii,** 535

Pillemar, L. (1955). Properdin system and immunity. *Science,* **122,** 545

Ruddy, S. (1975). Human complement metabolism. *Medicine,* **54,** 165

Ruddy, S., Gigli, I. and Austen, K.F. (1972). The complement system of man. *N. Engl. J. Med.,* **287,** 642

Ruley, E.J. *et al.* (1973). Hypo-complementaemia of membranoproliferative glomerulonephritis. *J. Clin. Invest.,* **52,** 896

Antigens and nephritis

Barabas, A.Z. and Lannigan, T. (1974). Autologous immune complex glomerulonephritis in the rat. *Br. J. Exp. Pathol.*, **55**, 282

Richard-Mendes da Costa *et al.* (1974). Tumour antigen in membranous nephropathy. *Clin. Nephol.*, **2**, 245

Fillit, H.M., Read, S.E., Sherman, R.L., Zabriski, I.J.B. and van de Rijn, I. (1978). Reactivity to glomerular basement membrane. *N. Engl. J. Med.*, **298**, 861

Koffler, D., Schur, H. and Kunkel, H. (1967). Antigen cannot be detected without prior elution of antibody. *J. Exp. Med.*, **126**, 607

Mallick, N.P. and Williams, R.J. (1972). Cell-mediated immunity in nephrotic syndrome. *Lancet*, **i**, 507

Miyakawa, Y. (1976). Demonstration of human nephritogenic antigen in membranous nephritis. *J. Immunol.*, **117**, 1203

Treser, G.M. *et al.* (1970). Streptococcal antigen. *J. Clin. Invest.*, **49**, 762

Yoshizawa, N. (1973). Streptococcal antigen. *Am. J. Pathol.*, **70**, 131

Zabriskie, J.B. *et al.* (1971). Streptococcal antigen. *J. Exp. Med.*, **134**, 3, pt. 2 suppl., p. 180

Zabriski, J.B. *et al.* (1973). Streptococcal antigen. *Kid. Int.*, **3**, 100

Experimental glomerulonephritis

Cochrane, C.G. and Koffler, D. (1973). *Adv. Immunol.*, **16**, 185

Unanue, E.R. and Dixon, F.J. (1967). *Adv. Immunol.*, **6**, 1

Masugi nephritis (heterologous antiGBM antibody nephritis)

Cochrane, C.G., Unanue, E.R. and Dixon, F.J. (1965). Polymorphs and complement in N.T.S. nephritis. *J. Exp. Med.*, **122**, 99

Couser, W.G. and Stilmont, M. (1973). *Lab. Invest.*, **29**, 236

Shigematsu, H. (1970). Role of mononuclear cells. *Virchow's Arch. Abt. B.*, **5**, 187

Unanue, E.R. and Dixon, F.J. (1964). First and second phases. *J. Exp. Med.*, **119**, 965

Steblay nephritis (autologous antiGBM antibody)

Steblay, R.W. (1962). *J. Exp. Med.*, **116**, 253

Heymann's nephritis (autologous membranous renal tubular antigen nephritis)

Edgington, T.S. *et al.* (1968). *J. Exp. Med.*, **127**, 555

Heymann, W. *et al.* (1959). *Proc. Soc. Exp. Biol. Med.*, **100**, 660

Glomerulonephritis

Acute serum sickness nephritis

Dixon, F.J. (1958). *Arch. Pathol.*, **65**, 18

Germuth, F.G. (1953). *J. Exp. Med.*, **77**, 257

Chronic serum sickness nephritis

Dixon, F.J., Feldman, J.D. and Vasquez, J.J. (1961). *J. Exp. Med.*, **113**, 899

SLE models

Hicks, J.B. and Burnet, F.M. (1966). NZB mice. *J. Pathol. Bacteriol.*, **91**, 467

Lemmell, E. *et al.* (1971). Differential effects of 6MP and cyclophosphamide in NZB mice. *Clin. Exp. Immunol.*, **8**, 355

Mellors, R.C. (1969). *J. Exp. Med.*, **133**, 1045

Porter, D.D. *et al.* (1969). Aleutian disease of mink. *J. Exp. Med.*, **130**, 575

Other viruses

Oldstone, M. and Dixon, F.J. (1971). LCM virus. *J. Exp. Med.*, **134**, 32

Viruses and renal disease. *Am. J. Med.*, 1967, **43**, 897

Malaria (Plasmodium)

Boonpucknavig, S. *et al.* (1972). *Arch. Pathol.*, **94**, 322

Wing, A.J. and Hutt, M.S.R. (1972). *Q. J. Med.*, **41**, 273

5
Clinical varieties and treatment of nephritis

Post-streptococcal glomerulonephritis

This is common in children of school age, but also in adults and even the elderly, as a sequel to sore throat or skin sepsis. Biopsy reveals a diffuse proliferative and exudative nephritis. The infecting organism is usually a beta-haemolytic streptococcus of Griffith's M protein type 12. One week after a sore throat, or even earlier in some cases, the patient starts to pass brown 'smoky' urine which is indicative of haematuria. Collection of the urine volume will reveal oliguria. Facial oedema is minimal, although there can be striking facial pallor, and the blood pressure rises in some two-thirds of patients. Hypertensive encephalopathy is rare but can appear as headache, vomiting, convulsions and temporary loss of vision. Congestive heart failure is also rare, although, depending on fluid intake and the urine output, there may be evidence of fluid overload in the form of raised jugular venous pressure, a dilated heart and some pulmonary oedema.

It is clear that with glomerular inflammation there is a reduction of GFR and renal plasma flow, and that hyperreninaemia and secondary aldosteronism will contribute to the salt and water retention and to the hypertension. The result is circulatory congestion without reduction of the cardiac output and also secondary haemodilution. In fact the generalized vasoconstriction will redistribute the blood volume towards the central veins and the atria. In addition an increased permeability of the skin capillaries to small molecules explains the oedema, even though the protein content of the exudate is hardly increased.

Characteristically the urine contains some protein and red cells, white cells and granular casts.

The outcome is in brief:

(1) 80–90% recovery (children); 50–80% recovery in adults;
(2) rarely death due to anuria, heart failure, hypertensive encephalopathy;
(3) sometimes rapidly progressive nephritis leading to uraemia in 16–18 months;
(4) sometimes heavy proteinuria and the nephrotic syndrome.

In children the nephritis is mild and resolves. Penicillin therapy clears the primary infection and prevents recurrences, but is probably of little use once a nephritogenic streptococcus has been *in situ*.

Pathogenesis
There are three mechanisms to be considered:

(1) Localization of *streptococcal antigen* in the glomeruli, with subsequent local antibody interaction at these sites.
(2) Deposition in the glomeruli of circulating *antigen–antibody complexes*—this is the principal mechanism. Indeed immunofluorescence studies show the presence of IgG, C3 complement, fibrin and even streptococcal antigen. Streptococcal M protein has been shown in the mesangial cells, and it is known that M protein will cause fibrin deposition.
(3) Since some streptococci share antigens with the glomerular basement membrane, production of antibody to the bacterial antigen will also result in *antiglomerular* basement membrane *antibodies*. Likewise the patient's lymphocytes become sensitized to his own glomerular basement membrane.

In reality the offending antigen of the streptococcus appears not to be the polysaccharide of the cell wall but the cellular membrane of types 5 or 12. Indeed sensitization of the lymphocytes to these antigens has been shown and immediate hypersensitivity reactions with streptokinase—streptodornase occur in patients.

Histological changes and functional abnormalities

Circulating antigen—antibody complexes are the favoured mechanism, and in keeping with this it is possible to demonstrate the following histological changes:

(1) endothelial and mesangial proliferation: the latter persists even though there may be good clinical resolution;
(2) endocapillary proliferation in patients with hypertension;
(3) in adults mesangiocapillary or crescentic nephritis: in these the prognosis is bad;
(4) at any age endothelial proliferation leading to glomerular sclerosis.

The following functional abnormalities are also expected:

(1) Circulating complexes by the C1q inhibition technique.
(2) A lowering of the components of the classical complement pathway, namely C3 and C4, and also of total haemolytic complement (CH_{50}) at the time of active nephritis. In fact it is said that C1q and the components C1, 4, 2 are not so depressed as is the terminal sequence $C3 \rightarrow C9$. This means that the alternate pathway must also be activated, and it has been shown that a 'nephritic factor' is detectable and that it triggers this path (Figure 52).

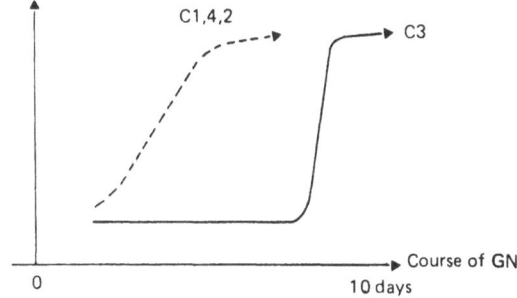

Figure 52. Lowering of complement in streptococcal nephritis

(3) A slight lowering of the platelets at the onset of the illness.
(4) Increased consumption of radiofibrinogen, the presence of cryofibrinogen in plasma (which precipitates in the cold), or of its counterpart high molecular weight fibrin products (HMWS). The latter appear as a high molecular weight peak, which separates in front of the normal fibrinogen peak, when a plasma fibrinogen chromatogram (Figure 53) is performed on Biogel 5 M agarose gel.

The result of the deposition of antigen—antibody complexes in the renal

121

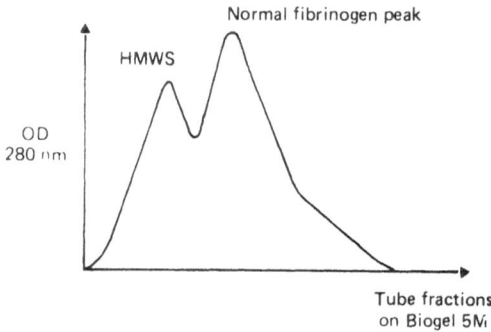

Figure 53. **A fibrinogen chromatogram**

glomeruli, in a subendothelial or subepithelial position causing a 'lumpy-bumpy' pattern of fluorescence, is that there is endothelial and mesangial proliferation and some polymorph exudation. Capillary obliteration explains the fall of creatinine clearance. Later the process resolves except when crescent formation leads to a progressive nephritis. Otherwise the only sign of previous nephritis is persisting mesangial hyperplasia. Even though microscopic haematuria and proteinuria resolve in 6–12 months, some cases may later develop hypertension and insidious chronic renal failure, marked by glomerular sclerosis. Persistent autoimmune damage is suggested by the finding of linear fluorescence.

Bacterial endocarditis

When there is a focus of infection on the heart valves, on a Spitz–Holzer valve or anywhere in contact with the circulation, then bacterial antigen has free access to the blood. Classically endocarditis gives rise to either focal embolic nephritis or to a diffuse proliferative nephritis (Bell, 1932). It was in 1962 that Williams and Kunkel noted a lowering of the serum complement and the appearance of cryoglobulins and rheumatoid factor during the 'immunological phase' of endocarditis. At this stage antibodies are being produced to bacterial antigen but also rheumatoid factors to the patient's own altered gammaglobulins. Current thinking is that rheumatoid factors are antipeptidoglycans. This prolonged phase of the illness, characterized by circulating immune complexes, continues until antigen production has been arrested by adequate antibiotic therapy.

The important features of this *immunological phase* are:

(1)   Persistent anaemia and a raised ESR.
(2)   Raised IgG and IgM serum immunoglobulins, together with the

122

cryoglobulins which are usually of mixed IgG–IgM type, and often cold agglutinins.

(3)   Evidence of autoantibody formation to the patient's own denatured gammaglobulins in the form of rheumatoid factors.

(4)   Accelerated radiofibrinogen catabolism or even more florid evidence of intravascular coagulation.

Figure 54 shows the sequence of events. In the case of 'focal embolic nephritis' there is necrosis and luminal obliteration of glomerular capillaries causing intraglomerular granuloma formation and ischaemia of parts of the glomerular tuft. This lesion is the result of a small infected embolus.

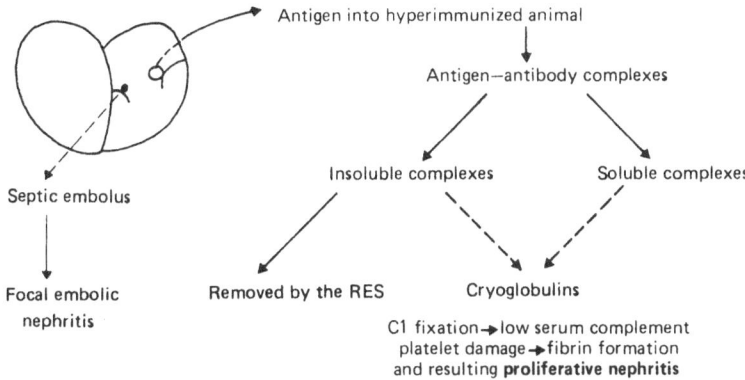

Figure 54.   Events in bacterial endocarditis

Proliferative nephritis may follow any bacteraemia or septicaemia and there can be a nephritis as part of lobar pneumonia, since there are enormous quantities of pneumococcal antigen in the lungs and it is released into the circulation. This serum antigen can be detected by countercurrent electrophoresis. So there will be intravascular coagulation which is caused in part directly by the pneumococcal polysaccharide and partly by the immune complexes.

Staphylococcal septicaemia
Staphylococcal septicaemia deserves special mention as it can cause not only crescentic glomerulonephritis but also acute renal failure and renal cortical necrosis. There is often a florid endarteritis due to the depostion of fibrin and also some immune complexes on the arteriolar walls. Both staphylococcal coagulase and its alphatoxin are known to cause intravascular coagulation. Additionally staphylococcal A-protein will precipitate IgG, for it binds to the Fc portion of the antibody molecules.

Henoch–Schönlein purpura

It was in 1782 that Heberden described two children with purpuric rash, bloody diarrhoea and haematuria. The disease has a peak incidence between 2–5 years and it affects boys. The classical triad consists of purpura, joint pains and abdominal colic; the first two features were described by Schönlein and the latter by his pupil Henoch. The term has become synonymous with *anaphylactoid purpura,* as described by Osler, although the rash may also be nodular, or even an erythema with a wheal and accompanied by eosinophilia. Often there is haematuria indicative of a nephritis. Those cases without nephritis resolve within 1 month.

The glomerular lesion is proliferative but can vary from a focal nephritis to a severe crescentic nephritis with some accompanying vasculitis. It is said that subepithelial humps indicative of class I complexes are uncommon. Typically the lesion involves the mesangium as a 'mesangiopathic nephritis' and is due either to large class II complexes or to localization of aggregated antigen with IgA in the mesangial cells.

Mild cases have microscopic *haematuria* and some proteinuria; these account for 30% children and 50% adults. More severe cases are *nephritic* with oliguria and hypertension, or *nephrotic.* The progressive form often causes mixed nephritic and nephrotic features. Patients may recover or the disease may progress rapidly to renal failure; in those with focal renal lesions it is anticipated that two-thirds will recover, but older patients are more likely to have persistent renal disease. When there are gastrointestinal complications, the worst that can happen is that haemorrhage or intussusception occurs.

Inherent in the term anaphylactoid purpura is the assumption that the condition is a hypersensitivity reaction. Allergy to foods has been proven on occasions, or allergy to drugs such as sulphonamides (possibly microscopic polyarteritis) but commonly there is a preceding bacterial infection. The reaction is basically an acute necrotizing vasculitis with polymorphs in the arteriolar walls and is the counterpart of the Arthus reaction (Figure 55). It can be precipitated by streptococcal infection and possibly by *Staphylococcus albus, Escherichia coli* and other bacteria. IgG globulin, complement, fibrinogen and sometimes the bacterial antigen can be shown in the affected vessel walls.

When antigen and antibody precipitate together in a vessel wall, there is complement activation and attraction of polymorphs. In the experimental situation one of the reactants has to be in the circulation (usually the antibody) and the other is injected locally (as when antigen is disseminated first). Although the platelet count may be lowered, and there is some evidence for diffuse intravascular coagulation, serum complement levels are usually normal.

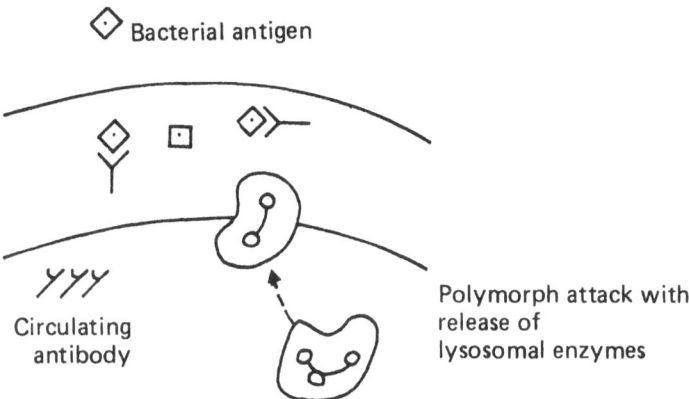

Figure 55.   The Arthus reaction

In the kidney there is a wrinkled scalloped basement membrane with deposits above it on the subendothelial side and in the mesangium; fluorescence reveals mesangial IgA.

Although steroid therapy will relieve joint pains and swelling, there is no specific treatment for Henoch's purpura. Antibiotics should only be used for specific pathogens. When giving analgesics it is important to enquire about aspirin which might itself be a cause of the reaction or exacerbate the bleeding tendency due to inhibition of platelet reactions. Immunosuppressive agents have been tried but are not guaranteed to be successful; in fact immuno-stimulation might be required.

In those cases progressing to chronic renal failure and dialysis, recurrence has often been reported after transplantation.

Recurrent haematuria and mesangial IgA nephritis

In patients who have recurrent haematuria after upper respiratory tract infection and who are found to have IgA–IgG deposits in the mesangial cells of their glomeruli (Berger, 1969), the probability is strong that this syndrome forms part of a spectrum of disease which is the same as the Henoch–Schönlein syndrome. Indeed biopsy of even normal skin will show IgA–IgG deposits. Moreover, the presence of IgA distinguishes this group from post-streptococcal mesangial proliferation, isolates of streptococci are uncommon and serum complement levels do not fall. This mesangial IgA disease leads on to a progressive nephritis with hypertension and terminal renal failure.

In all, some 50% of mesangioproliferative nephritides prove to have IgA deposits. It is not in fact certain that these are immune deposits because the

IgA C3 deposits have an homogeneous structure, although sometimes there are small granulations. Since serum IgA levels are often elevated the possibility is raised that an abnormal IgA might be deposited in the mesangium either alone or in response to a bacterial antigen, and then serve as auto-antigen for an Arthus-type of mesangiopathic reaction. It is quite likely that this IgA also serves to activate the alternate complement pathway.

Polyarteritis nodosa

This is the clinical counterpart of the classical Arthus reaction producing a focal necrotizing arteritis with polymorph infiltration of the arterial walls, and thus areas of weakening of the musculature which develop into small aneurysms. *True polyarteritis* affects medium-sized arteries but there is also a *microscopic hypersensitivity angiitis* involving small blood vessels. Four stages can be distinguished: (a) fibrinous exudation into the media of the artery, (b) neutrophil infiltration, (c) fibroblast proliferation with granulation, and (d) fibrosis and weakening.

Involvement of the renal vessels is usual, so that there is a resulting hypertension and small renal infarcts. The acute glomerulitis can cause an acute renal failure which histologically will be a rapidly progressive glomerulonephritis. Yet usually the glomeruli show mild to moderate proliferative changes. Additionally in scattered glomeruli there are segmental areas of necrosis that are seen to be due to fibrin thrombi in those capillaries affected by vasculitis (Figure 56).

Two facets of the renal disease, which may present as no more than a hypertension with proteinuria, help with the diagnosis. First, as in SLE there is a 'telescoped urinary sediment' which means that features of acute, subacute and chronic nephritis are incorporated. In effect the outstanding finding is red cells with red cell casts. Secondly a renal arteriogram shows the

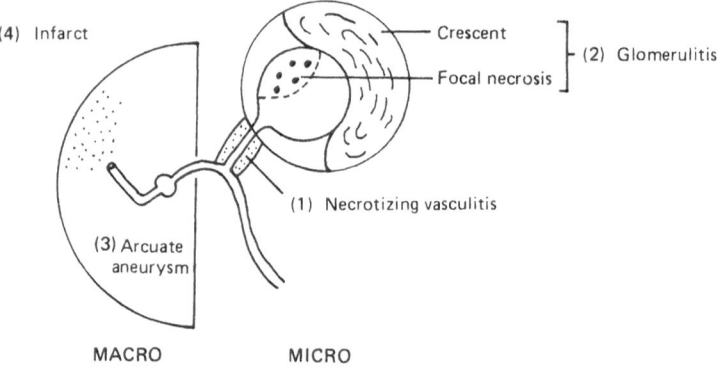

Figure 56. Features of polyarteritis

small aneurysms on the arcuate vessels; this is often a better way of proving the diagnosis than biopsy of kidney or muscle.

Polyarteritis affects arteries of the skin, muscles, nerves, gut, kidneys and central nervous system, as well as the bronchial mucosa, and therefore has many manifestations, such as:

(1)   vasculitic lesions, purpura, urticaria, maculopapular lesions;
(2)   hypertension and renal failure;
(3)   coronary arteritis with angina and infarction;
(4)   hemiparesis, convulsions, mononeuritis multiplex;
(5)   transient or progressive necrotizing pneumonitis.

As in the case of SLE (see below) treatment is with high dosage corticosteroids and either azathioprine or cyclophosphamide. Some cases are hepatitis B-antigen positive. However, a variety of drugs, sulphonamides, iodides, penicillin and propyl-thiouracil—may cause the 'microscopic angiitis' which affects small arteries, veins and capillaries.

Wegener's granulomatosis

This is a variant form of vasculitis in which there are obvious granulomata indicative of a type IV allergic reaction. There is granulomatous inflammation of the upper respiratory tract, granulomatous disease of the lungs and a necrotizing glomerulonephritis. Serum IgE is characteristically raised.

Systemic lupus erythematosus (SLE) and nephritis

Immune mechanisms

When New Zealand black (NZB) and New Zealand white (NZW) mice are crossed, it is found that the NZB x W hybrids are prone to early death on account of the development of a Coomb's positive haemolytic anaemia together with a lethal glomerulonephritis. Since the condition is accompanied by the development of antinuclear antibodies (ANA), this syndrome is the counterpart of human SLE. It is known further that these mice harbour murine leukaemia virus (MuLV) in their spleen, kidneys and thymus. Additionally there is a defect in suppressor T cells and for this reason there are heightened antibody responses mediated by the B cells against both external viral and autoantigens. There is thus a haemolytic anaemia due to antibody formation against red cells (the cytotoxic type II allergic response), and a circulating immune complex disease causing nephritis (classified as a type III allergic reaction). It is in fact possible to demonstrate, among the immune complexes on the glomerular basement membrane, antigenic components of the MuLV virus. Not only envelope glycoprotein, but also double-stranded DNA and a reverse transcriptase which will form RNA–DNA hybrids, can all be shown. Furthermore the nephritis can be exacerbated by injection of soluble DNA into animals which already have antiDNA antibodies, or by active immunization of young animals with DNA-methylated bovine serum albumin aggregates (Figure 57).

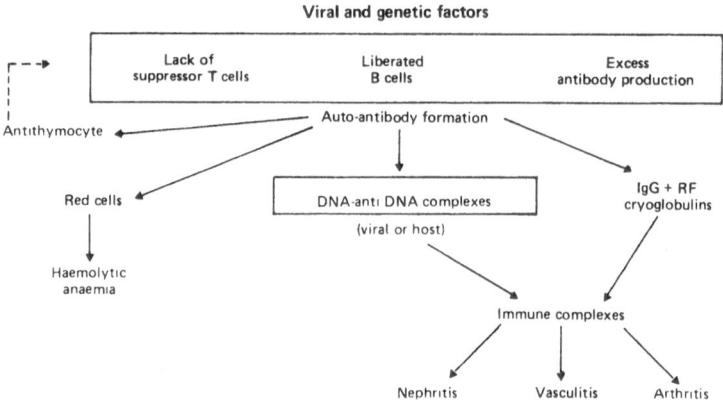

Figure 57.   The SLE syndrome

In human SLE it is thought that there is activation or *de novo* infection with a C-type virus, which is responsible for some leukaemias and cancer. In the mouse it is known that the C-type oncornavirus is transmitted vertically, that is, from mother to foetus.

It must be considered how it is that DNA is continuously liberated into the circulation, giving rise to the formation of DNA–antiDNA complexes. In view of the LE cell phenomenon in which the nucleus of a degenerate polymorph is seen to be ingested by another, it seems likely that leucocytotoxic antibodies play a major role. Indeed one of the accepted criteria for SLE is a leucocyte count below 4000 per mm^3. Release of polymorph nuclei as haematoxylin bodies will keep up the titre of antiDNA antibodies.

There are phases in SLE when large amounts of free DNA antigen can be found in the circulation, as after exposure to sunlight, and other phases when high titre antibodies to double-stranded DNA are found. At interim times there will be DNA–antiDNA complexes which are deposited in the renal glomeruli. The *histology* of SLE nephritis is, in fact, highly variable. From an immunopathological viewpoint certain fundamental variables can be foreseen:

(1)   availability of DNA antigen;
(2)   the rate of immune complex deposition in the glomeruli;
(3)   the affinity of antibodies;
(4)   the rate of complex dissolution;

(5) the intermediary role of antiglobulin rheumatoid factors, which in general bind to immune complexes so that they become larger and are therefore removed from the circulation by the RES—this should result in less glomerular localization;

(6) in addition antiglobulins are anticomplementary because they may attach to the Fc tail of antibody molecules to which C1q component would normally bind; in so doing they may interfere with immune complex phagocytosis by polymorphs.

Therefore if a case of SLE is investigated sequentially it may be found that the appearance of free DNA in the circulation will be followed by antibodies to double-stranded DNA and immune complex formation. At this stage there are often cryoglobulins, and also a positive C1q precipitin test which indicates that there are circulating large 19S complexes. Hence the complement components C3 and C4 are depressed at this time (Figure 58).

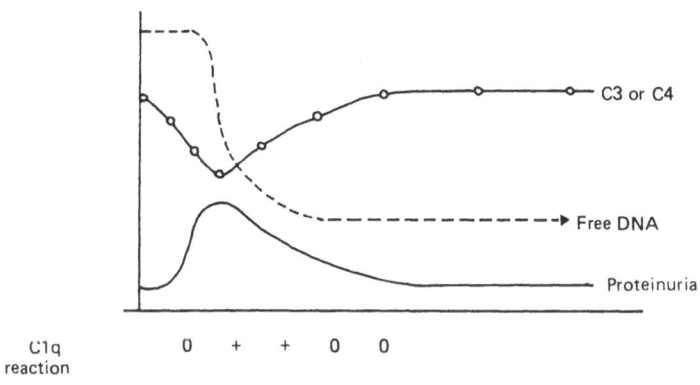

Figure 58. Sequence of events in SLE exacerbation

On the whole there is a reasonable correlation between lowering of the serum C3 and elevation of the DNA *binding capacity* (the antibody activity). So when the course of the disease is progressing favourably there is a return of the serum C3 to normal at 100 mg %, and a fall of the DNA binding capacity to less than 40%. Note that whilst antibodies to double stranded DNA do decline, antinuclear factors as determined by immunofluorescence do not. The amount of light chains (Bence Jones) excreted in the urine also bears some relation to the activity of SLE as does the urine output of E-type prostaglandins.

The principle of the DNA-antigen binding capacity technique is that antibodies to ds-DNA will bind to such antigen that has been labelled by incorporation of tritiated actinomycin D or by tritiated dimethyl sulphate.

The DNA that becomes complexed with antibody is easily measured as it is precipitated by 50% ammonium sulphate (the Farr test), whereas unbound free DNA remains in the supernatant.

There are a variety of possible *nuclear antigens:*

(1)   native or double-stranded DNA;
(2)   nucleoprotein (DNA-histone);
(3)   saline extractable antigens—either the ribonucleoprotein antigen (nRNP) which is RNAse sensitive, *or* the carbohydrate-containing protein, Sm antigen, which is RNAse resistant;
(4)   RNA nucleolar antigens (as are found in scleroderma);
(5)   viral antigens of the C-type oncornavirus.

Another SLE-like syndrome called 'mixed connective tissue disease' is characterized by swollen hands with Raynaud's phenomenon and myositis. Such patients have antibodies to nuclear ribonucleoprotein antigen (nRNP), little antiDNA and seldom have renal disease. Conversely when there are antibodies to the Sm antigen this usually signifies that SLE is responsive to conventional therapy. It is said that those patients with SLE nephritis unresponsive to therapy have antiDNA antibodies but that they lack the antiSm antibodies.

More will be heard in the future about *antibody affinities*. Already it has been found that patients with membranous-type SLE nephritis have non-precipitating antibody (cf. page 96), that is poor at the immune elimation of antigen. Conversely those with a diffuse proliferative SLE nephritis, or with no clinical renal disease at all, are those whose response is vigorous with high-affinity precipitating antibody.

Pathology

The frequency of the various histological types of SLE is as follows:

(1)   nil lesions—5% (good prognosis)
(2)   mesangial prominence—15% (good prognosis)
(3)   focal proliferative nephritis—5% (can be bad prognosis)
(4)   mesangiocapillary—35% (bad prognosis)
(5)   mild, moderate or severe proliferative nephritis—25% (bad prognosis)
(6)   membranous nephritis—15% (good prognosis).

When deposits are found only in the mesangium, the prognosis is good, but it is poor when deposits are subendothelial. There is little relation between histology and the finding of intramembranous or subepithelial deposits. What is more certain is that the proliferative types of SLE nephritis (focal, mesangio-capillary or diffuse proliferative) have a poor prognosis. These are the patients who usually have lowered C3 and C4 complement levels and who have increased DNA-binding capacities. In such patients one may see the typical 'wire-loop' lesion due to the deposition of 'fibrinoid' on the endothelial side of the basement membrane; it is strongly eosinophilic, and superimposed hyaline thrombi often occur in the capillary lumina. Indeed SLE can form part of a spectrum with thrombotic thrombocytopenic purpura (TTP) in which thrombosis occurs as a result of antiendothelial antibodies.

The histology of SLE may change with time, usually for the worst so that renal failure develops. Unfortunately there seems to be no way as yet of predicting this, even though it depends on the nature of the individual's immune response. Actually studies of coagulation or of the turnover of radiofibrinogen may be more helpful. It is of note that azathioprine has been known to cause a transition from subendothelial to subepithelial deposits (*Medicine* (1972), **51**, 393) and this should be beneficial.

The membranous lesion carries a favourable outcome. It has been suggested that it reflects the production of low affinity non-precipitating antibody, but in part it may also be caused by the local attachment of antibody to free DNA that has become bound to the basement membrane.

Clinical features
The American Rheumatism Association criteria, (as shown below with approximate incidence), were intended to distinguish SLE from rheumatoid arthritis and other 'collagen diseases'.

(1)   Facial erythema (60%)
(2)   Discoid lupus (35%)
(3)   Raynaud's phenomenon (15%)
(4)   Alopecia (40%)
(5)   Photosensitivity (50%)
(6)   Oral or nasal ulceration (20%)
(7)   Arthritis without deformity (60%)
(8)   LE cells (70%)
(9)   False position WR (8%)
(10) Proteinuria >3.5 g/day (20%)
(11) Cellular casts (70%)
(12) Pleuritis or pericarditis (30%)
(13) Psychosis or convulsions (40%)
(14) Haemolytic anaemia (10%)
(15) Leucopenia <4000 per mm^3 (40%)
(16) Thrombocytopenia <100000 per mm^3.

IgG antinuclear factors (ANF) are found by the immunofluorescent technique in practically all (90%) patients with SLE. Should the result be negative the diagnosis is doubtful, but IgM ANF is found in some 20–30% of patients with rheumatoid arthritis. Certain drugs such as hydralazine, isoniazid, diphenyl hydantoin and a-methyl-dopa can all cause the appearance of ANF.

Antinuclear antibody will alter the nuclei of neutrophils so that they become homogeneous 'haematoxylin bodies' which are then ingested by other leukocytes giving rise to the typical LE cell appearance. Such cells are best found in a buffy coat smear.

Clinical syndrome of renal SLE
This may present in the following ways:

(1) as acute nephritis;
(2) as nephrotic syndrome;
(3) as rash/arthritis/hypertension and proteinuria.

On account of the variable morphology the renal sediment is often 'telescoped' as in polyarteritis. This means that it contains red cells and granular casts, and fatty and hyaline casts just as if acute, subacute and chronic nephritis were blended.

In fact, some 50–70% of patients with SLE have clinical evidence of renal involvement and 95% have biopsy evidence. Only 50% of the membranous cases are actually nephrotic. Those patients with subendothelial deposits have the worst prognosis. Although remissions occur, it is usual for renal failure to be unrelenting and this is a common cause of death (Figure 59).

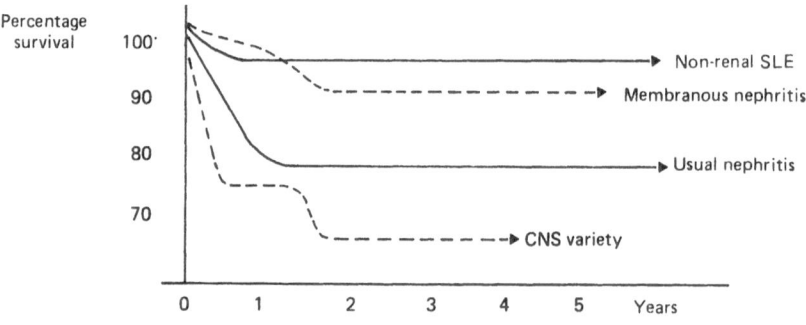

Figure 59.   Prognosis and type of SLE

It is clear, therefore, that nephritis can severely curtail survival in SLE. Some patients have minimal glomerular lesions in spite of haematuria or proteinuria and are likely to follow a benign course, although adverse transitions can occur. The present vogue for aggressive therapy with immunosuppressive drugs and use of high dose steroids appears valuable and some patients with an initial nephritic or nephrotic syndrome can do well. The later clinical picture can be indistinguishable from chronic glomerulonephritis and death occurs in renal failure, unless there is dialysis or transplantation. Hypertension is more often absent than present. At times there may be acute renal failure due to a necrotizing vasculitis and ischaemia of the tubules.

Treatment
The essential treatment is with high dosage corticosteroids, starting with prednisone at an initial daily dose of 45 mg/day, and usually 60 mg/day. In order to reduce side-effects it may be better to give the dose on an alternate-day basis. Steroid sparing can be achieved by the combination of steroids with azathioprine or cyclophosphamide. Azathioprine 50 mg t.i.d. or cyclophosphamide 100 mg t.i.d. is added in order to reduce the steroid to 15–30 mg/day. Steroid treatment must always be continued in a minimal dosage as withdrawal nearly always results in relapse.

When relapse does occur there is some value in the use of pulse therapy with very large doses of methyl-prednisolone (Solumedrone, 1 g) given intravenously. Two pulses are given 48 h apart for relapses of nephrotic syndrome due to diffuse proliferative lupus nephritis, which is notably refractory to therapy. In part steroid prevents the release of DNA from damaged cells and thereby reduces immune complex formation. Additionally steroid can block the production of circulating lymphotoxins, and damp down complement-mediated reactions.

Rapidly progressive glomerulonephritis (extracapillary proliferative nephritis)

Cases of nephritis which deteriorate over a few weeks due to uraemia or congestive heart failure without hypertension, turn out to have either epithelial crescents obliterating Bowman's spaces or endocapillary proliferative nephritis. Three types of lesion are seen in the glomeruli, (a) partial glomerular collapse due to ischaemia, (b) necrotic lesions, (c) thrombotic lesions.

The following entities have to be considered as part of the differential diagnosis, so that a careful clinical evaluation and renal biopsy are essential.

Acute post-streptococcal
The features of this proliferative nephritis are polymorphs in the glomeruli, subepithelial humps, and a low complement and raised antistreptolysin titre.

Bacani type
This is a rapidly progressive nephritis. There is little proliferation but many crescents and a linear fluorescence is seen on the basement membrane. Complement is normal.

133

Goodpasture's syndrome

This is true antibasement membrane antibody disease, in which there is a linear pattern of IgG and C3 deposition. It may follow an attack of influenza or inhalation of hydrocarbon solvents. There is pulmonary haemorrhage which makes a fine distinction from pulmonary haemosiderosis. In haemorrhage, as opposed to pulmonary oedema, the transfer factor for carbonmonoxide is actually increased.

Lupus nephritis

There is an acute form which causes glomerular necrosis in young women.

Henoch's purpura, polyarteritis and Wegener's granulomatosis

Here the associated clinical features usually make the diagnosis clear.

Scleroderma

The appearance of the skin with its rigidity and telangiectasia is telling. There is an arthropathy and also malignant hypertension, which is the result of small renal infarcts caused by the intimal hyperplasia and occlusion of small vessels.

Malignant hypertension

There is fibrinoid necrosis of vessel walls leading on, after adequate lowering of the blood pressure so as to allow healing, to fibrointimal hyperplasia. Areas of focal glomerular necrosis are common but crescent formation is limited.

Thus the syndrome of rapidly progressive nephritis embraces those nephritides with the worst prognosis. In the classical Goodpasture's syndrome the linear fluorescence in the glomeruli is also seen in the alveoli of the lungs. Antibasement antibodies are demonstrable. The lung fluorescence is important because experimentally it has been shown that immune complexes can produce a granular pattern in the lungs. This latter syndrome produces a rapidly progressive nephritis with a pneumonitis.

Cryoglobulinaemia

Cryoglobulins are a heterogeneous group of immunoglobulins, which through their interaction form a precipitate when serum is cooled from 37 °C to 4 °C. Although the precipitate may appear as early as 6 h in the cold, for the purpose of quantitation it is normal to wait for 48 h. Cryoglobulins can have the following constitution:

(1) IgG or IgA or IgM cryoglobulins;
(2) Bence Jones cryoproteins;
(3) Mixed IgG + IgM (frequent);

(a) IgG + IgA;
(b) IgG + IgM + complement components;
(c) IgG + lipoprotein cryoglobulins.

The common type of cryoglobulin is a mixed IgG–IgM type, in which the IgM has rheumatoid factor (antiglobulin) activity and reacts with an IgG₃ subclass. Circulating immune complexes of this type lead to a vasculitis and rapidly progressive nephritis. Thus in the original syndrome described by Meltzer and Franklin the patients had purpura, arthralgia, vasculitis, hepatosplenomegaly and a progressive nephritis. There may also be a renal tubular acidosis (Lo Spalluto, 1962). The serum complement is commonly reduced.

In nephritis research one would hope to find an antigen in the cryoglobulin complex. This is so with the DNA complexes of lupus, but search for the bacterial antigens has been negative. Obviously this might be due to the technical difficulty of identifying small amounts of antigen. However, antibody activity in the complexes has been shown since there can be rheumatoid factor activity, antinuclear antibodies, antithyroglobulins, anticomplementary activity and antierythrocyte antibodies (cold agglutinins).

Haematological or autoimmune disease and cryoglobulins
Cryoglobulinaemic syndromes complicate the haematological malignancies and those 'collagen diseases', infections or autoimmune conditions such as the liver diseases where the serum globulins are very high. The patients have cold-hypersensitivity with Raynaud's phenomenon and purpura, arthralgia or hyperviscosity symptoms. The syndrome is seen typically when caused by the raised IgM of Waldenström's macroglobulinaemia.

The nephrological interest is in:

(1)   glomerular endothelial deposits and proliferative retinopathy;
(2)   renal amyloid;
(3)   coincident renal tubular acidosis;
(4)   occasional acute renal failure or rapidly progressive crescentic nephritis.

Nephritides
Cryoglobulins in nephritis are of considerable interest since they may represent immune complexes. They are certainly related to disease activity. They have been found in diffuse proliferative and rapidly progressive nephritis, in membranous and membranoproliferative nephritis, and in patients with focal segmental lesions or even benign haematuria. Such cryoprecipitates are in antibody excess and so far detection of bacterial antigens has been unrewarding. In reality antigen may not be present since a cryoglobulin is largely an

135

artefact produced by the cold and in this situation immunoglobulins interreact. On the other hand all the recognition sites on a small amount of antigen could be masked by antibody coating.

Vasculitis

Most patients with vasculitis have cryoglobulins. The lesions are basically a venulitis involving the capillary-venules of the upper dermis, since these vessels are spread out horizontally so that they are exposed to cooling. Thus inevitably there is an increase in the viscosity of the blood. Immune complexes within the circulation are therefore likely to become localized here. Alternatively the same vessels can be the site of an Arthus reaction to bacterial antigen which has localized in their walls (Figure 55).

Cold causes exacerbation of the purpura in at least 30% of cases. Certainly there are some antiglobulins which are more reactive in the cold. Other antibodies, IgA class in particular, are also known to react so as to cause complement fixation at low temperatures.

The classification of the vasculitides overlaps with that of nephritis. A modification of the classification of Zeek (1952) still has practical advantages:

Necrotizing vasculitis akin to polyarteritis

(1)   Classic polyarteritis nodosa;
(2)   Henoch–Schönlein disease;
(3)   hypersensitivity, serum sickness, drug allergy;
(4)   rheumatic diseases, SLE, rheumatoid arthritis, rheumatic fever;
(5)   other immune complex disorders, ulcerative colitis, hepatitis B, endocarditis and other infections.

Paraproteinaemias

(1)   Essential cryoglobulinaemia;
(2)   macroglobulinaemia, multiple myeloma.

Respiratory diseases

(1)   Loeffler's syndrome;
(2)   asthma (Churg–Strauss syndrome);
(3)   Wegener's granulomatosis.

Temporal arteritis or polymyalgia rheumatica

(1)   Aortic arch arteritis.

Hyperglobulinaemic purpura

This is a rare condition in which there are circulating intermediate-sized complexes of IgG–IgG type causing purpura on the legs. The prognosis is good; renal disease does not usually occur, although there may be renal tubular acidosis.

Renal tubular acidosis in immune conditions

Renal tubular acidosis occurs in a wide variety of hyperimmunoglobulin-aemic states as in chronic active hepatitis, primary biliary cirrhosis, Sjögren's syndrome and myeloma. Patients are identified by their hyperchloraemic acidosis and hypokalaemia. There may be changes of membranous or proliferative nephritis, but in particular one should be on the look out for antibodies to tubular basement membrane and an associated interstitial nephritis.

Mesangiocapillary (membranoproliferative) glomerulonephritis (MCGN)

This histological type has a variety of aetiologies, which supports Germuth's theory that histology is really a reflection of the physicochemical state of the immune complexes. Thus it can be seen with streptococcal or pneumococcal infections, in SLE, with hepatitis B virus infection and in persistent hypocomplementaemic membranoproliferative nephritis. The latter was described by West and Gotoff in 1965, although, in fact, the original Bright's kidneys are said to show this condition.

The typical finding is of mesangial proliferation. This gives rise to the interposition of mesangial matrix between the endothelium and the basement membrane, so that there is an apparent capillary wall thickening or under high magnification an apparent splitting of the basement membrane. The glomerulus is often lobulated, although MCGN is not the only cause of a lobular nephritis. When crescents are seen, the prognosis is bad.

This condition is an important cause of chronic nephritis in children and adults. It usually arises between the age of 8–30, more commonly in the female, and nearly half the patients have had an upper respiratory tract infection. At the onset there may be a nephritic passing on to a nephrotic phase, or it may appear as a nephrotic syndrome in which there is some haematuria. Sometimes there is only asymptomatic proteinuria and haematuria. Hypertension develops as the nephritis progresses.

The lobulation of the glomeruli is consequent on mesangial hyperplasia; in the periphery of the lobules there is striking deposition of C3 and properdin (factor B) and of fibrinogen. (see Figure 47, Immunofluorescence patterns) IgG and IgM are often present though they can be unimpressive. Electron microscopy shows that the immune deposits are mesangial and subendothelial.

When there are dense intramembranous deposits (DIMD) the picture is distinctive, as described by Berger and Galle (1963). There is some doubt as to whether these patients do differ clinically from other types of MCGN but they tend to have persistent nephrotic syndrome and haematuria. Those with

DIMD also possess the 'nephritic factor' and therefore have a persistently low serum C3.

It is now certain that both the classical pathway and the alternate pathway are activated in mesangiocapillary nephritis. In the *intramembranous* type (DIMD) properdin factor B is lowered and C3NeF is always demonstrable, whereas in the *subendothelial* deposit disease C1q and C4 can be appreciably low. In both conditions C3 and C5 are equally depressed. It is wise to avoid living donor kidney transplantation when the histology is that of dense deposit disease and when C3NeF is present.

This C3NeF or nephritic factor came to light in 1968 when Pickering and Gewurz showed that there is in the serum of such patients a factor which inactivates guinea-pig complement. The nephritic factor activates the alternate complement pathway so that there is continuous catabolism of complement component C3 (see below). Thus it promotes C3 convertase.

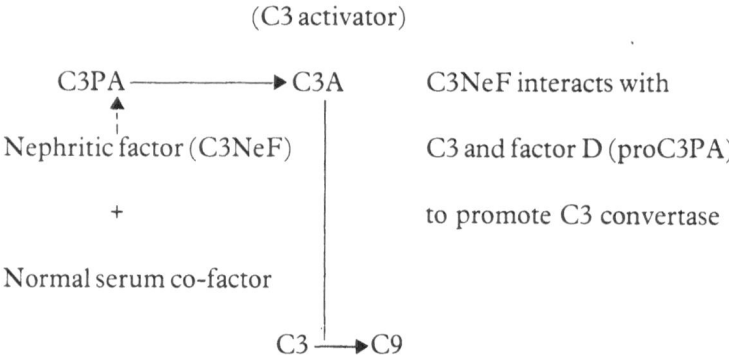

(C3 activator)

C3PA ⟶ C3A   C3NeF interacts with

Nephritic factor (C3NeF)   C3 and factor D (proC3PA)

+   to promote C3 convertase

Normal serum co-factor

C3 ⟶ C9

It is accepted that the nephritic factor is an intrinsic part of the alternate pathway of complement activation, but some think it could be a bacterial antigen. Only certain patients with MCGN appear to have it.

Various types of assay are now available:

(1)   Assay based on the conversion or loss of C3PA (B antigen);
(2)   Direct demonstration of either C3PA or C3 cleavage products by means of counterimmunoelectrophoresis;
(3)   Nephritic factor induced lysis of glutathione-treated human erythrocytes that is, (PNH-erythrocytes), since these are known to be exquisitely sensitive to fluid phase C3 activation;
(4)   Assay based on a reduction of total haemolytic complement utilizing EGTA which, since it absorbed Ca^{2+} ions rather than Mg^{2+}, blocks the classical complement pathway but allows the alternate pathway to proceed. Thus nephritic factor will use C3PA, C3PAse and Mg^{2+}

and thereby cause consumption of C3. The assay therefore depends on accurately quantitated red cell haemolysis.

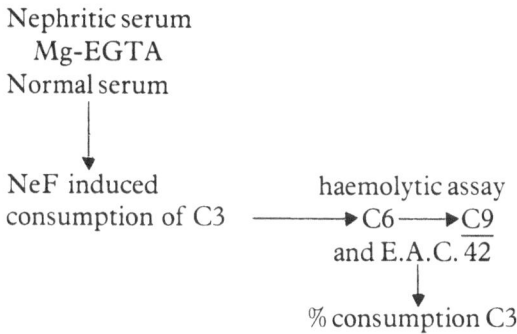

Much work has been devoted to elucidation of the complement anomaly in MCGN. It appears that there is not only increased complement consumption, but also defective C3 synthesis—patients vary of course. In some the hypocomplementaemia is persistent and in others it fluctuates. The indications are that sometimes the disease burns out and that in these serum C3 levels return to normal.

There is one striking clinical association, namely with partial lipodystrophy. In distinction to congenital lipodystrophy in which there is muscle hypertrophy, hepatomegaly and diabetes, patients with *partial lipodystrophy are* females who after an illness such as measles or whooping cough, develop a rather sudden change in their appearance. Their faces are distinctly thin due to atrophy of the subcutaneous fat and yet their legs can be fatter than normal. They may also have glucose intolerance and hepatomegaly or even thyroid disease.

Mesangiocapillary glomerulonephritis is said to recur frequently in the renal transplant. The problem is that the histology is rather similar to that of chronic rejection itself. However, there is no doubt that, even if the original kidneys are removed, the nephritic factor can persist after transplantation and be a cause of persistent hypocomplementaemia. Such patients do have a predictable recurrence. This is not necessarily an absolute contraindication to transplantation, for the graft kidney may still survive for some time.

Membranous nephropathy

This is a chronic stable glomerular disease (previously called Ellis Type II nephritis) characterized by *thickening of the basement membrane* of the capillary walls.

Causation

A variety of potential causes have been recognized:

(1) idiopathic—this appears to be an autoimmune response to nephritogenic tubular antigen;

(2) infections—syphilis, filariasis, schistosomiasis, hepatitis B antigen, allergy;

(3) exposure to heavy metals—penicillamine, gold, mercury, thiouracil, CCl_4, penicillin;

(4) SLE;

(5) neoplasms;

(6) renal vein thrombosis;

(7) diabetes.

Although nephritogenic tubular antigen can be found in the serum and urine of normal individuals, it now appears that its deposition in the basement membrane as part of an autoimmune nephrosis will account for cases of 'idiopathic' membranous disease. This idiopathic form follows a variable course. On the one hand some 25% of patients progress to renal failure and hypertension, but another 25% show spontaneous remission. Thus the patient is either nephrotic or has progressive nephritis with some haematuria. Renal function rarely deteriorates suddenly, unless there is superimposed *renal vein thrombosis.*

Although membranous disease can be found in children, the adult age range is 40–60 and the male:female ratio is 3:1. Since there is a 5% incidence of membranous nephropathy in cancer patients, investigation on these lines is necessary. Occasionally a remission can be induced by resection of the cancer.

A similar lesion can be produced experimentally by constriction of a renal vein, so as to mimic renal vein thrombosis. The result is a heavy proteinuria with deposition of protein in the capillary walls giving rise to the thickened appearance. Indeed it is also known that patients with extreme obesity can have proteinuria, which resolves when there is loss of weight. This may be caused likewise by a high pressure in the renal veins.

Treatment

Most cases do not respond to steroids, although an occasional case may remit whilst on steroid therapy. Clearly this possibility makes the interpretation difficult. Trials of cyclophosphamide or chlorambucil for relapsing nephrosis are now in progress, but one has to be aware of the potential toxicity of these agents.

Minimal change nephrosis

Nephrotic preschool children commonly turn out to have no glomerular lesion that can be detected by light microscopy, which means that they have 'minimal change' nephrosis. In this condition there is no nitrogen retention, no hypertension and no haematuria, but there is an increased permeability of the basement membrane to relatively small molecules (70 000–150 000) so that differential protein clearance shows a 'selective proteinuria'. Hypercholesterinaemia gradually develops and the lipaemia accounts for the term 'lipoid nephrosis'.

Boys predominate by 2:1 and due to the finding of low IgG and IgA but raised IgM levels it has been suggested that the condition can be an X-linked immunodeficiency syndrome. Of course hypogammaglobulinaemia with susceptibility to infection is a result of the urinary protein loss but the supposition is based on the finding of persistently low immunologlobulin levels even after resolution. This work has to be confirmed!

On the other hand, association of minimal change nephrotic syndrome with pollen allergy and other *atopic conditions* has led to the finding that steroid-responsive nephrotic children are commonly atopic, and that HLA-B12 is predominant. Atopy is based on a history of hay fever, positive skin tests to grass pollen and raised serum IgE levels.

Pollen and milk allergies

There are only a few recorded cases of seasonal nephrotic syndrome associated with *pollen allergy* (Figure 60) but the course of events is impressive. At the time of exacerbation there is an elevated serum IgE, especially that IgE which is specific for grass pollen as determined by RAST. Grass

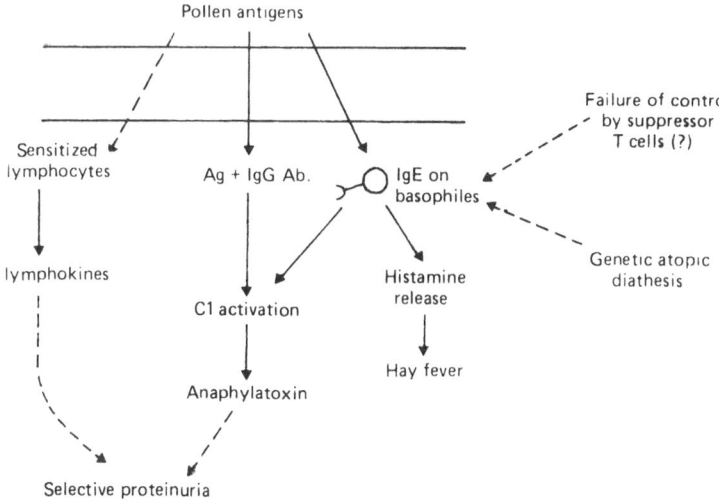

Figure 60. Postulated sequence of events in pollen allergy nephrosis

141

pollen IgG (which is really blocking antibody) is found in the serum throughout the year. Indeed successful desensitization vaccine therapy, which lowers the IgE and raises the IgG, leads to resolution.

Milk allergy is yet another relatively common possibility, which has been revealed by placing children on an elemental liquid diet in the form of Vivonex or Flexical 1800–2400 kcal/day, until such time as their proteinuria has lessened to less than 500 mg/day and then challenging with 30 g cow's milk. When milk allergy is the cause, there is a decrease of the urine volume and a return of proteinuria and oedema.

Other cases have been described as the result of bee stings, drugs, toxins or other food allergies.

Mechanisms

The current hypothesis is that in minimal change nephrosis the lymphocytes are producing lymphokines which act as basement membrane permeability factors. The evidence is not yet absolute but it is as follows. First, using the leucocyte migration test with either adult kidney basement membrane or neonatal kidney as antigen, sensitization of the lymphocytes of the patients with minimal change nephrotic syndrome has been shown. Second, Lagrue has found that when lymphocytes are taken from minimal change patients and are stimulated with PHA or concanavalin A, they release a factor which increases the permeability of the guinea-pig skin.

Also it is known that (a) there is no evidence for humoral antibody (other than perhaps IgE) acting in minimal change nephrosis, (b) that remission can occur during measles which acts as a T cell immunosuppressant, (c) that both steroids and cyclophosphamide which are lymphocyte inhibitors are known to control minimal change, and (d) that minimal change nephrosis is a particular feature of Hodgkin's disease which is itself a T cell malignancy. Thus the indications are that minimal change nephrosis is closely related to an abnormality of the T lymphocytes.

Treatment

It is normal to treat minimal change nephrosis with a high dose of corticosteroids, that is reduced once a response is achieved; 60% achieve complete remission, 20% show a resolution of the nephrosis although the proteinuria persists, and another 20% are steroid-resistant. If the steroid-sensitive but relapsing cases are treated by cyclophosphamide, the relapses become less frequent. Thus the policy now is to induce a remission with steroids, and then to give cyclophosphamide (3 mg/kg per day) for 8 weeks, and when the steroids are withdrawn the tendency to relapse is reduced. The alternative approach is to use chlorambucil in combination with prednisone.

Variant conditions

(1) When in minimal change nephrosis the juxtamedullary glomeruli show *focal and segmental sclerosis,* hypertension appears and the prognosis is poorer; haematuria may also occur. The sclerosis is the result of an initial hyperplasia of the mesangial cells; it is commoner in adults and older children and does not respond to steroids. In aminonucleoside nephrosis of rats the same phenomenon is seen and is dependent on the duration and severity of the proteinuria. It is thus a secondary phenomenon.

(2) *Focal global sclerosis* is yet another variant in which one glomerulus in a group is sclerosed. In this case minimal change nephrosis is relapsing but non-progressive.

(3) *Familial nephrosis.* Cases with infantile onset have a variable histology but it is often focal glomerulosclerosis and there is haematuria and a poor prognosis. In this group congenital nephrotic syndrome can be selected prenatally because of the high alphafoetoprotein levels in the serum and amniotic fluid.

Cases of familial nephrosis with a juvenile onset have a typical minimal change histology.

THE TREATMENT OF NEPHRITIS
General measures

Antibiotics
If the patient has a preceding steptococcal sore throat or other infection, such as bacterial endocarditis, then the use of antibiotics to achieve antigen elimination is mandatory.

Bed rest and diet
Bed rest until after the initial fever and illness have gone, is no longer regarded as essential for acute nephritis. A low protein diet is important for uraemia and additionally does appear to benefit children with acute nephritis. Conversely the nephrotic patient who is losing large amounts of protein in the urine will need protein supplementation. If the serum gammaglobulin is low, injections are required to prevent infection.

Salt and water balance
This is important when the patient is oliguric or nephrotic and has a low colloid osmotic pressure of the plasma. Diuretics are often required and hypertension must be controlled.

Cortisone

This anti-inflammatory compound with diuretic potential is most useful for minimal change but also for membranous nephropathy, SLE, polyarteritis and almost any nephrotic syndrome.

For children the starting dosage is 2 mg/kg of prednisone for 10 days, followed by a reduction when diuresis occurs. If there is relapse, a course of 2 mg/kg for 5 days is repeated and later reduced. Prolonged treatment is necessary if there are frequent relapses or when there is persistent proteinuria of more than 1 g/day. The same regime applies to the adult nephrotic.

Cortisone reduces both the permeability of the basement membrane and lymphocyte-mediated reactions and it tends to increase the glomerular filtration rate. It is always indicated when there is a 'selective' differential protein clearance, but steroid side-effects can be severe and dangerous, and in children there is a particular risk of growth retardation. Alternate day dosage, utilizing the same total dose in all, is now an accepted alternative; in this way there are fewer side-effects and the method carries a greater guarantee of continued integrity of the hypothalamo–pituitary–adrenal axis. For the same reason consideration should be given to the use of ACTH or synacthen injections.

Specific immunosuppression

Since much experimental work indicates that a poor antibody response is detrimental to the course of class I complex nephritis, immunosuppression must be viewed with caution. It is clearly appropriate, however, for situations in which there are heightened antibody responses to circulating antigen as in SLE and other causes of mesangiopathic class II complex nephritis. It has to be stressed that the benefit seen with cytotoxic agents such as azathioprine (Imuran), cyclophosphamide (Endoxana) or chlorambucil could be simply consequent on inhibition of polymorphs and proliferative cell responses within the renal glomeruli.

In lupus nephritis there is depressed T cell function but increased antibody formation to virus antigens and to DNA, so that it is the classic autoimmune disease. The standard therapy, therefore, is prednisone 40–60 mg/day, and when a steroid sparing effect is required the dose is tailed by adding azathioprine (Imuran) 2–3 mg/kg according to patient tolerance. Azathioprine reduces polymorph numbers and therefore inflammatory responses, and produces a modest depression of cellular and humoral immune responses. If it is not tolerated, cyclophosphamide is substituted.

When using immunosuppressant drugs it is important to have some measure of the granulocyte reserves. After taking a basal white blood cell count, aetiocholanalone 0.1 mg/kg is administered and the rise of the white

144

cell count is recorded up to 12–20 h. Those patients who mobilize white cells feebly so that the blood count rise is less than 3000 per mm³ can easily develop leucopenia and they should be given half-normal dosages of the cytotoxic drugs. In general this is a feature of patients with SLE.

Cyclophosphamide with steroids can be a successful combination for Wegener's granulomatosis, and azathioprine with steroids is used for Good-pasture's syndrome. Trials of these agents in other types of proliferative nephritis have not given clearcut results, and clearly it is necessary to identify the causative antigens so as to be able to measure the relevant antibody responses. Additionally cyclophosphamide can be used as an adjunct to steroid therapy in minimal change nephrosis. One should therefore enquire further into the specific properties of these drugs.

Corticosteroids
The action of corticosteroids can be briefly summarized:

(1)   They cause lysis of T and B lymphocytes since there is inhibition of RNA and protein synthesis.
(2)   They stabilize polymorph lysosomal membranes.
(3)   They depress the phagocytic function of polymorphs and macrophages.
(4)   They have anticomplementary effects.
(5)   They reduce the permeability of the glomerular basement membrane.

Cyclophosphamide
The action of cyclophosphamide is as follows:

(1)   Since it interferes with cell replication of antigen-reactive and antibody-producing cells during the period of maximum cell proliferation after antigen exposure, it causes early suppression of an antibody response.
(2)   This immune depression is linked to a depression of circulating lymphocytes.
(3)   It has the special property of being able to facilitate '*immune tolerance*' to an antigen. Tolerance can be achieved in the adult animal, if a suppressive drug is present when antigen is being presented to a new population of lymphocytes that are gaining immunological competence. Apparently under the influence of cyclophosphamide there is antigen inhibition of reactive lymphocytes.

It is therefore instructive to compare the actions of these two agents, and also to compare their action with that of other cytotoxic drugs. Thus, combined cyclophosphamide with cortisone therapy will reduce the mortality from nephritis of NZB/NZW mice. However, whereas cyclophosphamide will reduce the proteinuria, azathioprine does not.

Table 14 Comparative effects of cyclophosphamide and cortisone therapy

Cyclophosphamide	*Cortisone*
Antigen clearance is impaired	Antigen clearance by macrophages is retarded
Maximum sensitivity is during cell proliferation after receipt of the antigen	Maximum sensitivity is prior to antigen exposure
Increasing the dose of antigen actually increases the immunosuppression	Increasing the antigen mitigates against effective drug action
Timing of the drug is not critical	Cortisone has to be present before the antigen is presented
Effective antibody suppression occurs	If the cortisone is given after antigen exposure (as is normal clinically), then there may be some antibody suppression

N.B. Cyclophosphamide will produce severe side-effects such as cystitis, alopecia, or azoospermia and ovarian fibrosis when given long term. It suppresses polymorphs short term.

The agents to be used in nephritis control must, therefore, be viewed critically, especially when available drugs have widespread non-specific effects on many cell systems. It is hoped that in time there will be a better scientific definition of the principles to be followed. Meanwhile it has to be remembered that each patient presents an individual problem and should be assessed accordingly. The possible modes of treatment are as follows.

Modes of treatment

Antigen specific treatment

(1)   Antigen avoidance, for example, in grass pollen hypersensitivity;
(2)   antigen administration,
    (a) to produce tolerance (page 95)
    (b) to dissolve away immune deposits; (page 92)
(3)   antigen elimination by antibiotics, antimalarial therapy, etc.

Immunosuppressive and anti-inflammatory agents—these have to be chosen with care.

(1)   These are cytotoxic drugs with little specificity which are used to suppress antibody production, such as alkylating agents (cyclophosphamide, chlorambucil); antimetabolites— (azathioprine);

(2)   chloramphenicol;

(3)   lysosomal stabilizers, such as chloroquine, gold and cortisone;

(4)   the lymphocytolysis inducer—cortisone;

(5)   anti-inflammatory—indomethacin and other prostaglandin synthetase inhibitors.

Inhibitors of platelet aggregation

(1)   Aspirin, dipyridamole (Persantin), or antihistamines such as cyproheptidine;

(2)   drugs which are also inhibitors of complement and promote fibrinolysis, such as indomethacin, flufenamic acid and salicylaldoxime.

Anticoagulants—heparin and warfarin.

Stimulation of macrophages—for example, by levamisole or clofazimine.

(1)   As a means to processing antigen; or

(2)   to promote removal of immune complexes from the circulation.

Means of removing either immune complexes or antibody from the circulation

(1)   Plasmapheresis;

(2)   perfusion over an immunoadsorbent such as C1q for removal of immune complexes.

Treatment in Goodpasture's syndrome

A particular challenge is posed by the patient with Goodpasture's syndrome or an immune complex-mediated rapidly progressive nephritis who is still passing adequate urine but who is likely to deteriorate. In the case of Goodpasture's disease, plasmapheresis to remove the antibody within the circulation combined with immunosuppression to reduce further antibody production is now the vogue and good results are shown. Patients are given combined therapy with prednisone 60 mg/day, cyclophosphamide 3 mg/kg per day or azathioprine 2 mg/kg per day, aspirin 300 mg/day or Persantin 200 mg three times a day, and they are anticoagulated with heparin. Plasma exchange is performed on a Haemonetics cell separator and the plasma removed is replaced by purified protein fraction (PPF); 4 l/day of plasma can be removed but the procedure is expensive. Fortunately antiGBM antibody production in the Goodpasture's patient seems to be of limited duration. Indeed formerly such patients were dealt with by bilateral nephrectomy followed by a 'rest period' on dialysis and thereafter transplantation.

A similar technique is being applied to SLE and other forms of rapidly progressive nephritis, and also for transplant rejection.

Assessment of therapy

One has to be aware of the natural course taken by the average case of a particular type of nephritis. Mesangiocapillary nephritis progresses only slowly at first so that survival is normally relatively good. Such considerations mean that any trial must proceed for a long time during which there are bound to be spontaneous variations in disease activity. Actuarial survival curves are applied to this type of analysis (Cutler and Ederer, 1958).

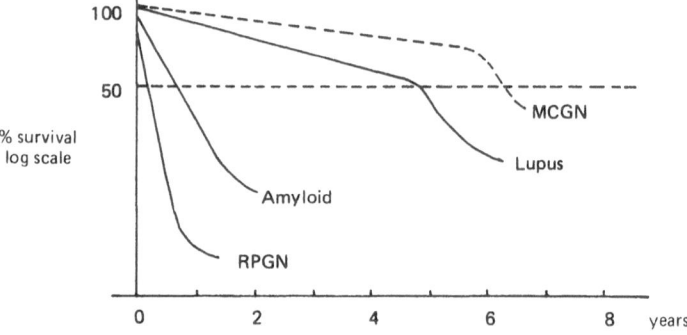

Figure 61.   Survival in nephritis

In one trial of patients with MCGN the therapy consisted of cyclophosphamide 1.5–2.0 mg/kg per day, dipyridamole (Persantin) 100 mg q.i.d., and anticoagulants (*Med. J. Aust.* (1972), **2**, 587). At 30 months it appeared that the 16 treated patients had better survival curves than those who were untreated. Since this is a short period of follow-up, time will show whether this is valid. Usually in MCGN 50% patients have a serum creatinine 72 mg% at 6 years and then rather suddenly 85% have renal insufficiency by 8 years.

In many ways a better appraisal of drugs can be obtained from short-term assessment regimes of about 12 months. This can only be done if in this time

148

maximum use is made of dynamic tests such as quantitation of immune complexes, complement levels, radiofibrinogen catabolism and the urinary excretion of FDP. Lipid levels, plasma fibrinogen, the differential protein clearance and the endogenous creatinine clearance all give information on how the kidneys are behaving. The kidneys, however, cannot be thought of in isolation and attention ought to be paid to the performance of white cells and to the activity of the reticuloendothelial system. One has always to remember that obsessional control of hypertension is the one factor known to restrain a nephritic process.

Transplantation in nephritic patients

There has been much concern about any possible recurrence of nephritis in a transplant, although the incidence is relatively low at 5–20%. When the cost of a transplant is considered both in economic terms and in human endurance, it is a serious matter. The types which recur frequently are dense deposit MCGN, focal sclerosis, mesangial IgA disease and antiGBM antibody disease. When a patient after transplantation still has the circulating immune complexes or the 'nephritic factor' that caused the original disease, then a recurrence is to be expected.

Since there is a very close morphological resemblance between chronic allograft rejection and, for example, mesangiocapillary nephritis, it is not surprising that the operative mechanisms are still being hotly debated.

(1) The simplest situation is when there is a direct *recurrence* due to circulating immune complexes, nephritic factor or antiglomerular basement membrane antibody. On the one hand there has been a vogue for removing the original kidneys, since they might be a source of autoantigen, and on the other it is said that they should be left in place in the hope that they will serve as a 'dump' for immune complexes. Certainly a period of dialysis is often thought to have been successful in allowing the original immunological process to subside. This can actually happen both in SLE and in Goodpasture's syndrome.

(2) The *de novo* development of glomerulonephritis in the transplant kidney of a patient who did not previously have nephritis is quite common. Indeed it has been shown that there is a correlation between presensitization to HLA-antigens and the presence of glomerular transplant disease. Likewise there is a close relation between recurrence of glomerular disease and incompatibility of the host and donor as shown by lymphocyte typing. In other words the nephritis may be an integral part of the *rejection* process. There is

149

also the possibility of a humoral mechanism, for graft-derived HLA-antigen can enter the circulation to elicit immune complex formation, and alloantibodies are formed to membrane-associated antigens as on the GBM itself.

(3)   Since transplant patients suffer many *infections*, a new nephritic process may arise on this basis. Thus it is quite possible for patients to develop a new post-streptococcal nephritis, or viral antigen–antibody complex nephritis on account of hepatitis B or cyto-megalovirus (CMV) antigens.

Additionally there is considerable scope for the occurrence of an autologous immune complex disease that can be caused by the release of antigen from damaged renal tubular epithelium and thereby cause formation of complexes containing renal tubular antigen.

Therefore, recurring glomerular disease can be accounted for by:

(1)   recurrence;
(2)   chronic rejection;
(3)   *de novo* nephritis based on infection or autoimmunity to renal tubular antigen.

In order to diagnose the persistence of nephritogenic mechanisms, new approaches will have to be developed. Already assays for immune complexes are established. At present the evidence is assimilated from:

(1)   The occurrence of linear patterns or granular immune deposits in the transplant kidney that have the same immunofluorescent morphology as in the original kidneys.
(2)   Elution of linear-reacting antiGBM antibody, so as to be able thereafter to confirm that it does in fact bind directly to GBM.
(3)   Elution of antigen–antibody complexes in the hope that a procedure will become available for the detection of the relevant antigens. So far this has been unrewarding.

Two clinical points have to be stressed. The first is that some degree of proteinuria is usual after transplantation. One has to consider this, and the possibility of the rejection process itself, in deciding whether a suspected recurrence of nephritis is benign, is causing the nephrotic syndrome, or is progressing rapidly to renal insufficiency. The second point is that renal vein thrombosis of an allograft is relatively common, and that on occasions it may be causing the nephrotic syndrome. It must not be overlooked.

REFERENCES

Post-streptococcal nephritis

Baldwin, D.S. (1974). Post-streptococcal nephritis. *Ann. Intern. Med.*, **80,** 342

Baldwin, D.S. (1977). Post-streptococcal nephritis. *Am. J. Med.*, **62,** 1

Baldwin, D.S. and Schacht, R.G. (1976). Late sequelae of post-streptococcal nephritis. *Ann. Rev. Med.*, **27,** 49

Dodge, W.F. *et al.* (1972). Post-streptococcal nephritis prospective study in children. *N. Engl. J. Med.*, **286,** 273

Gill, D. (1977). Post-streptococcal nephritis. *Arch. Dis. Child.*, **52,** 423

Hinglais, N. (1974). Post-streptococcal nephritis. *Am. J. Med.*, **56,** 52

Jennings, R.B. and Earle, D.P. (1961). Histopatholology and clinical studies of post-streptococcal nephritis. *J. Clin. Invest.*, **40,** 1525

Kushner, D.S. *et al.* (1961). Acute glomerulonephritis in the adult. *Medicine*, **40,** 203

Lee, H.A. *et al.* (1966). Glomerulonephritis in the elderly. *Br. Med. J.*, **2,** 1361

McCluskey, R.T. and Baldwin, D.S. (1963). *Am. J. Med.*, **35,** 213

Rodriguez-Iturbe, B. (1976). Post-streptococcal nephritis. *Clin. Nephrol.*, **5,** 197

Schacht, R.G. (1977). Post-streptococcal nephritis. *N. Engl. J. Med.*, **295,** 977

Bacterial endocarditis

Bayer, A.S. *et al.* (1976). Circulating complexes in infective endocarditis. *N. Engl. J. Med.*, **295,** 1500

Gutman, R.A. *et al.* (1972). The immune complex nephritis of bacterial endocarditis. *Medicine (Baltimore)*, **51,** 1

Weinstein, L. and Schlesinger, S. (1974). Correlations in endocarditis. *N. Engl. J. Med.*, **291,** 1122

Mesangiocapillary,nephritis

Davis, B.K. and Cavallo, T. (1976). Morphology and complement. *Am. J. Pathol.*, **84,** 283

Galle, P. and Mahieu, P. (1975). Dense deposit disease. *Am. J. Med.*, **58,** 749

Habib, R. (1975). Dense deposit disease. *Kidney Int.*, **7,** 204

Jones, D.B. (1977). Membrano-proliferative nephritis. *Arch. Pathol.*, **101,** 457

Limmermann, S.W. (1974). Transplant recurrence. *Ann. Intern. Med.*, **80,** 169

West, C.D. (1970). Hypocomplementaemic nephritis. *Nephron*, **7**, 193

West, C.D. (1976). Complement studies: classical versus the alternate pathway. *Kidney Int.*, **9**, 1.

West, C.D. *et al.* (1965). Hypocomplementaemic nephritis. *J. Paediatr.*, **67**, 1089

Levy, M. (1973). Hypocomplementaemic nephritis. *Biomedicine*, **19**, 447

Williams, D. (1974). Complement studies: classical versus the alternate pathway. *Clin. Exp. Immunol.*, **18**, 391

Lipodystrophy

Eisinger, A.J., Shortland, J.R., and Moorhead, P.J. (1972). *Q. J. Med.*, **41**, 343

Senior, B. and Gellis, S.S. (1964). *Paediatrics*, **33**, 593

Membranous nephropathy

Gluck, M.C., Gallow, G. and Lowenstein, J. (1973). Clinical and pathological features of membranous nephropathy. *Ann. Intern. Med.*, **78**, 1

Pollack, V.E., Rosen, S. and Pirani, C.L. (1968). Natural history of membranous nephropathy. *Ann. Intern. Med.*, **69**, 1171

Rosen, S. (1971). Pathology of membranous nephropathy. *Human Pathol.*, **2**, 209

Renal vein thrombosis

Llach, F. *et al.* (1975). Renal vein thrombosis in adults. *Ann. Intern. Med.*, **83**, 8

McFarland, J.B. (1951). Renal vein thrombosis in children. *Q. J. Med.*, **34**, 269

Schwartz, M.M. (1973). Renal vein thrombosis in adults. *Am. J. Med.*, **54**, 528

Trew, P.A., Biava, C.G., Jacobs, R.P. and Hopper, J. (1978). Renal vein thrombosis in membranous nephropathy. *Medicine*, **57**, 69

Henoch–Schönlein purpura

Gairdner, D. (1948). Henoch–Schönlein purpura. *Q. J. Med.*, **17**, 95

Meadow, S.R. (1972). Henoch–Schönlein purpura. *Q. J. Med.*, **41**, 241

Oliver, T.K. and Barnett, H.L. (1955). Henoch–Schönlein purpura. *Am. J. Dis. Child.*, **90**, 544

Philpott, M.G. (1952). Henoch–Schönlein purpura. *Arch. Dis. Child.*, **27**, 480

Anaphylactoid purpura

Urizar, R.E. (1968). Anaphylactoid purpura. *Lab. Invest.*, **19**, 437

Urizar, R.E., Herdman, R.C. (1970). Anaphylactoid purpura. *Am. J. Clin. Pathol.*, **53**, 258

Recurrent haematuria

Van de Putte (1974). Recurrent haematuria. *N. Engl. J. Med.*, **290**, 1165

IgA-nephritis

Laurance, D.C., Mullims, J.D. and McPhaul, J.J. (1973). IgA associated nephritis. *Kid. Int.*, **3**, 167

Mauer, S.M. and Sutherland, D.E.R. (1973). Acute immune mesangial injury. *J. Exp. Med.*, **137**, 553

Vernier, R.L., Resnick, J.S. and Mauer, S.M. (1975). Recurrent haematuria and focal nephritis. *Kidney Int.*, **7**, 224

Polyarteritis nodosa

Rich, A.R. (1942). The role of hypersensitivity. *Bull. Johns Hopkins*, **71**, 123

Rich, A.R. and Gregory, J.E. (1943). The role of hypersensitivity in polyarteritis. *Bull. Johns Hopkins*, **72**, 65

Zeek, P. (1932). Periarteritis: a critical review. *Am. J. Clin. Pathol.*, **22**, 777

Vasculitis syndromes

Bjornberg, A. and Gisslen, H. (1965). Thiazides as a cause of necrotising vasculitis. *Lancet*, **2**, 982

Christian, C.L. and Sergent, J.S. (1976). *Am. J. Med.*, **61**, 385

Gocke, D.J. (1970). Polyarteritis and Australia antigen. *Lancet*, **ii**, 1149

Parish, W.E. (1970). Studies on vasculitis. *Clin. Allergy*, **1**, 97

Trepo, C.G. (1974). Hepatitis B antigen–antibody complexes. *J. Clin. Pathol.*, **27**, 863

Cryoglobulinaemia

Bengtsson, U. (1975). Monoclonal IgG cryoglobulinaemia and nephrotic syndrome. *Q. J. Med.*, **44**, 491

Brouet, J. *et al.* (1974). Cryoglobulinaemia. *Am. J. Med.*, **57**, 775

Feizi, T. Gitlin (1969). *Lancet*, **ii**, 873

LoSpalluto, J. (1962). Cryoglobulinaemia. *Am. J. of Med.*, **32**, 142

Meltzer, E. and Franklin, M. (1966). Cryoglobulinaemia. *Am. J. Med.*, **40**, 828

Thrombotic thrombocytopenic purpura

Levine, S., Shearn, M.A. (1964). TTP and SLE. *Arch. Intern. Med.*, **113,** 826

Lukes, R.J. (1961). Thrombotic thrombocytopenic purpura. *Blood,* **17,** 366

Taub, R.N. (1964). Thrombotic thrombocytopenic purpura. *Blood,* **24,** 775

Lupus nephritis

Appel, G.B. and Silva, F.G. (1978). Natural history of SLE. *Medicine,* **57,** 371

Baldwin, D.S. *et al.* (1970). Proliferative and membranous forms of lupus nephritis. *Ann. Intern. Med.,* **73,** 929

Bardana, E.J. *et al.* (1975). DNA–anti DNA antibody complexes in SLE. *Am. J. Med.,* **59,** 5151

Grigor, R.R. *et al.* (1973). Outcome of pregnancy in SLE. *Proc. Roy. Soc. Med.,* **70,** 99

Koffler, D. *et al.* (1971). SLE as an immune complex nephritis. *J. Exp. Med.,* **134,** 3, pt. 2 169 s

McCluskey, R.T. (1970). Lupus nephritis classification. *Pathol. Ann.,* 125

Mixed connective tissue disease

Sharp, G.C. (1972). Mixed connective tissue disease. *Am. J. Med.,* **52,** 148

Rapidly progressive glomerulonephritis

Bacani, R.A. (1968). Rapidly progressive glomerulonephritis. *Ann. Intern. Med.,* **69,** 463

Rosen, S. (1975). Crescentic glomerulonephritis. *Pathol. Ann.,* 37

Goodpasture's syndrome

Lewis, E.J. *et al.* (1973). Goodpasture-like syndrome. *Am. J. Med.,* **54,** 507

Proskey, A.J. *et al.* (1970). Goodpasture's syndrome. *Am. J. Med.,* **48,** 162

Seigel, R.R. (1970). Pulmonary disease resolution after nephrectomy. *Am. J. Med., Sci.,* **259,** 201

Immune renal tubular acidosis and interstitial nephritis

Andres, G.A. and McCluskey, R.T. (1975). Interstitial nephritis. *Kidney Int.,* 7, 271

Baldwin, D.S. *et al.* (1968). Interstitial nephritis. *N. Engl. J. Med.,* **279,** 1245

Bergstein, J. and Litman, N. (1975). Interstitial nephritis. *N. Engl. J. Med.,* **292,** 875

Bridi, G.S. *et al.* (1972). Renal tubular acidosis in chronic active hepatitis. *Am. J. Med.,* **52,** 267

Lehman, D.H. (1974). Interstitial nephritis. *Kidney Int.,* **5,** 187

Ooi, B.S. (1974). IgE levels in interstitial nephritis. *Lancet,* **i,** 1254

Simenhoff, M.L., Guild, W.R. and Dammin, G.J. (1968). Interstitial nephritis. *Am. J. Med.,* **44,** 618

Minimal change nephrosis

Eyres, K. (1976). Cell-mediated immunity in minimal change. *Lancet,* **ii,** 1158

Hayslett, J.P. (1969). Lipoid nephrosis to renal insufficiency. *N. Engl. J. Med.,* **281,** 181

Lim, V.S., Sibley, R. and Spargo, B. (1974). Adult lipoid nephrosis. *Ann. Intern. Med.,* **81,** 314

Sandberg, D.H. (1977). Nephrotic syndrome and milk allergy. *Lancet,* **i,** 388

Wittig, H.J. (1970). Nephrotic syndrome and inhaled allergens. *Lancet,* **i,** 542

Focal sclerosis

Habib, R. (1973). Focal sclerosis. *Kidney Int.,* **4,** 355

Hyman, L.R. and Burkholder, P.M. (1973). Focal sclerosis. *Lab. Invest.,* **28,** 533

Nash, M.A., Greifu, I. *et al.* (1976). Focal sclerosis. *J. Paediatr.,* **88,** 806

Saint-Hillier, Y. *et al.* (1975). Focal and segmental hyalinosis. *Adv. Nephrol.,* **5,** 67

Nephrotic syndrome

Adams, D.A. (1960). Nephrotic syndrome in children. *Arch. Intern. Med.,* **106,** 117

Blainey, J.D. *et al.* (1960). Diagnosis by renal biopsy and immunological analyses. *Q. J. Med.,* **29,** 235

Bohle, A. *et al.* (1970). Renal biopsies. *German Med., Monthly* **Jan,** 32

Bolton, W.K. *et al.* (1977). Alternate day steroids. *Am. J. Med.,* **62,** 60

Churg, J. *et al.* (1970). Nephrotic syndrome in children. *Lancet,* **i,** 1299

Hallman, N. (1959). Congenital nephrotic syndrome. *J. Paediatr.,* **55,** 152

Kark, R.M. *et al.* (1958). Nephrotic syndrome in children. *Arch. Intern. Med.,* **49,** 751

Michael, A.F. (1967). Immunosuppressive therapy. *N. Engl. J. Med.,* **276,** 817

Miller, R.B. *et al.* (1969). Long term results with steroids. *Am. J. Med.,* **46,** 919

Pearl, M.A. *et al.* (1963). Nephrotic syndrome in children. *Arch. Intern. Med.*, **112**, 716

Robson, J.S. (1972). *Nephrotic Syndrome in Renal Disease.* Ed. D.A.K. Black. (Oxford: Blackwell)

Stokke, K.T. (1976). Nephrotic syndrome with ulcerative colitis. *Scand. J. Gastroenterol.*, **11**, 571

Yamauchi, H. *et al.* (1964). Shock and volume depletion. *Ann. Intern. Med.*, **60**, 242

Lipids in nephrotic syndrome

Baxter, J.H. (1962). Hyperlipoproteinaemia in nephrosis. *Arch. Intern. Med.*, **109**, 742

Baxter, J.H., Goodman, H.C. and Shafrir, E. (1959). Glucose infusion and serum lipids in nephrotics. *J. Clin. Invest.*, **38**, 986

Chronic renal failure, triglycerides and degenerative disease. *Nutr. Rev.*, 1977, **35**, 10

Treatment of nephritis (immunosuppression)

Basu, D. (1972). Regulation of heparin therapy. *N. Engl. J. Med.*, **287**, 324

Booth, L.J. and Aber, G.M. (1970). Immunosuppressive therapy in adults with proliferative glomerulonephritis. *Lancet*, **2**, 1010

Cade, R. *et al.* (1973). Azathioprine, prednisone and heparin alone or combined in lupus nephritis. *Nephron*, **10**, 37

Cameron, J.S. (1975). Treatment and natural history of glomerulonephritis. *6th. Int. Congress Nephrology*, 492

Cameron, J.S. (1977). Appraisal of nephritis therapy. *Br. Med. J.*, **1**, 1457

Clarkson, A.R. and Robson, J.S. (1972). Drugs for immunological disease. *Prog. Biochem. Pharmacol.*, **7**, 427

Colman, R.W. (1970). Regulation of heparin therapy. *Am. J. Clin. Path.*, **53**, 904

Cutler, S.J. and Ederer, F. (1958). Actuarial survival curves. *J. Chron. Dis.*, **8**, 699

Denman, E.J. *et al.* (1970). Cytotoxic drugs are not necessarily immuno-suppressive. *Ann. Rheum. Dis.*, **29**, 220

Dukor, P. and Dietrich, F.M. (1968). Immunosuppression by steroids and cytotoxic drugs. *Int. Arch. Allergy*, **34**, 32

Ibels, L.S. Cyclophosphamide for nephritis. In Edwards, *Drugs and The Kidney. Prog. Biochem. Pharmacol.*, **9**, 65

Kincaid-Smith, P. (1972). Anticoagulation in nephritis. *Med. J. Aust.*, **2**, 587

McAdams, A.J. (1975). High alternate day prednisone. *J. Paediatr.*, **86**, 23

Paulus, H.E. (1972). Guide lines for drug dosage. *Arth. Rheum.,* **15,** 29

Sharpstone, P. (1969). Prednisone and azathioprine in nephrotic syndrome. *Br. Med., J.,* **2,** 535

Swenson, M.A. and Schwartz, R.S. (1967). Immunosuppressive therapy—anti-inflammatory action is more evident. *N. Engl. J. Med.,* **277,** 163

Vanrenterghen, Y. (1975). Does anti-inflammatory drug treatment modify nephritis? *6th. Int. Congress Nephrology,* 500

Plasma exchange

Lockwood, C.M. (1976). Plasma exchange. *Lancet,* **i,** 711

Perfusion over immunoreactive collodion membranes

Terman, D.S., Ogden, D. and Petty, D. (1976). Perfusion over immunoreactive collodion membranes. *FEBS Lett.,* **68,** 89

6
Nephropathies

Normal urine contains less than one red cell per high-power field. Macroscopic haematuria causes a brown-red discolouration of the urine but microscopic haematuria is only found by routine microscopy.

Haematuria can be looked at in various ways:

(1) *According to anatomical site of the blood leak into the urinary tract* (Figure 62).

(2) *According to distribution of the blood in the voided urine.* This is assessed by means of the three glass fractionated micturition test of Guyon;

    (a) *initial haematuria* must come from the urethra or prostate;

    (b) *terminal haematuria* indicates an origin from the bladder or posterior urethra;

    (c) *total haematuria* is when all three glasses contain blood—it is in any case inevitable whenever haematuria is profuse.

(3) *According to sympatomatology.* Haematuria due to surgical conditions is characteristically intermittent, and that due to a tumour appears suddenly, stops within one to two days and then recurs at a later date. Haematuria with renal pain can occur with TB, pyelitis,

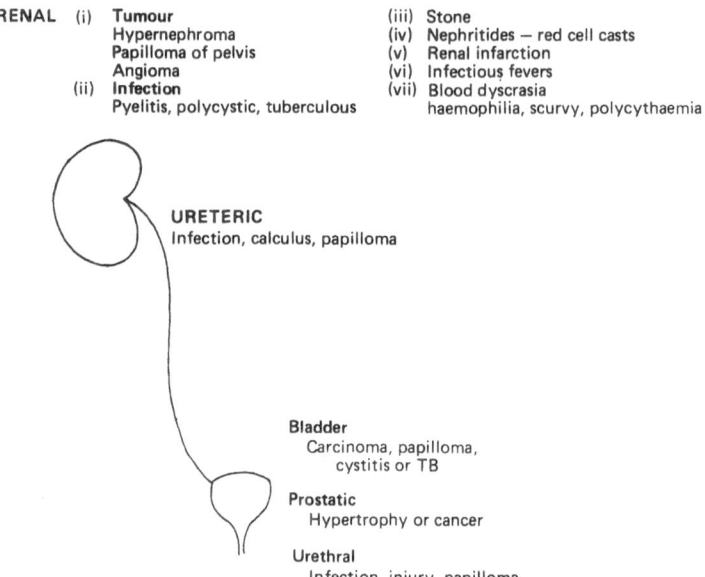

RENAL (i) **Tumour**
                  Hypernephroma
                  Papilloma of pelvis
                  Angioma
    (ii) **Infection**
                  Pyelitis, polycystic, tuberculous

  (iii) Stone
  (iv) Nephritides — red cell casts
  (v) Renal infarction
  (vi) Infectious fevers
  (vii) Blood dyscrasia
             haemophilia, scurvy, polycythaemia

URETERIC
Infection, calculus, papilloma

Bladder
   Carcinoma, papilloma,
      cystitis or TB

Prostatic
   Hypertrophy or cancer

Urethral
   Infection, injury, papilloma

Figure 62.   Sites of blood leak into the urinary tract

polycystic kidneys, or with renal infarction, renal stone or renal tumour. Haematuria with dysuria indicates a bladder problem such as cystitis, TB, stone, tumour or prostatic hypertrophy.

(4)   *According to age*

Child   1–10 pyelonephritis and cystitis, or glomerulonephritis;
            15–40 nephritis, pyelitis, stone or papilloma;
            40–50 stone, neoplasm or inflammation;
            50–70 prostatic hypertrophy or cancer, vesical neoplasm.

Benign recurrent haematuria

This can be a problem in the younger age group; 50% of these cases occur below the age of 15 and the episodes may go on for 2–5 years. It is often asymptomatic and found only on routine examination and yet at other times it will be noted that brown urine is passed after exercise, following a sore throat or after tonsillectomy or dental extraction.

When the patient is first seen the possibilities are numerous and the following are the steps in investigation:

(1)   Urine microscopy for assessment of pyuria, red cell casts and so on. Pyuria with some haematuria indicates either bacterial infection or TB. Red cell casts indicate glomerular involvement as in renal

infarction or acute tubular necrosis, vasculitides or nephritides, and hypertension.

(2) Urine culture for bacteria and tubercle bacilli.

(3) Renal function—blood urea and creatinine clearances are required.

(4) Twenty-four hour urinary protein and studies of selectivity of the proteinuria.

(5) Nephritic serum tests such as AST 'O' titre, C3 and C4, antinuclear factor, rheumatoid factor.

(6) IVP and cystoscopy; renal arteriograms are often indicated and also ultrasound scanning for tumours.

(7) Renal biopsy.

(8) Basic haematology to exclude thrombocytopenia, haemophilia and von Willebrand's disease should not be overlooked.

The renal biopsy result should give a definitive diagnosis in those cases which are thought to be due to a form of nephritis. The possibilities are:

(1) normal renal histology—this might only mean that the renal changes are patchy;

(2) typical focal nephritis;

(3) diffuse proliferative nephritis;

(4) other nephritides, such as focal embolic nephritis, Henoch-Schönlein purpura or a vasculitis such as PN, SLE, or Alport's hereditary nephritis.

It remains only to emphasize those features which differentiate a focal nephritis from a typical post-streptococcal nephritis; they are summarized in Table 15 below.

Table 15

	Acute post-streptococcal nephritis	*Focal nephritis*
Sore throat	+	Sometimes
Haematuria	++	+
Latent period	7–21 days	1–3 days
Oedema/hypertension	+	0
Glomerular filtration	Reduced	Normal
Antistreptolysin	Raised titre	Normal
C3 Complement	Can be low	Normal or raised
Outcome	Clears	Active sediment persists

161

Alport's syndrome

This is an hereditary nephropathy accompanied by nerve deafness, and is more severe in males. Because it is associated with an abnormality of the anterior capsule of the lens, it is worth considering when a patient with haematuria wears glasses. Indeed it is possible that the glomerular basement membrane and the basilar membrane of the organ of Corti share a common abnormality. Occasionally there is a nephrotic syndrome.

The electron microscope reveals a characteristic splitting of the basement membrane into many thin layers with an accumulation of small dense particles between. In early years, in fact, the basement membrane may appear normal, then more thick than usual, and then finally it has this shredded appearance. Likewise the tubular basement membrane shows splitting and an accumulation of lipid vacuoles. Therefore it is possible that lipid is being filtered through the glomeruli and is then reabsorbed by the tubular cells with an accumulation in the tubular basement membrane. There are also interstitial foam cells. Additionally, the permeability of the basement membrane leads on the one hand to a fusion of the foot processes of the epithelial cells as in any proteinuric syndrome, and on the other to a mesangial hypertrophy and sclerosis.

Since an Alport's syndrome is known to be associated with anomalies of metabolism of those amino acids prominent in collagen, it seems likely that an enzyme defect in the synthesis of basement membrane collagen will be found. In fact hyperprolinaemia, hyperhydroxyprolinaemia and hyperglycinaemia have all been described in association with Alport's syndrome.

PROTEINURIA AND ITS INVESTIGATION

The normal daily loss of protein in the urine is very small, 40–80 mg/day. When such small amounts have to be detected the urine first has to be concentrated by means of a Diaflo ultrafiltration membrane or by absorption of water by means of 60% polyethylene glycol (PEG) or Carbowax 20 M. Thereafter assay of total protein can be achieved by the Lowry or Folin colour reactions, by the biuret reaction, or by protein precipitation with recording of the turbidity produced by 3% trichloracetic acid or by sulphosalicylic acid. The latest immunoprecipitation techniques, which utilize antisera specific for proteins (such as albumin) and recording of the turbidity change, enable quantitation of small amounts of a defined protein.

The pores in the basement membrane are mainly 30 Å in size with a range from 20 Å to 55 Å. Additional restriction to the passage of proteins is given by the slits between the foot processes of the epithelial cells and likewise the gaps between the endothelial cells. These normally carry a negative surface charge due to the sialic acid of the cell surfaces.

The several types of proteinuria are classified as follows.

Glomerular proteinuria

This occurs in nephrosis and the nephritides, renal transplant rejection or acute renal failure, and indeed in any process which disorganizes the glomerular basement membrane; it can result in heavy proteinuria. If only small molecules leak through the proteinuria is said to be 'selective', whereas if molecules of all sizes and shape pass through it is termed 'non-selective'.

Tubular proteinuria

Normally a high proportion of the proteins that do filter through the glomeruli are reabsorbed by the renal tubular epithelium. Thus if the protein of the filtrate is 2 mg/l then with a GFR of 180 l/day this amounts to 360 mg protein, of which 95% is reabsorbed, so that ultimately 18 mg albumin and 18 mg low molecular weight protein are lost in the urine.

The protein reabsorbed by the tubules can increase considerably. Thus in nephrotic patients their increased fractional catabolic rate for albumin has been found to correlate with the degree of proteinuria. This is explained by catabolism within the tubules.

However, in certain diseases there is specific damage to the tubular epithelium which causes failure of reabsorption and a 'tubular proteinuria'. The bulk of the protein lost is of low molecular weight (20000–30000), for example, beta-2-microglobulin. It cannot be detected by heating the urine but is precipitated by the acid denaturants such as TCA. Causative conditions include chronic pyelonephritis, Wilson's disease and the Fanconi syndrome as well as damage by cadmium, phenacetin, vitamin D poisoning, or chronic hypokalaemia.

Other causes of proteinuria

Postural

This is when proteinuria is present in the upright position only, so that protein is not detected when the patient first passes urine in the morning but is present later in the day. Clearly in the upright position vasoconstriction is acting to increase the protein of the filtered fraction. Many of these cases have some evidence of nephritis on biopsy.

Exercise proteinuria (athletic proteinuria)

This is proteinuria with cast excretion which appears after vigorous exercise. It is presumed that a combination of vasoconstriction and vasopressor amine release causes slowing of blood flow through the glomeruli and an increased leakage of protein. A similar proteinuria is seen after emotional stress, exposure to cold or during fever. These types of proteinuria are 'non-selective' and probably reflect a failure of protein reabsorption by the renal tubules.

The type of proteinuria can be clarified by *starch gel electrophoresis* of concentrated urine. Figure 63 shows the diagnostic patterns.

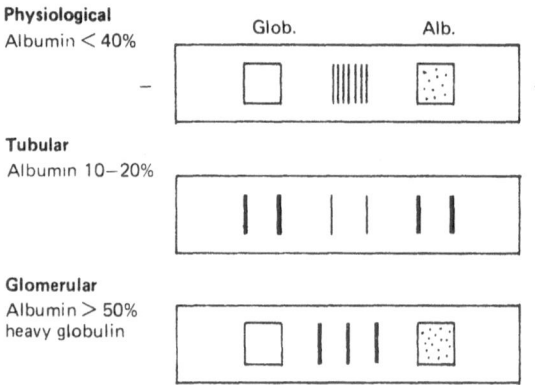

Figure 63.   Types of proteinuria on starch gel

Selectivity is quantitated most accurately by measuring the concentration of a particular protein in relation to the urinary content of either albumin (molecular weight 70000), transferrin (molecular weight 90000) or IgG globulin (molecular weight 150000). In fact the ratio of IgG concentration to that of transferrin is most easily and accurately quantitated on *immunodiffu-*

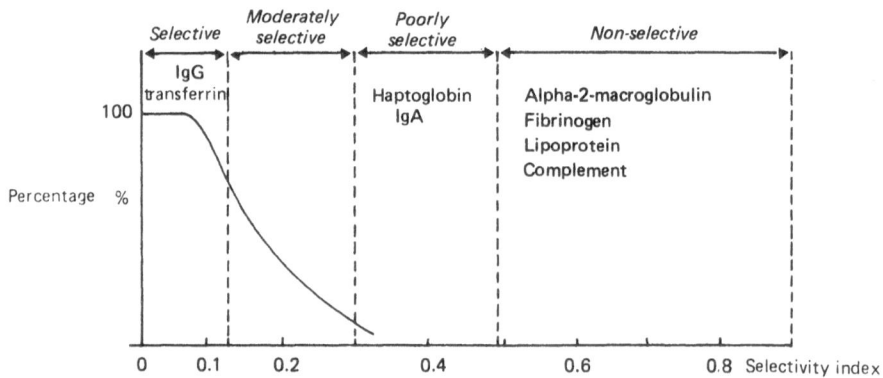

Figure 64.   Steroid response and selectivity of proteinuria

sion plates. A selective proteinuria indicates that there has been little leakage of IgG compared with transferrin (IgG/transferrin ratio 0.2). The other definitions are as shown in Figure 64, which also stresses those proteins whose presence in urine gives an immediate indication of the severity of a proteinuria—alpha-2-macroglobulin indicates a non-selective proteinuria, haptoglobin and IgA a poorly selective proteinuria and IgG and transferrin only a selective proteinuria.

Measurement of DPC (the differential protein clearance) is important as a means of gauging prognosis; normally a highly selective proteinuria responds to steroid therapy.

Quantitation of selectivity
In many publications the amounts of proteins of specified molecular weight in urine are related to the percentage loss of those proteins compared with the creatinine clearance, and the values are plotted so as to give a slope. When the angle of the line is acute ($0 = 75°$) the proteinuria is said to be 'selective', but when the slope is extended because of the occurrence in the urine of high molecular weight proteins (and the angle is $35°$), the proteinuria is 'non-selective' (Figure 65).

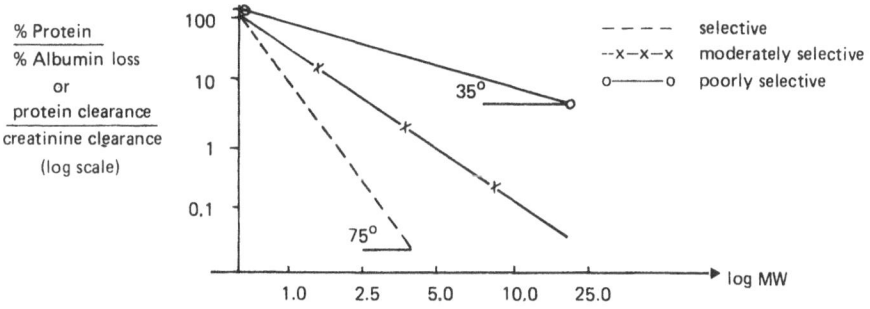

Figure 65. **Immunochemical determination of 'differential protein clearances'**

It is not appropriate to extend this discussion to the immunochemistry of proteins but it is nevertheless of help to have an overall idea of the sizes of proteins and thus what their appearance in urine actually means (Table 16).

Small amounts of the low molecular weight proteins are found normally, but of course large quantities can appear when there is damage to the tubular epithelium. In any type of renal disease light-chain losses in the urine are increased, and the κ/λ ratio is then raised. With renal insufficiency the light-chain content of the serum rises owing to the reduced glomerular filtration.

165

Table 16   The proteins of normal urine

>90 000	40 000–90 000	<40 000
Non-selective [index 0.9]	albumin (69 000)	post-γ-protein
	a_1-antitrypsin (60 000)	gamma R
a_2-Macroglobulin (820 000)	a_1-acid glycoprotein (44 000)	β component
Fibrinogen (350 000)	β_2-glycoprotein (40 000)	a_2-component
Poorly selective [index 0.45]	IgG light-chain dimer (45 000)	post-albumin
		pre-albumin (61 000)
IgA (160 000)		IgG light chain monomer
Haptoglobin (100 000)		β_2-microglobulin (11 800)
Selective [index 0.15]		a_2-microglobulin
		(these are the proteins of
IgG (150 000)		tubular proteinuria)
Transferrin (90 000)		

The approach to trace proteinuria

At the present time proteinuria is being sought routinely by means of Albustix, which detect 10–20 mg%; a level of 30 mg% may certainly have clinical significance. However, it is important to confirm the finding by means of the sulphosalicylic acid quantitation because false-positive Albustix reactions occur in alkaline urine.

Proteinuria can be an indication of, but is not invariably present in, urinary tract infection, for which bacterial cultures are regarded as a more reliable indicator of active disease. If the patient has proteinuria the coincident finding of red cells points to a glomerular lesion, but otherwise one has to be continually aware of postural proteinuria and testing of diurnal urine samples becomes necessary. Protein is present in urine *de jour* but not *par nuit*.

It is important:

(1)   to measure the blood urea and creatinine clearance (GFR);

(2)   to measure the selectivity of the proteinuria;
(3)   to distinguish between glomerular and tubular leaks;
(4)   to perform a renal biopsy when glomerular disease is suspected;
(5)   to exclude urinary tract infection including tuberculosis.

A family history of renal disease, hypertension or of deafness can be of considerable importance. In children, asymptomatic proteinuria occurs in some 2% of boys and 6% of girls. Most turn out to have normal biopsy findings, although some may show segmental or focal nephritis, and there is always a suspicion that it is a harbinger of long-term renal disease. Such proteinuria often lasts for at least 3 years.

After an acute nephritis a normal urinary pattern can be established between 2 weeks and 3 months later. Yet there can be a long intermediate period when alpha-2-macroglobulin persists in the urine. The same applies to anaphylactoid purpura. If biopsied, such patients are more likely to have some glomerular abnormality. Similarly, of course, a highly selective minimal change nephrosis may turn up as 'trace proteinuria'. So also may cases of acute tubulointerstitial nephritis, although in this situation the proteins are of low molecular weight and typical of 'tubular proteinuria'.

Increased light-chain excretion is normally associated with the Bence Jones protein of myeloma. It is not detectable by Albustix. It is best detected not by the heat test but by layering the urine onto concentrated hydrochloric acid, when a deposit of precipitated protein will appear at the interface. In fact light-chain excretion is now readily quantitated by means of urine concentration, followed by immunodiffusion against specific anti-λ and anti-κ antisera. Increased excretion occurs in neonates up to 1 year, in many inflammatory disorders and in monoclonal gammopathies and SLE.

Molecular chromatography of urinary proteins on Sephadex gels has, of course, received some attention. Molecules pass through a Sephadex column at rates inversely proportional to the fluid volume available to them (the K_{av}). Thus large molecules which are 'excluded' from the gel pass straight through the column in the 'elution volume', while smaller molecules are eluted according to how much they have become mixed with the interstices of the matrix. Good separation of the urinary proteins is obtained with a long narrow column of G-75 which excludes molecules above 110 000 daltons and which filters molecules according to size in the range 70 000 down to 2000 daltons.

The types of pattern found are shown in Figure 66. Thus a good differentiation can be obtained.

DIABETIC NEPHROPATHY

The clinical problem

The small vessel disease of diabetes results in retinopathy, nephropathy and

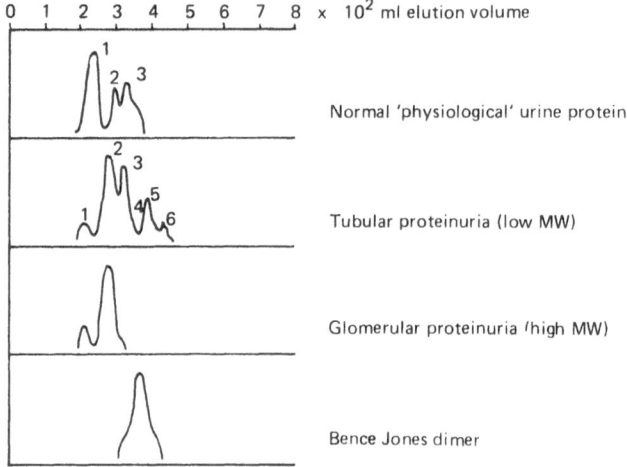

Figure 66.   Elution of urinary proteins on Sephadex G-75

neuropathy in all juvenile insulin-treated diabetics of some 15–20 years duration. Although the maturity-onset diabetic has only relative insulin deficiency and clinical manifestations apart from the obesity are variable, some of these patients can also have marked retinopathy and nephropathy, presumably because they have had undiscovered chemical diabetes for some years before clinical presentation. In fact, at the Joslin clinic, 10% of all diabetics die on account of renal disease; the development of proteinuria signals the onset of a steady downhill course. Among the patients who die between the age of 20–40 years nodular or diffuse glomerulosclerosis is present in 5%, but if they have had diabetes for 15–20 years then it is present in 100%.

The renal presentation is insidious with benign low-grade proteinuria which may increase over the years to the stage at which the patient develops ankle oedema, which is indicative of a low serum albumin, and anaemia, which is indicative of renal insufficiency. During this time the blood urea and serum creatinine will rise slowly; the blood pressure may also rise.

In patients who have only attended for treatment sporadically presentation may be dramatic when they appear with hypertension, ischaemic heart disease, stroke, disabling neuropathy, terminal uraemia or with the nephrotic syndrome.

It is a clinical maxim that the grade of retinopathy as assessed by the ophthalmoscope correlates with the degree of renal abnormality as indicated by the degree of proteinuria, by renal biopsy or by subsequent autopsy. This is because there is a basic underlying abnormality of the microcirculation and of the basement membranes whose severity reflects the duration of the diabetes. The one common factor is an increased permeability of the endothelial cell junctions and of the thickened abnormal basement membranes to proteins. Whether this can be controlled or reduced by obsessional attention to insulin to be determined. Endothelial cell prostacyclin (PGI_2) deficiency has now been identified.

Pathology

The lesions which can be found in the diabetic kidney are as follows (see Figure 67).

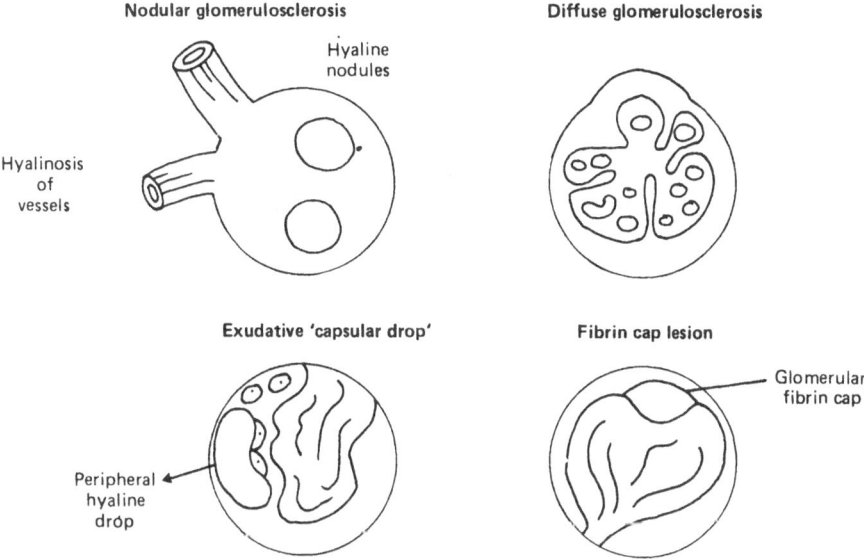

Figure 67. Summary of the pathological changes in diabetes

Nodular glomerulosclerosis (the Kimmelstiel–Wilson syndrome)
Eosinophilic laminated nodules appear in the periphery of a glomerulus as part of an expansion of the mesangium. Growth of the nodule together with local thickening of the basement membrane of the capillary loops results in progressive occlusion of glomerular capillaries and tuft ischaemia. Ultimately there is a large acellular mass.

Diffuse glomerulosclerosis
This is characterized by a diffuse accumulation of eosinophilic PAS-positive argyrophilic matrix material within the mesangium so that the initial impression is of thickening of the capillary walls as in a membranous nephropathy. The basement membrane thickening may vary from 2500–25 000 Å. Normal

basement membranes do thicken with age. They measure, on average, only 1330 Å in either sex at the age of 20. Diffuse glomerulosclerosis, therefore, has a double meaning, referring both to the basement membrane thickening and also to the overlying layer of mesangial matrix.

The exudative 'capsular drop'
This is an amorphous hyaline eosinophilic crescent of waxy consistency which is situated between the parietal epithelium and the basement membrane of Bowman's capsule. It is PAS-positive and rich in lipid. Later it becomes lost in connective tissue fibres as fibroblasts appear and lay down collagen.

Fibrin of 'lipohyaline' caps
The 'fibrin cap' is a collection of fibrinoid material situated in the periphery of a glomerular tuft.

The renal vasculature
As emphasized by Bell there is in diabetes a hyalinosis both of the afferent and the efferent arterioles. Thus when the *efferent* arteries show sclerosis and *hyalinosis,* this is specific for diabetes.

Renal tubular changes
  (1)   When glomeruli become ischaemic their tubules become atrophic and dilated. The proximal tubular damage is revealed by lysozymuria.
  (2)   Acute and chronic pyelonephritic changes are often found in diabetics, as also is papillary necrosis. In fact, if a policy of restricted catheterization is followed, although diabetics are susceptible to infection there should be little trouble until late middle age.

The immunofluorescent findings in diabetes are non-specific and are consequent on the increased permeability of the basement membranes to protein. Thus both albumin and IgG show as a linear pattern along the glomerular basement membranes, and often also along the tubular basement membrane. Both IgM and C3 complement appear as lumps in the mesangium, and typically it is IgM rather than fibrinogen that is found in the 'fibrin-cap'.

Pathogenesis

Ideas concerning the cause of diabetic nephropathy are closely linked to those concerning diabetic microangiopathy. There is undoubtedly a close relation between the severity of angiopathy and (a) the duration of diabetes, and (b) the adequacy of past metabolic control as judged by hyperglycaemia, quantitation of haemoglobin A_{ic} and collections for estimation of daily urine glucose loss.

170

There is now no support for the concept that basement membrane thickening is genetically determined and is present in prediabetes. In diabetes in animals basement membrane thickening is determined by the severity and duration of hyperglycaemia. The finding of haemoglobin A_{ic} suggests that it may all be explained by post-translational modification of glycoproteins.

Theories of diabetic microangiopathy
Insulin deficiency and inadequate metabolic control are paramount hence there is:
(1)   non-insulin-dependent glycoprotein synthesis and modification;
(2)   non-insulin-dependent collagen-linked disaccharide unit over-production;
(3)   impaired activity of pericytes and mesangial cells.

Poor metabolic control is reflected as:
(1)   raised growth hormone levels in plasma;
(2)   endothelial cell and basement membrane permeability to proteins;
(3)   an inverse correlation between ketones and alanine or lactate;
(4)   hyperglycaemia and raised plasma free fatty acids;
(5)   increased platelet aggregation together with raised HbA_{ic}
(6)   Prostacyclin deficiency in vascular endothelium.

Both hyperglycaemia and saturated fatty acids increase platelet aggregation. When platelets aggregate they release thromboxanes and lipoperoxides, which almost certainly are the explanation for the *increased endothelial cell junction permeability* of diabetic capillaries. Thus there is insudation of proteins into the arteriole and capillary walls giving rise to hyalinosis.

The basement membrane
The basement membrane of the renal glomerulus is synthesized by the epithelial cells. When weanling rats are given silver nitrate in their drinking water for a limited period, a line of silver deposit can be shown to move from the epithelial to the endothelial side, and on that side there is also impaired removal of effete membrane on account of the impaired phagocytic activity of the mesangial cells, which is found in insulin-deficient animals.

Basement membrane is a form of collagen, but glomerular membrane does not have the typical fibrillary appearance of normal collagen; this is explained by the high sugar content. In fact basement membrane is type IV collagen with the helical structure $(ai)_3$ and is characterized by a high content (10%) of sugar residues and increased 3-and 4-hydroxyproline and increased hydroxylysine. Spiro demonstrated that the increased hydroxylation is followed by increased glycosylation by means of glycosyltransferase enzymes so that typically there is an excess of glucopyranosyl–galactopyranosyl disaccharide units.

Growth hormone, insulin deficiency and glucose excess

It appears that glucose excess, insulin deficiency or perhaps excess growth hormone play a role in the assembly of the carbohydrate units. Certainly an increased number of these disaccharide units will interfere with the packing of the collagen helices into fibrils, so the diabetic basement membrane will be thickened and be more permeable. However, further studies are required, as not all authors agree on the biochemical abnormality; there is agreement on the fact that basement membrane thickness is related to the duration of diabetes, and that this also determines the amount of proteinaeous debris in the mesangial areas.

Whether growth hormone plays any role in this process is open to question. Growth hormone levels in uncontrolled diabetics are high and can be subject to wide fluctuation. Moreover experience has shown that they are normalized when there is adequate diabetic control. It is a fact that growth hormone is an insulin-antagonist in the sense that when it is elevated, free fatty acids are mobilized and by feedback inhibition excess citrate within the Kreb's cycle causes an inhibition of glucose utilization at the phosphofructokinase step. Hence when there is coincident insulin deficiency, glucose is not utilized and is available for diversion along non-insulin-dependent pathways towards glycoprotein synthesis. This accounts for elevation of glycoproteins in the blood of diabetics and possibly also for the abnormal basement membrane structure.

The kidneys of the diabetic animal or human are hypertrophied. Although this might be a growth hormone effect, it might also be the result of the increased glucose reabsorption in diabetic kidney together with increased gluconeogenesis and hence glycogen deposition.

Insulin deficiency certainly impairs the activity of leucocytes and phagocytes. The mononuclear phagocytic system (MPS) includes the mesangial cells of the renal glomeruli and also the pericytes which normally remove the basal lamina of capillaries. Vracko and Benditt have suggested therefore that it is pericyte dysfunction that results in a steady accumulation

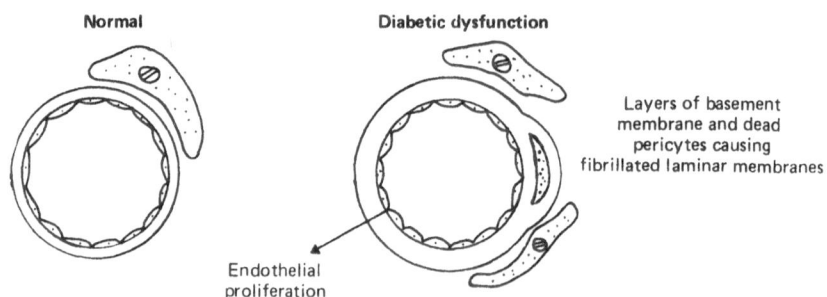

Figure 68. Pericyte dysfunction and the basement membrane

of effete basement membrane material (Figure 68). In the case of the glomerulus this would mean the accumulation of excess basement membrane on its upper surface, and thus ultimate basement membrane thickening.

Clinical management of the diabetic nephropathy patient

Certain points are of direct concern to the nephrologist.

(1) When faced with a diabetic with proteinuria who does not have an appropriate degree of retinopathy, it is important to think of glomerulonephritis. A renal biopsy becomes essential.

(2) It is clear that even patients with diabetes, nephropathy and hypertension can often have low renin levels. This can be accounted for (a) by volume expansion, (b) a result of hyalinization of the afferent arterioles, and (c) a decreased sympathetic drive or catecholamine stimulation of renin release owing to autonomic denervation. Many such diabetics never have hypertension but marked postural hypotension because of failure of their compensatory reflexes. It has been shown that when their blood pressure falls on standing, there is no compensatory rise of renin.

(3) One has to know how to manage uraemia and hypertension in the diabetic. Both will aggravate the retinopathy and lead to visual deterioration. The following features should be noted:

(a) Hypertension must be adequately controlled, but hypotension should be avoided as it leads to retention of nitrogenous products.

(b) The classical distal tubule-blocking diuretics cannot be used as potassium retention in the diabetic may give rise to hyperkalaemia and death, because potassium cannot enter the cells when insulin is in short supply.

(c) As chronic renal failure develops, insulin requirements tend to fall.

(d) As uraemia develops protein restriction takes precedence, so that when the GFR is 3 ml/min the patient will be taking 20–30 g protein and 80 g fat, and will therefore have to consume more carbohydrate (300 g) in order to maintain his calorie intake.

(e) Diabetics are not good candidates for dialysis, owing to their vascular problems and retinopathy with the liability to retinal haemorrhage, or for transplantation owing to their liability to infection even without the added burden of corticosteroids and immunosuppressants. However an occasional patient will be seen whose young age and responsibilities make the attempt a worthwhile proposition. Preliminary peritoneal dialysis using a Tenckhoff catheter (see p. 379), is recommended.

GLOMERULAR CHANGES IN NEOPLASIA

The general rules are quite simple: one expects to find *minimal change* nephrotic syndrome in the mixed-cell type of Hodgkin's disease, *membranous nephropathy* in association with cancer of lung or colon, and *proliferative disease* with lymphosarcoma or reticulum cell sarcoma.

Cancer

There seems to be a 5% incidence of membranous nephropathy in cancer patients, due to circulating tumour antigen–antibody complexes. Often the tumour antigens, such as CEA in colon cancer, can be shown in the basement membrane deposits. Moreover, occasionally a remission can be induced by resection of that cancer.

Hodgkin's disease

Minimal change nephrotic syndrome in Hodgkin's disease is not at all uncommon and the nephrotic syndrome can be gross. Urine protein clearances show high selectivity. Some 75% of these cases have Hodgkins of 'mixed-cell type'. It is therefore suggested, in keeping with theories concerning minimal change nephrosis, that there is an abnormality involving T lymphocytes which might be the source of a lymphokine which causes basement membrane permeability.

Additionally many of these cases have raised serum IgE levels which can be related to eosinophil infiltration of the tumour.

GLOMERULAR CHANGES IN SARCOIDOSIS

Typically the kidney of the patient with sarcoid may contain granulomata; it will also show nephrocalcinosis in those patients with hypercalcaemia due to vitamin D 'sensitivity'.

In addition, cases of membranous or proliferative glomerulonephritis have been described. It is always assumed that sarcoid is due to disseminated antigens, akin to that of Mycobacterium TB, and that these are of low solubility and cannot be adequately catabolized, causing a granulomatous reaction. Thus on occasions there might be circulating immune complexes. There is also hyperglobulinaemia, the rheumatoid factor test can be positive and there can be circulating cryoglobulins.

RADIATION NEPHRITIS

Unfortunately the kidneys may be irradiated as part of therapy aimed at tumours of the ovaries and uterus, as part of the field to be covered for proper therapy of seminoma of the testes, and in the treatment of tumours of the pancreas, retroperitoneal area or of the kidneys themselves. Damage to the epithelium of the tubules seems to be the primary lesion and with the tubular atrophy there develops an interstitial fibrosis and sclerosis of the blood vessels. Glomerular involvement is late and consists either of simple hyalinization or fibrosis, or of a lesion which simulates membranous nephropathy. This could be due to the production of a Heymann's type of autoimmune nephrosis. With the development of glomerulosclerosis hypertension appears and occasionally this will go on to a malignant phase. Such damage to the human kidney requires an exposure to over 2500 roentgens.

OTHER INFECTIONS AND CONDITIONS CAUSING DIFFUSE RENAL DAMAGE

Virus B hepatitis

Patients with serum hepatitis B can develop persistent antigenaemia with the viral coat antigen (HB_SAg) and this can give rise to a *nephritic* or *nephrotic* syndrome according to the localization of the immune complexes deposited in the kidneys. The nephritis varies from a mild, completely reversible form to an overt and progressive nephrotic syndrome associated with chronic active hepatitis. In this latter event the histology is likely to be that of a membrano-proliferative or epimembranous lesion. Circulating complexes containing B antigen are also known to cause *polyarteritis*. Yet another entity is *hepatic glomerulosclerosis* which is characterized by mesangial deposits in patients with acute hepatic necrosis or acute pancreatitis.

Other viruses which cause nephritis

In view of the immune complex formation that must occur at the time of viraemia or with the development of antibodies to those viruses which lodge in or on vascular endothelium, it is not surprising that many viruses may cause nephritis. This is usually of a transient benign type. Known agents include influenza, mumps, infectious mononucleosis. (EB virus) and also Echo, Coxsackie, pox and varicella viruses. Both varicella and infectious mononucleosis have been known to cause a nephrotic syndrome.

Syphilis

Congenital syphilis is rare and it is even rarer for it to cause nephrotic syndrome. Nevertheless this is a treatable lesion and should therefore not be forgotten. The serology will be positive; treatment is with penicillin.

A positive WR and a nephrotic syndrome suggest acquired syphilitic nephrosis, which will remit with penicillin therapy. The typical features are subepithelial humps, a perivascular mononuclear cell infiltration as in other organs, and foci of tubular damage due to direct damage by spirochaetes.

Malaria

The high incidence of nephrotic syndrome in some tropical countries has been shown to be due to quartan malaria. *Plasmodium malariae* is present on blood films; the peak incidence is in children aged 5–6 years and it is at this age that parasitaemia is common. Patients with the syndrome have very high IgM antimalarial antibody titres. Since the eradication of *P. malariae* in Guyana, the nephrotic syndrome has become rare. The lesion may be a mesangiocapillary, proliferative or (in adults) membranous nephropathy.

P. falciparum is traditionally the cause of 'blackwater fever', in which the patient has haemoglobinuria due to the plasmodium-induced haemolysis. On account of the hypercatabolism, dehydration and some degree of intravascular coagulation, an acute renal failure ensues. Both drug therapy and G6PD deficiency can be regarded as predisposing factors. The essential treatment is to clear the parasitaemia by means of intravenous quinine and to institute haemodialysis, which in this situation is more effective than peritoneal dialysis.

Additionally *P. falciparum* is the cause of a mild nephrotic syndrome. This is a typical immune complex disease with mesangial deposits in which the antigen can be identified. With drug therapy the erythrocytic form of *P. falciparum* is rapidly cleared from the circulation, whilst the extra-erythrocytic form of *P. malariae* persists longer so as to give a more prolonged antigenaemia. This is the probable explanation of the more severe nephrosis in the latter.

Leptospirosis

Weil's disease (or leptospirosis) presents typically with fever, myalgia and headache and is accompanied by a purpuric rash and impaired renal function at the time of the leptospiraemia. Severe renal failure is more common in those patients who have coincident jaundice, but the basic lesion is that of an interstitial nephritis as a result of damage to the tubular epithelium. Leptospira are demonstrable in the urine as well as in the renal tissue. The glomeruli show only a mild mesangial hyperplasia.

Interstitial nephritis

The pathology is either a diffuse or focal cellular infiltration of the renal interstitium with plasma cells and lymphocytes, and the tubules are separated by oedema. There is ischaemia of the cortex but congestion of the papillae on account of compression of the venules; in fact this is a comparable situation to that seen in renal transplant rejection. The collecting tubules showed the most marked ischaemic changes.

There are a variety of causes:

(1) infections with streptococci, leptospira, brucella;
(2) chronic paraproteinaemia;
(3) antibiotic allergy – penicillin, methicillin, ampicillin;
(4) allergy to thiazide diuretics and frusemide.

The latter possibility should be considered whenever renal failure is progressing more rapidly than would be anticipated. Categories (3) and (4) should each clear after removal of the offending agent. Those cases due to infection will likewise resolve when appropriate therapy is given, although there may be residual renal damage. A more refractory situation is when 'myeloma casts' are forming in the renal tubules due to deposition of paraproteins. The only hope here is to give primary cytostatic therapy and at the same time to promote a diuresis of an alkaline urine to try and wash out the tubular casts.

Chronic forms of interstitial nephritis occur with such conditions as gout, analgesic abuse, and when other irritants are deposited in the kidney as in oxalosis. Long-term transplant rejection, irradiation, poisoning by lead or cadmium, and pyelonephritis and hypertension all give rise to chronic changes in the interstitium.

Balkan nephropathy

The endemic nephropathy of Croatia, Serbia, Bosnia and Bulgaria is regarded as a primary chronic interstitial nephritis. It can affect families but perhaps only due to environmental factors in a peasant community living in poor conditions. The nephropathy may be discovered early on account of chance proteinuria, but unfortunately often not until there are small kidneys and symptoms of chronic renal failure.

Heavy metals such as lead have been blamed as a causative factor. Leptospirosis and brucellosis are endemic.

RENAL AMYLOIDOSIS

Renal amyloidosis usually causes a *membranous* thickening of the glomerular basement membranes and heavy proteinuria leading to the development of the *nephrotic syndrome*. This can be further complicated by superimposed thrombosis of the renal veins. On occasion involvement of the peritubular basement membranes by amyloid material can lead to a *nephrogenic diabetes insipidus.*

In actual fact the basement membrane is intact in renal amyloid. The apparent thickening is due to amyloid fibrils, which, although concentrated mainly in the mesangial areas (from which there may be local synthesis), lie above the basement membrane. Mixed with the fibrils is a deposit of plasma proteins, and the result is that the differentiation from idiopathic membranous nephropathy or from the diabetic KW kidney may have to depend on the special strains. Amyloid does occur in 3% of all renal biopsies and should always be looked for.

Amyloid was first described by Rokitanski in 1842 as an interstitial deposit found in the heart, tongue, liver, spleen, kidneys, adrenals and gut mucosa. On account of its starchy appearance and the fact that it stains with iodine it was named 'amylid' by Virchow. It demonstrates metochromatic staining with crystal violet or toluidine blue, and a green birefringence in the polarizing microscope after staining with Congo red. However, in 1959 Cohen recognized the fibrillary ultrastructure and this has led to intensive studies of the nature of amyloid. In fact it appears to be variable in composition but is a mixture of:

(1)   immunoglobulin related material, which is essentially Bence–Jones material (*light chains*);

(2)   a plasma component P, which forms periodic rods, and which is identical to an *alphaglobulin* present in normal human plasma;

(3)   amyloid *fibres,* called F-components.

Its immunoglobulin nature explains its association with multiple myeloma and with chronic infectious states such as tuberculosis, osteomyelitis, rheumatoid arthritis and ulcerative colitis. Therefore, in considering the pathogenesis one has to take into account:

(1)   That there is a plasma cell proliferation leading to excess light-chain formation.

(2)   That light chains are fixed in tissue together with a P-protein of plasma, whose precursor can be detected in serum. This serum component can be detected in increased quantities in the aged and in persons with carcinoma, lymphoma, myeloma, rheumatoid arthritis or TB. This P-component undergoes calcium-dependent binding to agarose, agar, sulphated polyacrylamide beads and other polyanions, so there can be selective uptake of calcium-seeking 99m-technetium diphosphonate into amyloid deposits.

(3)   That antigen–antibody complexes may, in fact, be processed by macrophages and be extruded as fibrils.

There is no specific treatment. Ascorbutic guinea pigs are more prone to amyloid and therefore vitamin C has been advocated. It is very important to control hypertension and improve life expectancy. The situation is also helped by the vigorous treatment of any associated chronic inflammatory disease. Since it has been noted recently that amyloid fibrillar substance appears in the urine when patients are given an intravenous dose of DMSO (dimethylsulphoxide), this may not only turn out to be a diagnostic test but also to have therapeutic potential.

THE KIDNEYS IN RHEUMATOID ARTHRITIS

Rheumatoid arthritis is a chronic synovitis and tissue immune complex disease. However since it is associated with the production of rheumatoid-factors to the body's autologous but altered gammaglobulin, a circulating immune complex process accounts for secondary features such as the vasculitis and glomerulitis.

(1)   *Glomerulitis* occurs in some 60% of patients. There is an increase of endothelial and mesangial cells. It can be a typical mesangiocapillary glomerulonephritis.

(2)   Thus *proteinuria* and cast formation is a feature of many patients.

(3)   The proteinuria may be much worse when there is some *toxic nephropathy* as can be induced by gold or penicillamine.

(4)   Since patients take large doses of analgesics, superimposed *analgesic nephropathy* might be found but it is extremely uncommon in this type of patient, possibly because the microsomal enzymes have been induced so as to detoxify analgesics.

(5)   *Amyloidosis* is found to account for proteinuria in some 20% cases. It has always been suspected that cortisone therapy will make amyloid worse.

SCLERODERMA / SYSTEMIC SCLEROSIS

This is a vascular disease which affects the interlobar, arcuate and interlobular arteries, which show narrowing due to hyperplasia of the intimal cells which lie in a mucoid or finely collagenous ground substance (Figure 69). The result is that there are areas of ischaemia and focal necrosis of the renal cortex. In other areas glomeruli show increased lobularity and mesangial hyperplasia. Fluorescent studies will show non-specific fibrin–fibrinogen deposition and sometimes vascular localization of IgM, other immunoglobulins and complement.

There is some question as to whether there is a neurogenic basis since typically scleroderma starts with Raynaud's phenomenon, and the skin

179

degeneration and thickening of the subepidermal collagen follow. It is said that there are reductions of renal cortical blood flow during cutaneous Raynaud's phenomenon, so that it is conceivable that small vessel vasoconstriction might be compounded by increased renin release and angiotensin II generation.

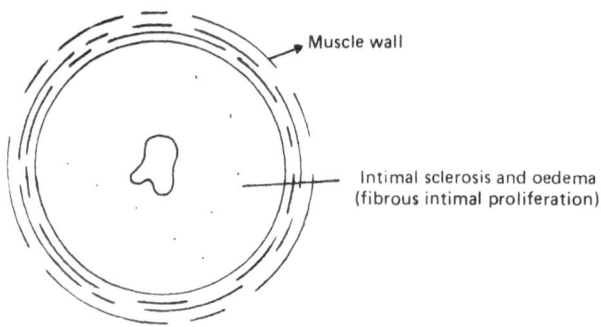

Figure 69. Arteriole in scleroderma

The resulting renal effects are:

(1)   a decrease of GFR;
(2)   renin release causing hypertension;
(3)   tubular injury causing proteinuria.

Antiglobulins and antinuclear antibodies together with hyperglobulin-aemia and an elevated ESR occur in patients, so that there seems to be an autoimmune background. There could also be complexes of nuclear antigens and antibodies in the vessel walls. The predominance of IgM must reflect the production of rheumatoid factors. The occurrence of antinuclear antibodies is especially typical of scleroderma and, in particular, there are antiRNA antibodies whose specificity can be shown to be directed against uracil moieties.

In time most cases develop hypertension and progress to oliguria in days or months. Others are found at autopsy to have renal disease. The nephrotic syndrome is exceptional. On account of the vascular narrowing microangio-pathic haemolytic anaemia can also occur.

Clinical features of systemic sclerosis

(1)   Raynaud's syndrome, polyarthritis, smooth shiny fixed skin with pigmentation and telangiectasia.
(2)   Reduced oesophageal and gut motility; causing dysphagia.

(3) Scleroderma cardiomegaly with heart failure.
(4) Renal failure and malignant hypertension.

It is refractory to all therapy. A trial of cyclofenil 300–600 mg/day is justified: this has an oestrogen-like effect. In the past cases have been subjected to nephrectomy followed by dialysis and/or transplantation on account of their high plasma renin levels and declining renal function. It is now thought that vigorous hypotensive measures, using minoxidil or the new oral converting-enzyme inhibitor captopril, to inhibit generation of angiotensin II will save many of these kidneys. Indeed prolonged peripheral vasodilatation may ameliorate the fibrosis of many organs.

SICKLE CELL DISEASE

In homozygous sickle cell anaemia (SS) there are a variety of renal functional and pathological changes which may be summarized as follows:

(1) Medullary/papillary damage resulting in
    (a) urine concentrating defect;
    (b) haematuria/papillary necrosis;
    (c) renal tubular acidosis.
(2) Cortical morphological appearances:
    (a) glomerular enlargement and peritubular capillary congestion;
or (b) nephrotic syndrome ? due to protein-iron complexes;
or (c) CRF—chronic glomerular sclerosis and interstitial scarring.

Sickle cell erythrocytes traversing the hyperosmotic medulla, where there are low rates of blood flow and a partial pressure of oxygen only 20% of that of the cortex, will naturally undergo sickling so causing increased viscosity and possible microthrombosis with obliteration of vessels. Functional studies suggest that the main damage is borne by the juxtamedullary nephrons which have long thin loops of Henle that descend into the renal papillae. These loops are only involved in concentration of urine at low rates of flow. The cortical nephrons (86% in all) with short loops of Henle restricted to the outer medullary zone are not involved, so there is relative preservation of the glomerular filtration rate, but the renal concentrating power does not rise above 400–450 mosmol.

Actual necrosis of papillae accounts for recurrent episodes of painless haematuria.

REFERENCES

Haematuria and proteinuria

Blainey, J.D. (1975). Trace nephropathy. *Advanced Medicine II,* Royal Coll. Phys., **II,** 317

Boyd, P.J.R. (1977). Haematuria. *Br. Med. J.,* **2,** 445

Cameron, J.S., White, R. (1965). Selectivity of proteinuria in nephrotic children. *Lancet,* **i,** 463

Davis, J.S., Flynn, F.V. and Platt, H.S. (1968). Gel filtration of urinary protein. *Clin. Chim. Acta.,* **21,** 357

Farquahar, M.G. (1961). Glomerular permeability: transfer of ferritin. *J. Exp. Med.,* **114,** 699

Ferris, T.F. (1967). Haematuria and focal nephritis. *N. Engl. J. Med.,* **276,** 770

Index of differential diagnosis of main symptoms. Ed. H. French, A.H. Douthwaite.

Gitlin, D. (1956). Metabolism of proteins in the nephrotic syndrome. *J. Clin. Invest.,* **35,** 44

Grant, G. (1968). Serological analysis in diagnosis. *Clin. Chim. Acta.,* **22,** 31

Hardwicke, J. (1972). Glomerular filtration of macromolecules. *Adv. Nephrol.,* **2,** 61/Clinical Nephrology (1975) **3,** 37

Laurent, T.C. (1964). Theory of gel filtration. *J. Chromatogr.,* **14,** 317

Maclean, P.R. and Petrie, J.J.B. (1966). Comparison of gel filtration and immunodiffusion in the determination of selectivity of proteinurua. *Clin. Chim. Acta.,* **14,** 367

Proteins in Normal and Pathological Urine. Ed. Y. Manuel, J.P. Revillard, H. Betuel. (Basel: S. Karger) 1970.

Petrie, M. (1966). Selectivity tests of proteinuria. *Clin. Chim. Acta.,* **14,** 367

Pesce, A.J. (1974). Methods for analysis of proteins in urine. *Nephron,* **13,** 93

Venkatchalam, M.A. (1970). Catalase for study of glomerular permeability. *J. Exp. Med.,* **132,** 1168

Protein chemistry

Laboratory notes for Medical Diagnostics. Behringwerke. No. 3. (1969)

Plasma Proteins in General Practice. *Ann. Gen. Pract.* (1971). Australian College

Diabetes and the kidney

Anderson, J. The kidney in diabetes. Ed. Oakley, Pyke, Taylor. *Clinical Diabetes.* (Oxford: Blackwell) 1968

Ashton, N. (1957). Relation of diabetic retinopathy to glomerulosclerosis. *Br. Med. J.*, **1**, 1002

Bell, E.T. (1953). Renal vascular disease in diabetes. *Diabetes*, **2**, 376

Dachs, S. and Churg, J. *et al.* (1964). Diabetic nephropathy. *Am. J. Pathol.*, **44**, 155

Farquhar, M.G. (1959). Glomerulosclerosis. *Am. J. Pathol.*, **35**, 721

Gellman, D.D. *et al.* (1959). Diabetic Nephropathy. *Medicine*, **38**, 321

Kefalides, N.A. (1974). Biochemistry of diabetic glomerular basement membrane. *J. Clin. Invest.*, **53**, 403

Kimmelstiel, P. and Osawa, G. (1966). Glomerular basement membrance thickness in diabetes. *American J. Clin. Pathol.*, **45**, 7

Lee, C.T. (1963). Renal disease in diabetes. *Med. Clin. N. Am.*, **47**, 1069

Miller, E.J. (1976). Types of Collagen. *Molec. Cell. Biochem.*, **13**, 165

Williamson, J.R., Volgler, N.J. and Kilo, C. (1969). Basement memorane thickness. *Diabetes*, **18**, 567

Urinary tract infection in diabetes

Barnard, D.M. (1953). *N. Engl. J. Med.*, **248**, 136

Huvos, A., Rocha, H. (1959). *N. Engl. J. Med.*, **261**, 1213

O'Sullivan, D.J., Fitzgerald, M.G. *et al.* (1961). *Br. Med. J.*, **1**, 786

Malaria

Dukes, D.C. (1968). Oliguria in blackwater fever. *Am. J. Med.*, **45**, 899

Gilles, H.M. (1963). Nephrosis in Nigerian children. *Br. Med. J.*, **2**, 27

Kibukamusoke, J.W. and Hutt, M.S.R. (1967). Nephrosis in Nigerian children. *J. Clin. Pathol.*, **20**, 117

White, R.H.R. (1973). Nephrosis in Nigerian children. *Nephron*, **11**, 147

Sickle cell disease

Levitt, M.F. (1960). Renal concentrating defect. *Am. J. of Med.*, **29**, 611

Schlitt, L.E. (1960). Renal manifestations. *Paediatrics*, **239**, 773

Statius Van Eps, L. (1970). Renal concentrating defect. *Lancet*, **i**, 450

Amyloid

Cohen, A.S. (1967). Renal amyloid. *N. Engl. J. Med.*, **277**, 522

Cohen, A.S., Cathcart, E.S. and Skinner, M. (1978). Pathogenesis of amyloid. *Arth. Rheum.*, **21**, 153

Glenner, C. (1972). The immunoglobulin origin of amyloid. *Am. J. Med.*, **52**, 141

Husby, G., Natvig, J.B. (1974). A serum component related to amyloid protein. *J. Clin. Invest.*, **53**, 1054

Isobe, T. (1971). Conditions associated with plasma cell dyscrasia. *Ann. N. Y. Acad. Med.*, **190**, 507

Kyle, R.A. (1975). Renal amyloid. *Medicine (Baltimore)*. **54**, 271

Ravid, M. (1977). The DMSO test. *Lancet*, **i**, 730

Shiraham, T., Cohen, A.S. (1967). Fine structure of the glomerulus in amyloid. *Am. J. Pathol.*, **51**, 869

Triger, D.S. (1973). Renal amyloid. *Q. J. Med.*, **42**, 15

Myeloma

de Fronzo, R.A. (1975). Renal failure in myeloma. *Medicine*, **54**, 209

de Fronzo, R.A., Cooke, C.R. Wright, J.R. and Humphrey, R.L. (1978). Renal failure in myeloma. *Medicine*, **57**, 151-166

Rheumatoid arthritis

Allender, E. (1963). Renal function in rheumatoid arthritis. *Acta Rheum. Scand.*, **9**, 116

Bacon, A.J. (1976). Penicillamine nephropathy. *Q. J. Med.*, **45**, 661

Dieppe, P.A. (1976). Renal function in rheumatoid arthritis. *Br. Med. J.*, **i**, 611

Missen, G.A.K. (1956). Amyloidosis in rheumatoid arthritis. *J. Pathol. & Bacteriol.*, **71**, 179

Reece, J.M. (1954). Amyloidosis in rheumatoid arthritis. *Am. J. Med. Sci.*, **228**, 554

Sarcoid nephropathy

Ford, M.J., Anderton, J.L. and Maclean, N. (1978). *Postgrad. Med. J.*, **54**, 416

Scleroderma

Cannon, P.J. *et al.* (1974). Progressive systemic sclerosis ... cause of hypertension and renal failure. *Medicine (Baltimore)*, **53**, 1

D'Agnelo, W.A., Fries, J.F., Masi, A.T. and Shulman, L.E. (1969). Pathology of systemic sclerosis. *Am. J. Med.*, **46**, 428

Fennel, R.H., Reddy, C.R. and Vasquez, J.J. (1961). Systemic sclerosis and malignant hypertension. *Arch. Pathol.*, **72**, 209

Norton, W.L. and Nardo, J.M. (1970). Vascular disease in scleroderma. *Ann. Intern. Med.*, **73**, 317

Oliver, J.A. and Cannon, P.J. The kidney in scleroderma. *Nephron*, **18**, 141

Alports syndrome

Churg, J. (1973). Hereditary nephritis. *Arch. Pathol.*, **95**, 374

Grünfeld, J.P. (1973). Hereditary chronic nephritis. *Kidney Int.*, **4**, 216

Kopelman, H., Asatoor, A.M. and Milne, M.D. (1964). Hyperprolinaemia and hereditary nephritis. *Lancet*, **ii**, 1075

Spear, G.S. (1970). Hereditary nephropathy with deafness. *Am. J. of Med.*, **49**, 52

Spear, G.S. and Slusser, R.J. (1972). *Am. J. of Pathol.*, **69**, 213

Nail patella syndrome

Hawkins, C.F. and Smith, O.E. (1950). *Lancet*, **i**, 803

Hoyer, J.R., Michael, A.F. and Vernier, R.L. (1972). *Kidney Int.*, **2**, 231

Glomerular changes in neoplasia

Couser, W.G. (1974). *Am. J. Med.*, **57**, 962

Kaplan, B.S. *et al.* (1976). *Ann. Rev. Med.*, **27**, 117

Ozawa, T. *et al.* (1975). Nephropathy and malignancy. *Q. J. Med.*, **44**, 523

Radiation nephritis

Levitt, W.M. (1957). Radiation nephritis. *Br. J. Urol.*, **29**, 381

Luxton, R.W. (1953). Radiation nephritis. *Q. J. Med.*, **22**, 215

Luxton, R.W. (1961). Radiation nephritis. *Lancet*, **2**, 1221

7
Urinary tract infection (UTI)

Symptomatic abacteruria

This is otherwise known as the 'acute urethral syndrome'. The implication is that there has been mild trauma, and the patient complains of dysuria. Recurrences are common but no organisms are grown. It is very important to exclude gonococcal infection, prostatitis or tuberculosis, and gynaecological disorders.

Non-specific urethritis (NSU)

Again there is dysuria but also a mucopurulent urethral discharge. It is called non-specific because for many years the agent was unknown, but it now seems likely that *Chlamydia trachomatis* (TRIC agent) causes most of the cases, and *Trichomonas vaginalis* or *Candida albicans* should also be considered. NSU usually responds to tetracycline therapy.

Bacteruria

This occurs when there are more than 100000 organisms/ml in the urine. When there is only contamination of the midstream or catheter specimen counts are usually below 10000 organisms/ml. Samples should either be cultured within 30 min or stored at 4 °C. For the benefit of patients at home, an agar slide (the dip-slide) is now available; it has only to be immersed in the urine, drained and then replaced in its plastic container for posting to the laboratory. Organisms grow in a small culture on the agar slide.

Bacterial quantitation can be performed by using urine diluted 1/100 in saline and pouring a given volume onto a nutrient agar plate so as to count the colonies which appear after incubation. Alternatively a platinum loop of 2 mm internal diameter holding 0.00176 ml urine can be used for all plate inoculations. It is known that when there are 100000 bacteria/ml the plate count is 175, but with only 10000 organisms/ml the colonies number only 20. Counts of 105/ml always indicate renal infection. Note that 20% of symptomatic patients do not have high bacterial counts.

Pus cell quantitation is also valuable since in renal infections there are more than 20000 pus cells/ml, whereas in bladder infection the count is less than that. When urine is strongly alkaline, however, the absence of pus cells does not rule out infection as the cells can die rapidly. *Pyuria* is simply defined as more than 10 leucocytes per mm^3 in an unspun sample of urine. Cells can be stained purple with Sternheimer–Malbin stain. White cell casts should be noted as these definitely indicate pyelonephritis (see below).

There are also simple chemical screening tests for bacteriuria. With the exception of *Streptococcus faecalis,* organisms that cause urinary tract infection reduce nitrates to nitrites. These can be detected by the Greiss reagent which consists of sulphanilic acid, acetic acid and napthylamine. A red colour develops due to the formation of aminonapthaline *p*-benzenesulphonic acid. Additionally actively respiring bacteria can reduce colourless 2,3,4–triphenyltetrazolium chloride to a red insoluble triphenyl formazan at alkaline pH.

The organisms involved in urinary tract infection are mainly motile bacteria that are the normal constituents of faecal flora and thus may soil the perineum. 85% of all infections are due to *Escherichia coli* and another 15% due to *Proteus, Pseudomonas* or *Klebsiella,* and sometimes the Gram-positive enterococci (*Streptococcus faecalis*). Infections with staphylococci, candida or tubercle bacilli are actually rare but should be kept in mind.

As defined above, more than 100000 bacteria/ml indicate clinical infection but a much lower count than this will do for the symptomatic patient.

Cystitis and pyelonephritis

Infection of the bladder (*cystitis*) is characterized by frequency and urgency of micturition together with pain on passing water (dysuria). Upper urinary tract infection, *pyelonephritis,* is more likely if the patient has fever and rigors, back pain and loin tenderness. But these symptoms are not as reliable as might be thought. When there is bladder infection the general policy is to treat with a short course of an effective antibiotic. At least one-third of cases recur and 80% of these are due to a new *E. coli* serotype! When there is pyelonephritis, as shown on the IVU by scarring and loss of renal substance, it is obligatory to exclude predisposing causes such as obstruction in the urinary tract or stones. Long-term antibiotic therapy is then required to eradicate organisms from the renal medulla; even so recurrence is common.

FACTORS PREDISPOSING TO INFECTION AND THEIR MECHANISMS

The age prevalence of urinary tract infection gives some clues as to the possible causes (Figure 70).

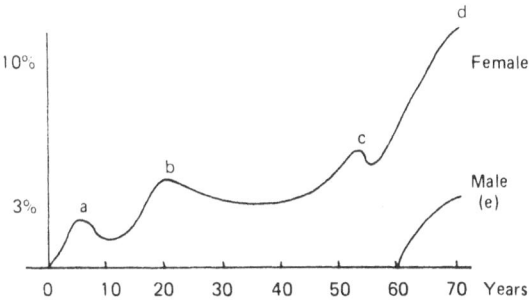

Figure 70. Urinary tract infections and age

Female infants under 2 years are at risk owing to soiling of the perineum (*a*), then there is a further peak as females achieve sexual activity (*b*), corresponding to the stage of 'honeymoon cystitis'. Contamination of the perineum with organisms from the bowel predisposes to trouble. The female is always at risk during pregnancy (*b*). In fact some 4% of pregnant women have bacteruria and yet only one-third of them have symptomatic pyelonephritis. In such women there is an increased incidence of fetal prematurity and loss, as well as pre-eclamptic toxaemia. Female infections increase after the menopause, especially as gynaecological problems such as prolapse and vaginitis become more common (*c–d*).

In the male, apart from some infections in early life associated with congenital obstructions in the renal tract or very early haematogenous infection in susceptible male infants, most infections tend to appear in later life with the advent of prostatic obstruction (*e*).

Urinary tract infection can occur in the following ways:

189

(1) through ascending infection by the natural passages; this is the most common means;

(2) more rarely, by bloodborne infection of the kidney, as in the case of staphylococcal abscesses;

(3) from reservoirs of infection within the urinary tract as in the case of prostatic infection in men or infection of the para-urethral glands in women.

Ascending infection

This is shown simply in Figure 71 and is self-explanatory.

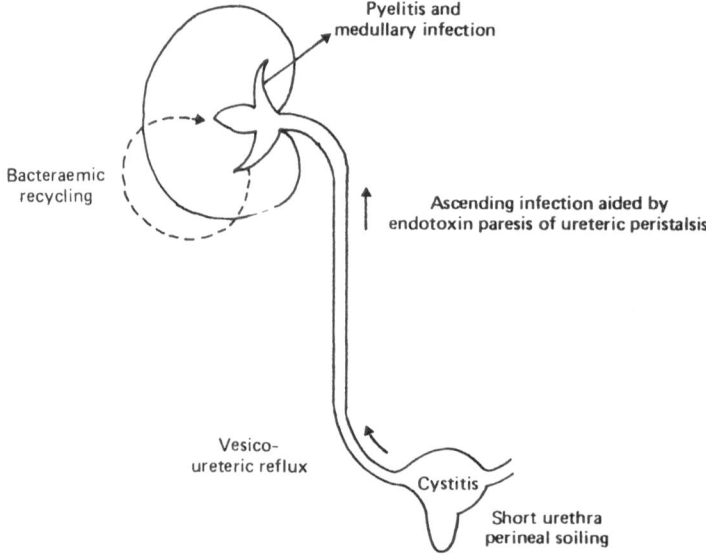

Figure 71. Ascending urinary infection

It is now appreciated that catheterization carries a 3% risk of causing urinary tract infection. The organism is often a pseudomonad. Particular care should be taken in patients with diabetes; indeed catheterization should normally be discouraged in them.

Soiling of the perineum in young infants and the direct introduction of infection during sexual activity is part of the female risk. There is normally bladder mucosal bactericidal activity and, of course, the downward flow of urine together with the voiding process form a protective mechanism. Those patients who are unable to empty the bladder fully due to paraplegia, neuropathy, bladder neck muscle dysfunction or simply normal nervousness have a great liability to infection in their residual urine. Some also have a vesicourethral reflux whereby urine that has entered the posterior urethra can then return into the bladder as a result of muscle dysfunction.

There are a variety of congenital lesions, particularly of the male, that obstruct the flow of urine and so give rise to stasis and thus a liability to infection. They are shown in Figure 72 according to their anatomical position.

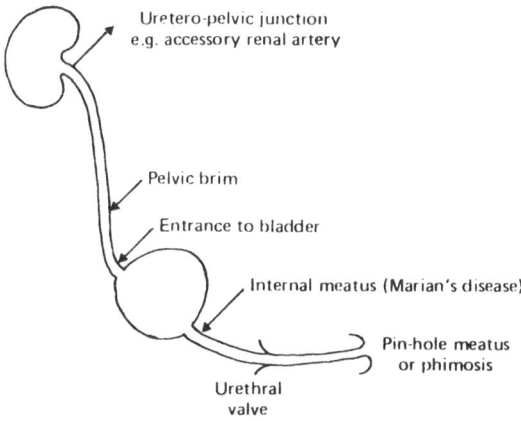

Figure 72. Congenital lesions causeing urinary tract stasis

Vesico-ureteric reflux

More important still are those conditions that give rise to vesicoureteric reflux, since this process causes kidney scarring and impairs renal growth. The causes are shown in Table 17.

Table 17 Causes of vesicoureteric reflux

Congenital	Acquired
Ureteric saccule	As a result of bacterial infection
Mega-ureter	Tuberculosis
Lower urinary tract obstruction or neuropathic bladder	Trauma by a calculus

The normal anatomy of the ureterovesical junction has to be kept in mind when considering the mechanism of reflux and possible corrective procedures (Figure 73).

191

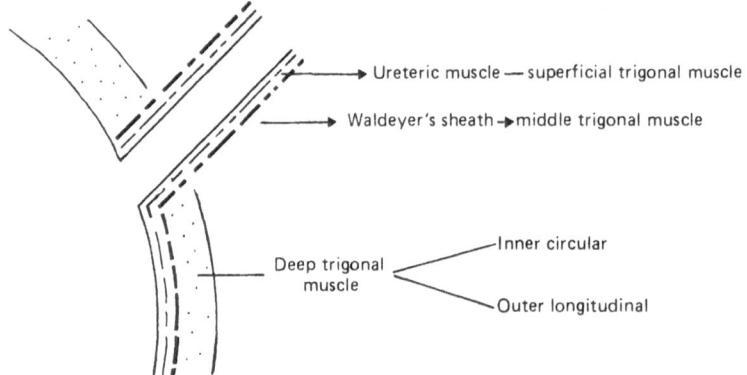

Figure 73.   Uretero-vesical junction

When the bladder muscle contracts in the process of voiding, the contraction closes the ureteric orifice. The tone of the muscle, the oblique arrangement of the ureterovesical valve, and the fact that the ureteric muscle is continuous with the superficial trigonal muscle all ensure adequate closing. Reflux is twice as common on the left side as the right, and is more commonly the result of infection causing the formation of fibrous granulation tissue that distorts the anatomy. The treatment therefore is to keep the urine sterile for six months in the hope that it will resolve. A revision operation on the ureterovesical junction is possible, but is often followed by a recurrence on the opposite side.

Once infection has reached the kidneys, there are various reasons why it becomes established. Papillary scars distort the tubules and give rise to stasis. They are seen as part of ageing but are, in fact, a reflection of pyelonephritic scarring. They may also occur on account of analgesic consumption, as part of diabetes, or sickle cell disease. Stones in the renal pelvis inevitably mean stasis and recurrent infection. The renal substance itself has its weakness: (a) the hypertonicity of the medulla means that leucocytes cannot phagocytose, and (b) the fourth component of complement is inactivated by ammonia. Furthermore if *Proteus* or *Klebsiella* organisms produce urease, the alkalinity caused by ammonia formation can initiate magnesium ammonium phosphate stones. In fact, in order to achieve the eradication of many organisms it is necessary to acidify the urine by oral administration of ammonium chloride or NaH_2PO_4.

Both diabetes and pregnancy constitute high-risk situations. In diabetes the leucocytes show dysfunction attributable to insulin deficiency or ketosis, the kidney itself suffers from arteriosclerotic degeneration, and later a neuropathy may embarrass bladder function. Catheterization should be avoided. In pregnancy there may be ascending infection because the ureters dilate, and the distended uterus puts pressure on them at the pelvic brim. At the time of delivery there is often bruising of the bladder neck and thereafter postpuerperal retention of urine.

Bacterial invasion of the kidney

In the more usual ascending infections a variety of predisposing causes have been enumerated. It should be pointed out that those Gram-negative organisms producing endotoxin give rise directly to a paresis of ureteric peristalsis. Once *Escherichia coli* organisms have entered the renal pelvis they can pass into the local veins, so causing bacteraemia, and recirculation of organisms back to the kidneys.

It is now realized that *E. coli* from the urinary tract can pass in the vertebral venous system of Batson up to the cranial venous sinuses and so miss the reticuloendothelial defence system. In this way Gram-negative endocarditis or osteomyelitis may occur. This is a special risk in immunosuppressed patients.

In animal experiments it has been shown that scarring in the kidneys is normally necessary to enable a bloodborne infection to become established as pyelonephritis. So only after local damage to the kidneys by oxamide feeding will an intravenous dose of bacteria cause pyelonephritis. In the particular case of *Staphylococcus* a suppurative pyelonephritis is simply a form of bloodborne micro-abscess formation.

LOCALIZATION OF URINARY TRACT INFECTION

When all infections are considered some 40% cases are pure cystitis, 30% are due to unilateral ureteric infection and the remaining 30% bilateral ureteric infection.

The classical features of *acute pyelonephritis* are dysuria and urgency of micturition (as in cystitis) but additionally there is back or loin pain, fever and chills and possibly haematuria. In children the symptoms are less specific and may consist of rigors, diarrhoea and vomiting, and in infants there is a meningitic syndrome. *Chronic pyelonephritis* is an insidious illness whose symptomatology is indefinite; there is often fatigue, anorexia and weight loss and anaemia; nocturia also occurs on account of the defect in urinary concentration. Children fail to grow, infants fail to thrive and bedwetting may be a feature.

Girls who develop infection early usually have some symptoms by their third birthday, and they are usually those who because of poor hygiene or anatomical defect have had early cystitis. Girls with duplex ureters are at special risk. Very often investigation will reveal 'non-obstructive atrophic pyelonephritis' and this may go on to cause hypertension. In boys obvious congenital defect is to be anticipated in the form of some type of obstruction (as depicted above), hypospadias, or a faecal fistula.

Techniques for localization

Much recent work has been devoted to the means of localizing the site of primary infection, and the available techniques are summarized in Table 18 below.

Table 18   Available techniques for localizing the site of primary infections

Direct	*Indirect*
Fairley bladder washout technique	Urinary concentration test
Ureteric catheterization	Urinary lysozyme or endotoxin excretion
Renal biopsy	Antibody-coated bacteria in urine
Suprapubic aspiration of the bladder	Serum antibodies to O-antigens, or to Lipid-A or CEA

The Fairley bladder washout technique consists of the insertion of a Foley catheter to drain the bladder urine, after which 100 ml saline containing 2 mg neomycin and 125000 units of streptokinase–streptodornase are left in the bladder for 30 min. The bladder is then washed out with 2 l of water and collections are made every 10 min for 1 h and then cultured. An upper urinary tract infection must be present if 100 bacteria/ml are found in at least four samples. The other direct techniques, namely ureteric catheterization or renal biopsy are to be discouraged but suprapubic aspiration is very helpful.

The urinary concentration mechanism is impaired when there is medullary disease, when the osmolality of a urine sample after water deprivation will be less than 700 mosmol/kg. Additionally, as there is tubular damage, there will be a tubular proteinuria (page 163). Coincident damage to proximal tubules, which arises because areas of ischaemia due to occlusion of arterioles complicate the pyelonephritic process, means that there is urinary loss of lysozyme.

When bacteria are resident in the renal parenchyma they elicit a systemic antibody response, and longstanding urinary tract infection may lead to amyloid. However, the point to be applied in diagnosis is that the presence of serum antibodies to specific O-antigens of *E. coli* serotypes means that these organisms are actually causing the pyelonephritis. Antibody titres to lipid-A or to the common enterobacterial antigen (CEA) of Kunin are always expected to rise and may be more specific. Additionally immunofluorescence techniques can be used in diagnosis: it is possible to identify IgG or IgM antibody-coated bacteria in the urine.

THE PATHOLOGY OF PYELONEPHRITIS

The evolution of pyelonephritis is best studied in the experimental animal. Early on there is a polymorph infiltration around the renal tubules, which show signs of destruction. Lesions are wedge-shaped with their base in the cortex and the apex at the pelvis. The glomeruli are normal at this stage. Within the medulla lymphocytes and plasma cells accumulate and the tubules become obstructed by hyaline casts giving rise to the 'thyroid-like areas' or 'intrarenal hydronephrosis' of de Navasquez. These thyroid-like areas are seen at their best in the barrier zone. Later, on account of the loss of nephrons, glomeruli become hyalinized or they may be surrounded by periglomerular fibrosis. They may also show the associated changes of hypertension (Figure 74).

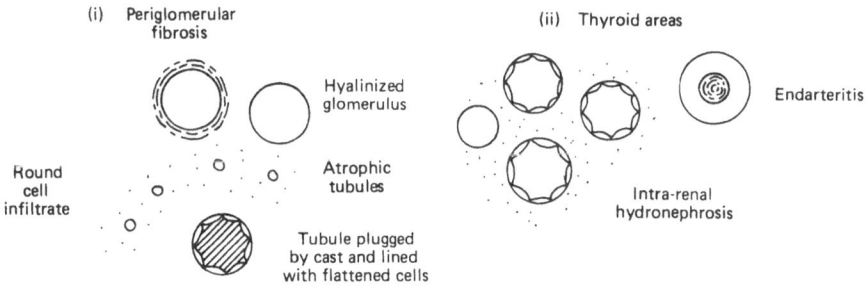

Figure 74. Histological features of chronic pyelonephritis

The original pyramidal lesions become converted into scars in which the contraction of fibrous tissue leads to a dilatation of the calyx and a shrinkage of the overlying cortex. This accounts for the characteristic radiological picture. Persistence of bacterial antigen in these areas can be shown by immunofluorescence. In the scar vessels become narrowed by endarteritis, and it is when interlobar and arcuate arteries become involved that areas of infarction occur. Such scars must be distinguished from those of atherosclerosis (benign nephrosclerosis) which are V-shaped. Yet actually scars appear in children of 4 years old when there is reflux (Figure 75).

195

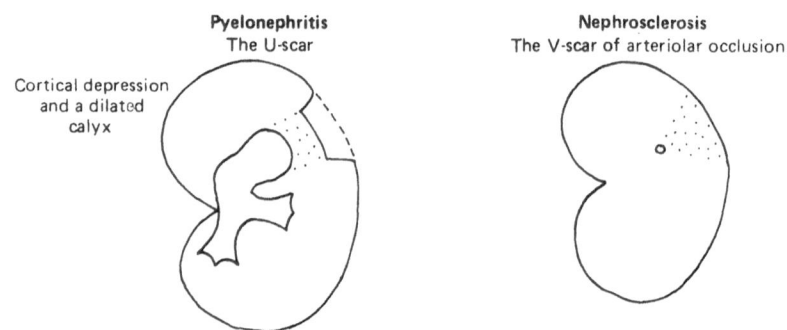

Figure 75. Scarring of pyelonephritis and benign nephrosclerosis

Pyelonephritis may often be unilateral, but even when bilateral it is seldom symmetrical. When in the advanced stage the kidneys are small and contracted, it may still be possible to distinguish the situation from chronic glomerulonephritis, for in fact an inflammatory infiltrate in the calyceal region is typical of pyelonephritis. In either condition there is likely to be an increase of the peripelvic fat as the kidneys shrink.

Table 19 summarises the factors that predispose to pyelonephritis.

Table 19   Factors predisposing to pyelonephritis

(a) Perineal soiling	Cystitis. Vesicoureteric reflux
(b) Urinary stasis	Obstructions
	Neurological and muscle disorders of the bladder
	Stones
	Polycystic disease
(c) Renal ischaemia	Glomerulosclerosis/diabetes mellitus
(d) Immune defects	—even induced by smoking or analgesic abuse

IMMUNOLOGICAL FACTORS AND PYELONEPHRITIS

Coliform organisms and virulence

The many *E. coli* serotypes have in all 150 O-antigenic groups. Some are found more commonly in urinary tract infections and this correlates with their presence in the gut. In fact a mixture of some eight O-antigens when absorbed onto the red cell surface can be used in indirect haemagglutination tests for the detection of antibodies (Andersen, 1967). The possession of greater than usual amounts of O-antigen renders organisms more resistant to the bactericidal effects of serum.

It is an interesting fact that symptomless infections occur with those *E. coli* that usually occur in the bowel (01, 02, 04, 06, 07, 018, 075) and that serum is normally bactericidal towards them. Conversely symptomatic infections occur with more unusual serotypes. The Kaufman, *K antigens,* are certainly related to virulence. They can be demonstrated by crossed immunoelectrophoresis. They make the organisms less sensitive to the action of complement and associated phagocytosis. These K antigens are in fact further subdivided into thermolabile L antigens and acidic polysaccharides A and B which are resistant to heat at 100°C. It is the acidic nature of the polysaccharide capsule that makes phagocytosis of such organisms difficult.

There is also a striking ability of virulent organisms to adhere to human uroepithelial cells, and this reflects the presence of pili. But in pili there can be acidic polysaccharides that carry a negative charge occurring among the hydrophilic O-antigens, so accounting for a repulsion by the negative charge of sialic acid on the epithelium of the urinary tract (Figure 76).

The body defences

The urinary tract is often colonized from the vaginal vestibule. Patients who are resistant have vaginal mucosal antibody to their own bacteria. Moreover it is known that in the urinary tract itself *secretory IgA and locally produced IgG* form part of the defence mechanism. It would be a particular advantage if the host were to produce IgM antibodies for they utilize complement in the lysis of bacteria. These antibodies are normally produced in the primary immune response and yet, of course, patients with recurrent urinary tract infection will inevitably be in their secondary immune response phase so that IgM levels will be less impressive. Worse still, it is theoretically possible for IgG antibody production to inhibit the formation of IgM antibodies or to block their action. Certainly there is less IgM than IgG during chronic urinary infection.

Patients with recurrent urinary tract infection often have *endotoxin tolerance,* so they do not suffer fever and rigors and their asymptomatic attacks may pass unrecognized. Endotoxin tolerance indicates pyrogenic resistance and increased endotoxin detoxification by the reticuloendothelial cells, whose main representative is the Kupffer cell system, rather than a particular titre of O-antibodies. Indeed there are so many O-antigens that antibodies to some common antigen might seem a more likely explanation.

197

Such an antigen exists as the common enterobacterial antigen (CEA) of Kunin. However this is often obscured by the more superficial O-antigens on the surface of the bacterium and blood antibody levels in patients to CEA tend to be low, unless there is chronic disease. There is some impression that antibody to CEA (measured by *E. coli* 014 antigen) does correlate with resistance to Gram-negative bacteraemia, yet it may also indicate persistence of bacterial antigen in the kidneys.

The common toxic moiety of all Gram-negative bacteria is the *lipid-A* which is actually attached deeply on the membrane of the bacterium so that there is doubt as to its immunogenicity (Figure 76). Although it does provoke antibodies, normal persons have low titres and this also may explain susceptibility to infection and endotoxinaemia. Lipid-A titres rise after urinary tract infection and they account for endotoxin tolerance! In *xanthogranulomatous pyelonephritis* there is nodular replacement of the parenchyma by lipid-filled macrophages, plasma cells and lymphocytes, which suggests an immune response due to local lipid-A. This type of reaction is seen (a) in association with stone, and (b) when there is a distorted calyceal system.

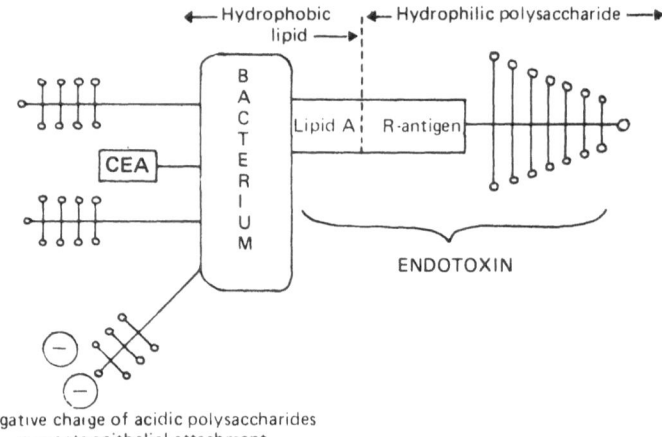

Figure 76. Diagram of a Gram-negative bacterium and its antigens

Features leading to chronic renal infection

There are several different factors to be considered:

(1) Persistence of *bacterial antigen*. Bacteria can transform into atypical variants called L-forms or spheroplasts which lack cell walls and which should therefore be susceptible to osmotic lysis, but they persist in the hyperosmolar environment of the renal medulla.

Additionally lipid-A material becomes deposited in the kidneys and will be the cause of a persisting cell-mediated immune response. Indeed it is recognized that endotoxin or its lipid-A can destroy tissue by activation of the alternate pathway of complement activation, and this is the reason why antigen surrounded by chronic inflammatory cells can be found at least 20 weeks after urine has been rendered sterile.

(2)   It is also likely that continued destruction of the kidneys by lymphocytic infiltration arises because there is a *cross-reaction* between *E. coli* antigens (of types 02, 022, and 014) with normal cellular components (see Holmgren *et al.*, 1975).

(3)   Escape of renal tubular antigen into the circulation or *E. coli* antigens might also give rise to a superimposed circulating *immune complex disease* leading to a glomerulonephritis. Certainly reflux of tubular Tamm–Horsfall mucoprotein into the circulation gives rise to autoantibody formation. However serum antiTamm–Horsfall antibody does not correlate well with vesicoureteric reflux or with kidney scarring.

(4)   It might be anticipated that cross-reacting antibodies to glomerular basement membrane could occur but in practice linear fluorescence patterns are not seen.

(5)   Finally, as a result of inflammation of the arterioles, there is a *superimposed ischaemia* which is very damaging to the renal substance.

THE RADIOLOGY OF PYELONEPHRITIS

The intravenous pyelogram

As can be deduced from the morbid anatomy the typical pyelonephritic scar gives rise to dilatation of a calyx associated with a U-shaped cortical depression. This can normally be distinguished from ischaemia in which there is a V-shaped cortical scar and the structure of the pyramids is normal. However, calyceal clubbing is not specific for pyelonephritis since it is seen in tuberculosis, whenever there is a small stone in the calyx, or in renal hypoplasia. Certain additional features can support one's impression of chronic pyelonephritis. The kidney is shrunken and in the case of unilateral disease the opposite kidney should show compensatory hypertrophy, so the size of the kidneys has to be judged in relation to the height and age. When there is medullary shrinkage autopsy examination will reveal an apparent increase of the peripelvic fatty tissue; this will appear on a film as coarse dark bands in the medulla and juxtamedullary cortex.

The normal renal size is 14 x 7 x 4 cm in the adult or three vertebral bodies in length. The kidney length in children is given by the Hodson formula $Y = 0.06X + 2.6$ where Y is the kidney length and X is the height of the child. In acute pyelonephritis the kidneys are swollen and can be some 2 cm larger than normal. Other conditions which may have to be distinguished from chronic pyelonephritis include polycystic disease in which the calyces are elongated and stretched out around cysts, and medullary cystic disease in which there is a characteristic blush caused by dilatation of the collecting tubules as they enter the minor calyces (Figure 77).

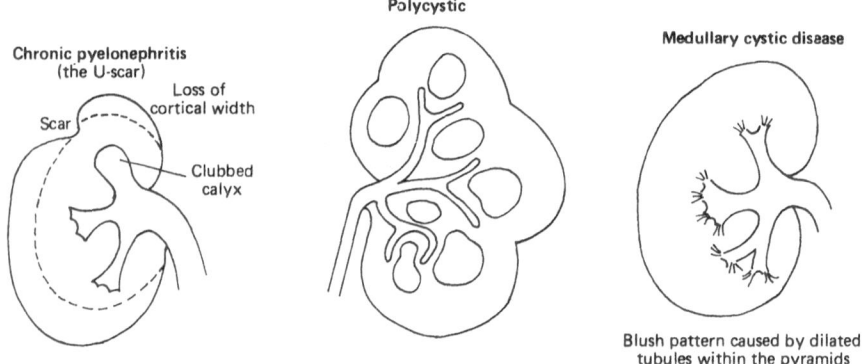

Figure 77.   Radiological features

When the pyelonephritic kidney is small, this indicates that the disease started in childhood. Then it is necessary to differentiate from congenital hypoplasia of the kidney, in which case a renal arteriogram will show a small hypoplastic artery supplying a small kidney. 'Segmental hypoplasia' is specifically a female disease and is often associated with hypertension and with other embryonic abnormalities; it might even be a form of pyelonephritis. It often occurs in the upper pole of a kidney. An arteriogram in this case will show a normal renal artery but the nephrogram phase shows a notching of the surface and a transverse avascular strip corresponding to the scar.

The micturating cystogram

This is required as a separate procedure in order to demonstrate vesicoureteric reflux. The bladder is overdistended with dye so that by fluoroscopy one can look for reflux at rest. Then films of the full bladder, lower ureters, bladder neck and urethra are obtained during micturition. Now that vesicoureteric reflux is well recognized, it is known that it is often accompanied by pain in the loin on micturition and by 'double micturition', whereby there is further urine to be passed as the refluxed urine returns to the bladder (Figure 78).

A collarlike impression protruding into the urethral lumen in association with dilatation of the distal urethra is typical of bladder neck hypertrophy. Furthermore when the bladder has been evacuated, trabeculation of the bladder wall and residual urine can be assessed.

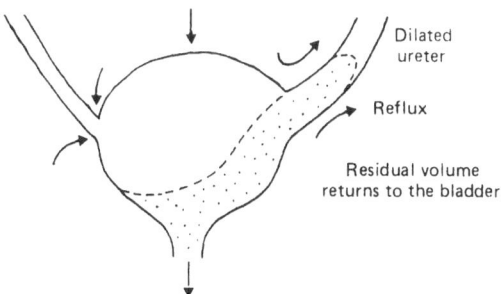

Dilated ureter

Reflux

Residual volume returns to the bladder

Figure 78. Vesico-ureteric reflux and double micturition

The renal scintigram

[197Hg]Chlormerodrin accumulates in the tubular cells of the inner two-thirds of the renal cortex, so 2 h after the intravenous injection of 100 μCi it is feasible to scan the kidney with a gamma counter so as to obtain a scintigram. This will not only indicate the renal size, but can also show up diffuse or localized image defects which may or may not be part of a lesion that is deforming the renal calyces; it is therefore a useful adjunct to investigations.

TREATMENT OF PYELONEPHRITIS

For acute urinary tract infections a 7-day course of antibiotic therapy will suffice, but if there is a relapse therapy should be continued for 2–3 weeks. Although bactericidal drugs are preferred for pyelitis, bacteriostatic agents are often just as effective in cystitis. A standard regime might be ampicillin 250 mg q.i.d., cotrimoxazole tabs, ii. b.d., tetracycline 250 mg q.i.d. or, for *Klebsiella*, cephalexin 250 mg q.i.d. All are given for 1 week. Due consideration must be given to the pH of the urine required for optimum drug action. Thus streptomycin has an activity 60 times greater at a urine pH of 8.0 than at pH 6.0, and the sulphonamides should be accompanied by urinary alkalinization to prevent precipitation in the urinary tract. When *Pseudomonas* is the infecting agent carbenicillin should be used at a dose of 1 g every 6 h, or gentamycin 80 mg t.i.d.; amikacin or ticarcillin can also be used. The mean cure rate for a single infection is about 80% whichever drug is chosen, but in patients who have recurrences only one-third remain free of infection for 6 months after a course of therapy, so a remission is not a cure. The treatment should include a high fluid intake of 3 l/day. Urine culture should always be obtained a week or less after therapy to ensure eradication and thereafter in those who relapse.

Cycloserine is a useful reserve drug for *E. coli* infections; negram is of value since it is actually concentrated in the renal substance. Conversely furadantin is ineffective and should probably be reserved for cystitis. It is also important to know that chloramphenicol is excreted as a glucuronide-conjugate which is an inactive form with no bacteriostatic activity. In the case of children tetracyclines are best avoided, since they stain the teeth. Table 20 shows the antibiotics used in treatment.

Table 20   Antibiotics for treatment of urinary tract infection

Orally (these are also used as prophylactics)	*Parenterally*
Ampicillin or amoxycillin	Sulphonamides
Cotrimoxazole or cephalexin	Ampicillin or high dosage penicillin V
Hippuric acid or mandelamine	Carbenicillin, cephalothin, colistin
Nalidixic acid or nitrofurantoin	Gentamycin, amikacin, ticarcillin

In general antibiotic selection should be determined by susceptibility as assessed by *in vitro* testing. The MIC (minimum inhibitory concentration) is the lowest concentration of antibiotic to prevent growth after overnight incubation. It may be measured either by a serial dilution technique in broth or by means of antibiotic-impregnated discs placed on an agar culture. In the latter situation it is important to realize that the size of the inhibition zone is not a direct measure of susceptibility, for it is influenced by the rate of diffusion of the antibiotic (see Ryan, 1976; and Sabath, 1976).

Antibiotic-susceptible bacteria may always be replaced by resistant mutants. If after 3–4 days of therapy there are still 100 000 organisms/ml it is likely that a resistant bacterium has proliferated and become dominant. Therapy should then be modified. Relapsing infection should prompt a search for stone or other form of obstruction. Asymptomatic bacteriuria persists in a variety of circumstances as in patients with indwelling catheters, ileal conduits or fistulae. Such patients tend to tolerate low-grade infection well, although there is an inevitable decline of renal function with time. Acidification of the urine together with the use of mandelamine 0.5 g q.i.d. is a good standby. Septrin can be used on a long-term basis but there is the risk of the development of sulphonamide hypersensitivity. In temperate climates it causes no deterioration of renal function.

Prophylactic therapy applies to particular circumstances. Some women develop post-coital bacteruria and they may take 50 mg nitrofurantoin or one cotrimoxazole nightly. On the other hand those who appear to have a traumatic form of urethral syndrome should not be so treated. Catheterization of diabetics or in pregnancy should always be covered by an antibiotic. When children have vesicoureteric reflux, they should have antibiotic therapy on a long-term basis, as also should patients with 'double micturition'. The control of such infection should favour the development of valve competence. Certainly the incidence of reflux should diminish with age, since growth of the base of the bladder favours continence.

BACTERURIA IN CHILDREN

This can be a problem even in neonates, particularly those who are delivered as a breech or by a Caesarian section from mothers who themselves are already infected during labour. There is pyrexia and failure to thrive, or more dramatic features such as jaundice (to be remembered as a result of UTI in infants) or convulsions. A persistent napkin rash should always raise the possibility of urinary tract infection.

There have been several studies of UTI or asymptomatic bacteruria in children. In the first attack two-thirds of children are symptomatic but with increasing age and with subsequent attacks infection is more likely to be asymptomatic. Apart from this the threadworm should be borne in mind as a cause of sterile urethritis in girls and a perianal cellophane test should be performed. Asymptomatic bacteruria in schoolgirls has a prevalence of 2.0% but only 0.2% in boys; it is not related to social class. Some 15% of children with bacteruria have renal scarring; this probably represents damage from vesicoureteric reflux during early childhood. Not surprisingly scarring is associated with anatomical defects such as saccules at the ureteric orifice, bifid and double ureters, or hydroureter. In fact bifid and double ureters are subject to hereditary and genetic factors, and ureterovesical incompetence itself can be inherited.

URINARY TRACT OBSTRUCTION

Obstructive nephropathy gives rise to stasis in the urinary tract and is a potential cause of superimposed infection.

Table 21 shows a simple classification into those causes which result in blockage of one renal pelvis or ureter and those which cause bilateral obstruction.

Table 21　Causes of unilateral and bilateral obstruction

Unilateral obstruction	*Bilateral obstruction*
Stone	Benign prostatic hypertrophy or prostatic cancer
Blood clot	Median bar hypertrophy (Marian's disease)
Carcinoma or papilloma	Urethral stricture
Tuberculosis	
Retroperitoneal fibrosis	
Aortic aneurysm	

BLADDER CANCER

Patients have symptoms of trigonal irritation and haematuria. A knowledge of the exogenous and endogenous carcinogens that predispose to this situation is of interest to physicians. They are summarized in Table 22.

Table 22

Endogenous causes	*Exogenous factors*
Recurrent inflammation	Industrial chemicals, rubber and plastics
Diverticulum or stone	Dye and cable industries
Schistosomiasis	Insecticides

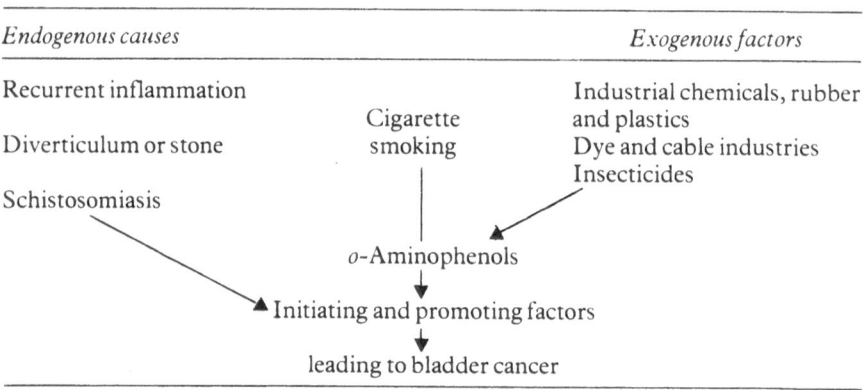

Carcinomata may either be papillary or pedunculated (such villous structures tend to occur around the ureteric orifices) or they are solid and sessile and infiltrate the mucosa. These spreading lesions can be regarded as (a) mucosal, (b) infiltrating the muscular layer, (c) perivesical and yet mobile, or (d) perivesical and fixed. The lesion is usually a squamous cell carcinoma or a transitional cell tumour, but occasionally there is an adenocarcinoma and this is highly malignant.

CONTROL OF MICTURITION

When tension receptors are activated in a distended bladder, the normal reflex through the parasympathetic nerve endings is to activate the detrusor muscle in the bladder wall. At this time the bladder outflow tract relaxes. The bladder controls are at the vesicospinal centre (S2, 3, 4 in Figure 79). However, this itself is regulated by sympathetic centres higher up the cord, and it is also the normal function of the brain to dampen down the enthusiasm of the bladder wall. In fact, the cerebral centres activate the sympathetic centres to cause inhibition of bladder wall contraction.

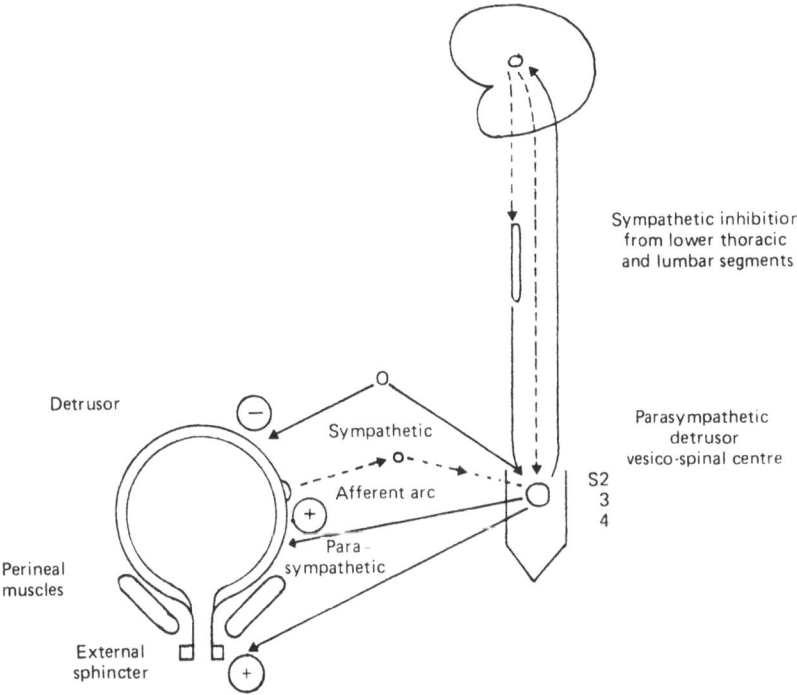

Figure 79. The normal micturition reflex

Voiding and continence

The act of micturition consists of contraction of the bladder detrusor muscle and at the same time relaxation of the bladder neck, urethral musculature and pelvic floor muscles. Continence is maintained because the urethral resistance (or pressure) is normally greater than the intravesical pressure. Three groups of muscles are involved in the sphincter mechanism (Figure 80)—(i) the bladder neck mechanism, (ii) the intrinsic urethral musculature, and (iii) the pelvic floor muscles and the external sphincter.

205

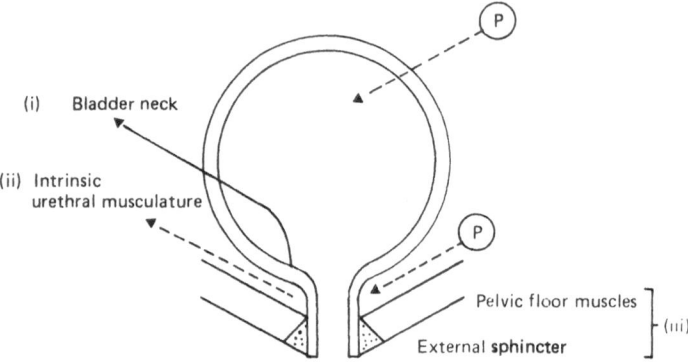

Figure 80. The bladder sphincters

An additional feature is that the proximal part of the urethra receives the rise of intraabdominal pressure since at all times the urethral resistance is greater than the bladder pressure, so even during micturition interruption of voiding is achieved by the combined contraction of the distal sphincter (intrinsic and external) and the muscle of the pelvic floor. Any urine which is proximal in the urethra is milked back into the bladder.

The urethral pressure profile
In practice this is not a very helpful investigation, but it demonstrates the mode of action of the sphincter. Changes in intraluminal pressure are recorded as a fine pressure recording catheter is withdrawn along the urethra. Figure 81 shows that there is a slight pressure rise at the internal meatus, which increases to some 50 cm water in the proximal third of the urethra and

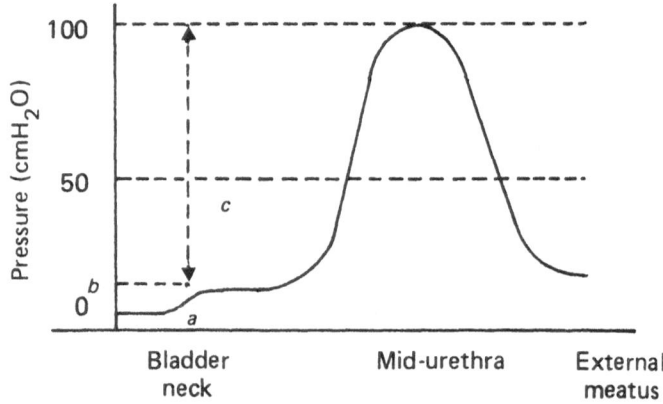

Figure 81. Urethral pressure profile

then rises sharply to a peak of nearly 100 cm water in the mid-urethra. The resting pressure in the bladder is 20 cm water. The voiding pressure in the female is 30–40 cm water, whereas in the male it is 40–60 cm water; this is because the female urethra offers much less resistance.

The cystometrogram

In the actual technique of cystometry combined with urethrography synchronous records are made of:

(1)   the filling volume of the bladder;
(2)   the total bladder pressure;
(3)   the rectal pressure (as a measure of the intraabdominal pressure);
(4)   the flow rate down the urethra as measured by a flow-rate meter.

The intrinsic bladder pressure (or *detrusor pressure*), is actually given by the total bladder pressure minus the rectal pressure. The performance is conducted as follows (Figure 82). During filling of the bladder the pressure is measured but, in fact, rises very little. Some 500 ml of fluid can be put into the bladder. At about 200 ml the patient experiences his first sensation (FS) of bladder filling, and at maximum filling he feels a strong desire (SD) to void. The patient then stands, or is tilted into the erect posture, and there is some rise of pressure in the bladder. The patient is then asked to cough so as to be able to test for stress incontinence. The cough shows on the total bladder pressure and the rectal (abdominal) pressure recordings but does not affect the intrinsic pressure of the bladder. Thereafter the patient starts to pass urine and when the flow rate has reached the peak, he or she is asked to 'hold'—this

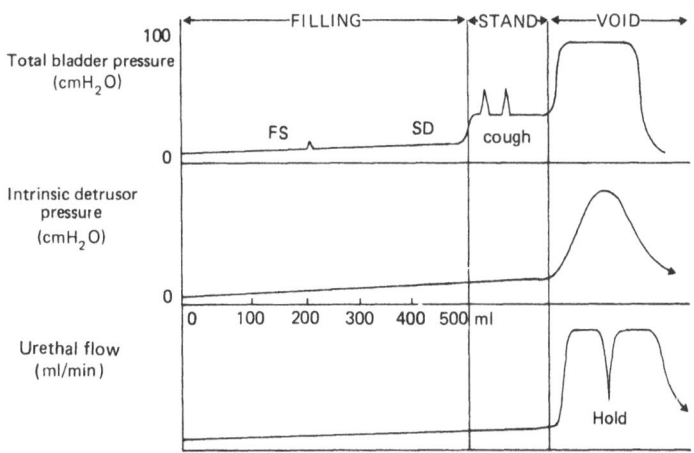

Figure 82. Pressure flow cystogram

207

tests the ability of the external sphincter to retain urine, producing a sharp rise in pressure in the mid-urethral segment, and micturition is thereafter completed.

The act of micturition therefore is initiated by contraction of the bladder muscle, and when this detrusor contraction is well under way the vesical orifice opens first and then the external sphincter relaxes. For coincidental fluoroscopic studies, as with a micturating cystogram, the bladder is filled with X-ray contrast so that when the patient is asked to void, descent of the bladder neck is first noted. The striated external sphincter contributes over 50% of the urethral resistance and determines the 'critical opening pressure', which in the normal female is 85–90 mmHg, and in the male is 100–105 mmHg. These pressures are actually so much higher than the pressures required to initiate micturition because the urethra is working as a coordinated functional striated muscle during the voiding process.

A normal flow pattern down the urethra can be seen in Figure 83. It is the product of the effective voiding pressure and the outflow resistance. A flow rate of 25 ml/min excludes significant outflow obstruction.

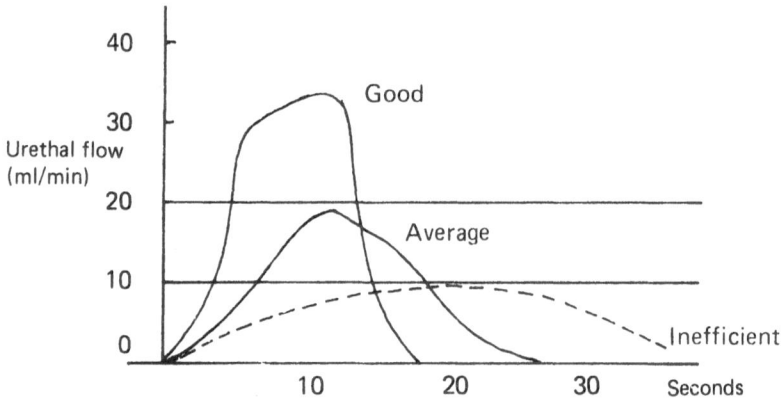

Figure 83.   Voiding flow rate patterns

URINARY INCONTINENCE

Urinary incontinence is symptomatic of a number of underlying conditions, all of which imply that the intravesical pressure is higher than the urethral sphincter can stand.

These voiding problems can be considered under three broad headings

(1)   *Detrusor abnormality*—the unstable bladder (detrusor instability); hypertonic bladder; and atonic bladder (neuropathic).
(2)   *Outflow obstruction*—in which the causes differ in the male and female.

Urinary tract infection (UTI)

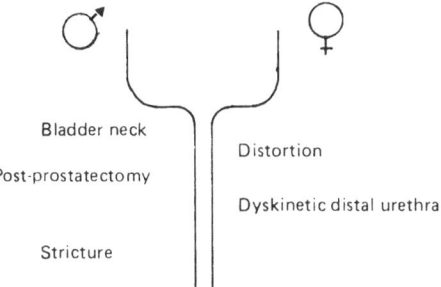

Figure 84. Sex differences in outflow obstruction

(3) *Sphincter dysfunction*—stress incontinence; enuresis; neurological—overflow incontinence/urge incontinence/frontal lobe incontinence.

In considering the above causes of urinary incontinence one also has to be aware that clinical symptoms and signs can be very misleading

(1) Stress incontinence does not always mean sphincter weakness.
(2) Urgency is not always due to unstable bladder contractions.
(3) Absence of residual urine does not exclude outflow obstruction.
(4) Presence of residual urine indicates an inability of the detrusor to overcome the outflow resistance but does not necessarily indicate an obstruction.

The pathological situations can be considered under the following headings.

Detrusor instability (the unstable bladder)

Normally the cystometrogram does not reveal any resting contraction because continence is maintained by inhibition of bladder muscle activity, but patients with an 'unstable bladder' have detrusor contractions that cannot be inhibited, and cause urgency, frequency and nocturia. The cause may be related to (a) enuresis or anxiety, (b) neurological disease, or (c) bladder outlet obstruction. Obstructive instability alone is reversible by operation. In other cases one chooses a drug such as Cetiprin (emepronium bromide 200 mg t.i.d.) or Urispas (flavoxate hydrochloride) 200 mg t.i.d.

Neuropathic bladder

Atonic bladder is suspect when there is a large residual urine and yet no mechanical obstruction. Ultimately one will see the urographic appearance of a heavily trabeculated firtree-shaped bladder with a wide-open neck. Atony is

209

due to a sacral or peripheral nerve lesion. Since the neurological control of the bladder is so delicate, a very minor failure in development may result in dysfunction and there will be no overt signs. Therapy should be with Myotonine (bethanechol chloride) 10 mg t.i.d. or Ubretid (distigmine bromide) 0.5 mg i.m.

Bladder neck obstruction

In the male
When there is prostatic obstruction the prostate may feel enlarged, the bladder is indented on routine urethrography and endoscopy will show median lobe enlargement. It is important at prostatectomy to preserve the distal sphincter mechanism. Persistence of symptoms after the operation signifies residual prostatic tissue, bladder neck contracture, urethral stricture or dyskinesia, or detrusor instability (Figure 84).

The intrinsic pressure required to empty the bladder is 40–50 cm water in the normal male, but is very much higher in outflow obstruction. Normal voiding is shown in Figure 83 above; the curve rises vertically and descends equally suddenly. Whereas the normal voiding rate can be 35 ml/min, when there is obstruction it is usually below 15 ml/min.

Bladder outlet symptoms need investigation not when there is obvious obstruction but (a) when there is a poor stream with delay and dribbling and yet the prostate feels normal, and (b) with recurrences of urinary tract infection. There can still be outflow obstruction even though the prostate is normal and even though there is no residual urine on the post-evacuation intravenous urogram films. Endoscopy does not help and urodynamic evaluation is necessary.

In the female
Outlet obstruction in the female is due to trouble in the distal urethra. Urethral distortion is common when there is prolapse. Less obvious trouble may arise from telescoping (Figure 84).

Stress incontinence

The urethra is normally situated above the bladder base and at an angle of 90–100°. Poor urethral tone can, however, result from (a) parturition damage to the supporting tissue, (b) menopausal atrophic changes, and (c) debilitation and loss of tissue turgor. The urethra may then lie directly at the base of the bladder where it receives the full force of the hydrostatic pressure and the result is a liability to incontinence. This is shown in Figure 85.

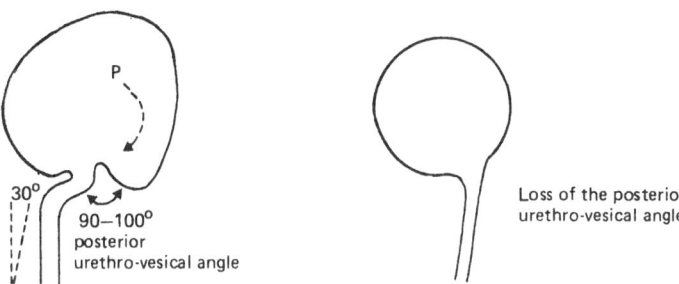

Figure 85. Urethro-vesical anatomy

The intact bladder neck is the first line of defence in the female and the distal urethra is only the second line of defence. In incontinence, therefore, one expects to find either that the bladder neck is open at rest or alternatively incompetent on coughing.

Urethral suspension procedures are designed to return the urethra and bladder neck to their normal retropubic position. The failure rate is likely to be much higher in cases of 'unstable bladder' than where there is pure sphincter weakness.

Enuresis (bed-wetting)

This is a special problem in children beyond the age of four. There are various causes:

(1) psychological and social problems and yet sleep that is too deep;
(2) immaturity due to delay in myelination of the central neurones;
(3) a persistent infantile bladder;
(4) mechanical obstruction to outflow with bladder hypertrophy and instability, or infection causing abnormal bladder behaviour.

Neurological sphincter disturbance

Overflow (dribbling) incontinence
This is a consequence of infranuclear bladder paresis, as is the case in a patient with a meningomyelocoele or a cauda equina lesion, or with a defect of the sensory nerves as in the case of diabetic or tabetic neuropathy. If sensation is intact as after polio or with acute prostatic obstruction, then the retention is painful.

Urge incontinence
This may be due either to a motor urge, which means an inadequate cerebral inhibition of the micturition centre, or due to a strong sensory input from the

211

bladder wall. The sensory urge is strong when there is inflammation, stone or tumour of the bladder.

Frontal lobe incontinence

This was originally recognized after prefrontal leucotomy. Although the patient is aware of his action, the lesion is such that he no longer cares.

ANALGESIC NEPHROPATHY

'Phenacetin nephritis' was reported first in the 1950s by Spühler and Zollinger in Switzerland, and also by researchers in Sweden and Australia. In fact, cases of chronic 'interstitial nephritis' had been on the increase since 1945 but it took some time to realize that its occurrence was linked to analgesic abuse, and that many patients were being diagnosed as having 'chronic pyelonephritis'. The particular problem was that necrosis of the papillae of the renal medulla, although common in phenacetin kidney, can also occur in any chronic interstitial nephritis or pyelonephritis. It is a chronic sclerotic process in contradistinction to the acute papillary necrosis of diabetes or urinary tract obstruction.

So analgesic nephropathy is marked by papillary necrosis, due to ischaemia of the vasa rectae, together with a diffuse interstitial nephritis. This appears as atrophy of the medullary tubular epithelia with secondary cortical scars but no infiltration of leucocytes as in a typical pyelonephritis. However, as a result of back-pressure there can also be atrophy of the loops of Henle and proximal tubules and often a superimposed bacterial pyelonephritis. Typically lipofuscin pigment is found in the kidneys, liver and brain and in the latter there are neurofibrillary degenerative changes and plaques.

The renal functional change is simply that of insidious chronic renal failure with associated anaemia and occasional hypertension, although on account of the medullary damage there is often a salt-losing nephritis. Since the damage is to the renal medulla rather than the cortex, there is a mild proteinuria with excess leucocytes in sterile urine, a failure of urinary concentration showing as polyuria and nocturia, and a failure of urinary acidification. At times episodes of haematuria may be indicative of papillary necrosis.

The intravenous urogram (IVU) findings can be absolutely typical. The kidneys tend to be smaller than normal but equal in size. The calyceal clubbing which remains after a papilla has been sloughed is seen typically in the mid-zones (as opposed to the polar regions in pyelonephritis). Here the renal cortex becomes very thin. The serial pathological changes in the renal papillae are as follows (Figure 86):

(1)   a failure of nephrogram 'blush' in the papillae on account of poor blood supply;

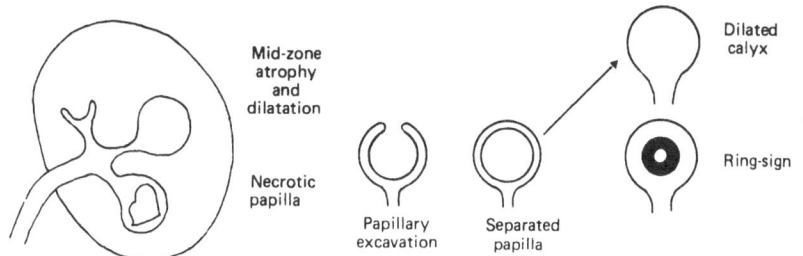

Figure 86.   Appearances in analgesic nephropathy

(2)   excavation and sloughing of papillae so that the kidney has the appearance of an intrarenal hydronephrosis and the separated papillae look like stones;

(3)   deposition of calcium on the surface of a necrotic papilla giving rise to ring calcification;

(4)   possible episodes of ureteric obstruction.

The typical clinical story is that of a person of unstable personality, possibly suffering from neurotic headaches, who resorts to consumption of mixed analgesics such as APC (aspirin, phenacetin and codeine). In order to develop renal damage the patient must have consumed some 2 kg phenacetin. Analgesic patients present either with peptic ulcer (after ingesting perhaps 7 kg phenacetin over 7 years), often having had a gastrectomy and an unexplained anaemia, or as patients with chronic renal failure following ingestion of 7 kg over 14 years.

There may be an iron deficiency anaemia caused by salicylate ingestion. Anemia due to phenacetin is a low grade haemolysis with Heinz bodies due to the accumulation of methaemoglobin (which can be reversed) and due to sulphaemoglobinaemia (which persists for the life of the red cell).

Much work has been devoted to study of the pathogenesis. It is clear that the primary insult is to the vasa rectae which supply blood to the renal papillae. This is likely to be caused by phenacetin, in particular by its toxic metabolite acetic-4-chloranilide, or by aspirin. Associated caffeine ingestion reduces the medullary blood flow and increases the local concentration of analgesic. The disease is always more florid in hot climates on account of the greater drug concentration within the kidneys.

The metabolism of phenacetin is shown in Figure 87.

The hydroxyl group in the *para* position is toxic, as also is the terminal amino. Both occur in acetanilide but are detoxified by alkylation and acetylation. Ingestion of phenacetin can be detected by the excretion of paracetamol in the urine.

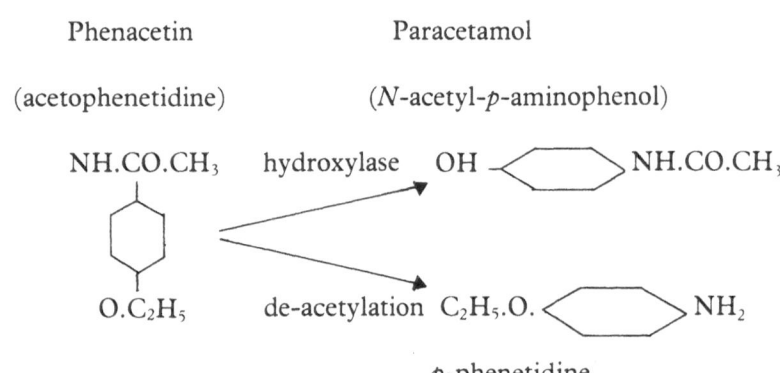

Figure 87. **Metabolism of phenacetin**

It has recently been suggested that one of the problems of the analgesic taker is an impairment of hepatic drug microsomal enzyme conjugating ability. Thus *N*-acetyl-*para*-amino-phenol is excreted in the free toxic form and is not conjugated as the glucuronide or sulphate.

One useful practical observation in the diagnosis of analgesic nephropathy is that the urine is dark brown and has the unusual property of reducing silver nitrate solution in the cold. After conc.HCl hydrolysis phenacetin metabolites can be detected by chromatography.

Aspirin has a pK_a of 3.5 so it is ionized in the proximal tubules, but when it is concentrated and acidified in the distal tubules non-ionized aspirin can be absorbed and will damage the tubular epithelium, whose cells are detected in the urine. Salicylate, is in fact known to be able to uncouple oxidative phosphorylation. It has also been shown that even a therapeutic dose of aspirin will lower renal plasma flow and glomerular filtration.

Another lesion which has been attributed to analgesics is ureteric obstruction due to a periureteral fibrosis in the middle third of the ureters.

Clearly nephropathy patients should be withdrawn from analgesics if they can be identified. If this is done the prognosis is good for there is an initial improvement in function that is often maintained, so that patients can live with glomerular filtration rates of 5–15 ml/min.

Carcinoma of the renal pelvis

Evidence from Sweden now suggests that phenacetin derivatives such as the 2- and 3-hydroxy-phenacetin forms cause a tumour of the renal pelvis in analgesic takers.

$C_2H_5.O$ ⟨ ₃   ₂ ⟩ $NH.CO.CH_3$
OH

The *ortho*-amino phenol configuration is similar to that of the naphthylamines which are known to be carcinogenic in the urinary tract.

RENAL TUBERCULOSIS

Tuberculosis of the urinary tract is often secondary to blood borne TB spread from a focus elsewhere in the body. This is usually from the lung but by the time the renal or bladder lesion is apparent, the chest X-ray may be normal in as many as one-third of the patients. On account of the haematogenous spread there are always some bilateral miliary foci, even though the gross finding may suggest unilateral fibrocaseous disease. Susceptible patients are working men aged 30–40, and the aged. Currently the death rate has declined considerably, and so has miliary TB, owing to the efficacy of modern chemotherapy. However caseous and cavitating lesions of the kidney are still quite common, and only some 20% of these lesions are actually found by the clinician.

The sequence of events in the establishment of genitourinary tuberculosis is therefore broadly as follows:

(1)   On account of bloodstream spread organisms lodge in the renal glomeruli and may there develop into caseous lesions which discharge into the renal tubules.

(2)   The bacilluria may lead to infection in the renal papillae, which are destroyed to give rise to the typical ulcerocavernous lesion. This is because the medulla is less vascular and the lesion is therefore more progressive. This lesion is sought on the IVU for it appears as a local abscess with associated caliectasis.

(3)   Spread of organisms down the urinary tract may then cause a focus of infection in a ureter and, as the granulomatous lesion fibroses, the result is a stricture which in turn causes hydronephrosis on that side. If there is still infection in that kidney, the result is a pyonephrosis.

(4)   Although the bladder is relatively resistant because of its stratified squamous epithelium, in due course nodules become established in the mucosa and ulcerate, and symptoms appear in the form of dysuria and frequency. At first the muscle wall hypertrophies but later it fibroses and contracts to give rise to the 'thimble bladder'.

(5)   The epididymis meanwhile may become involved by direct spread in the bloodstream, or by spread from the bladder along the vas, or along the perivasal lymphatics. There is pain and swelling in the epididymis, and a cold abscess may form and open through a sinus onto the skin.

(6)   Since the prostate has a rich blood supply, it is readily involved in

haematogenous spread or from the urinary passage, and the final result might be a urethral stricture or an abscess which discharges into the perineum.

The symptoms of urinary tract tuberculosis can, therefore, be anticipated. They comprise:

(1)   frequency and nocturia, fever and sterile pyuria;
(2)   loin pain;
(3)   epididymitis.

Note that at least 10% of cases will be asymptomatic and that another 15% will have pyuria only.

The actual pathological processes found in the kidneys are as follows:

(1)   miliary cortical lesions;
(2)   caseous or ulcerative lesions of the medulla with calyceal destruction;
(3)   hydronephrosis or pyonephrosis;
(4)   renal hypertension due to the TB lesion together with arteriosclerosis obliterans;
(5)   amyloidosis;
(6)   a microscopic (but not clinical) nephritis consisting of glomerular tuft hypercellularity with capillary wall thickening.

One should always remember that renal TB can remain dormant for a long time and then reappear coincident with depression of immunity due to intercurrent infection, with ageing or with reinfection.

The diagnosis depends on the finding of acid-fast bacilli which on culture have the morphology of *Mycobacterium tuberculosis*. For this purpose both early morning urine samples and 24 h urines must be examined. Drug therapy must *not* be started on the finding of a positive Ziehl Nielsen stain alone, for such a finding might be due to smegma bacillus (although this organism is non-alcohol fast). When attempting to exonerate a patient at least six E.M.U. samples must be carefully examined.

The IVU is of considerable value in showing parenchymal calcification, calculi, or a local or generalized caliectasis in association with a medullary abscess (the ulcerocavernous lesion).

Chemotherapy is on standard lines with streptomycin, PAS and isoniazid or with rifampicin, isoniazid and ethambutol. About 60% of urines will become sterile by 2 months and 80% by 4 months, but therapy must be continued until the urine has been sterile for at least 6 months.

If surgery is required this should be performed after about 8 weeks on therapy. The three vulnerable areas are the neck of a calyx, the pelviureteric junction and the lower end of the ureter. The possible operations are therefore:

(1)   Partial nephrectomy for an ulcerocavernous lesion. This is seldom required. Total nephrectomy is undertaken if the TB kidney is a cause of renal hypertension or a source of continuous infection of the lower urinary tract.

(2)   Cavernotomy to open up an obstructed calyx.

(3)   Plastic procedures at the pelviureteric junction are impractical on the whole owing to surrounding oedema and fibrolipomatosis. It is sometimes possible, however, to drain the kidney through a nephrostomy tube, while a plastic procedure is performed over a splinting catheter left in position for up to 6 weeks.

(4)   Excision of stricture at the lower end of the ureter or reimplantation into the bladder. If this does not work and a pyonephrosis ensues, nephrectomy will be inevitable.

RETROPERITONEAL FIBROSIS

The ureters become bound in dense fibrous tissue on the posterior abdominal wall, so that the patient may either present with unilateral or bilateral renal swellings indicative of hydronephrosis, or with a diminishing urine output and renal insufficiency. A third possibility is that there may be only vague backache or lower abdominal pain, a raised ESR and elevated serum globulins and a positive ANF in a patient who has been taking one of the known predisposing drugs such as methysergide, hydrallazine or amphetamine. In these cases it is possible that an allergic drug reaction has provoked the fibrotic process which involves the ureters from without so that they are occluded. A ureteric catheter, can however, be passed with ease.

The histology is pleomorphic but basically there are histiocytes, plasma cells and fibroblasts, which form an infiltrative mass that hardens to form a plaque. This fibrous tissue tends to occlude the ureters in their midcourse at L3/4 in the male, where in fact the ureters are often kinked and pulled medially, but in the female it occurs below the pelvic brim. The process can also involve either the bladder or the perirenal tissues. The diagnosis by biopsy is not easy owing to the variable histology, and differentiation from a retroperitoneal sarcoma may be impossible.

There is often an associated phlebitis or vasculitis. There can also be mediastinal fibrosis with swelling of the face, lymphadenopathy, a pericardial friction rub and also genital thrombophlebitis, hydrocoele and testicular perifibrosis, and occlusions of the femoral or iliac vessels.

Occasionally the back-pressure in the ureters may give rise to a diabetes-insipidus-like syndrome. At all times one must be aware that if, as commonly happens, only one kidney is involved at first, then the renal function may appear normal.

The IVU shows typical changes:

(1) extrinsic obstruction of the ureters in their midcourse giving rise to hydronephrosis;
(2) a tapering of the lower ends of those ureters at the level of the obstruction;
(3) some degree of medial deviation.

Lymphangiography can be helpful for it should show dilated lymphatics which are blocked at the level of L3/4, a delay in passage of the dye through the para-aortic nodes, and incomplete filling of the lymph nodes.

The patient has to be cystoscoped and retrograde catheters are passed. If a cine-retrograde examination is carried out, no peristalsis will be seen in the affected portions of the ureters.

The first line of treatment is a ureterolysis through a direct transperitoneal approach. It may even be necessary to bring out the ureters externally in the loins. The idiopathic variety can respond to high dose steroid therapy in the form of prednisone 40–60 mg/day. Sometimes there is some spontaneous resolution.

REFERENCES

Urinary tract infections

Aoki, S. (1969). Abacterial and bacterial pyelonephritis. *N. Engl. J. Med.*, **281,** 1375

Asscher, A.W. (1966). Urine as a medium for bacterial growth. *Lancet,* **2,** 1037

Asscher, A.W. (1977). Natural history of significant bacteruria. *Proc. Roy. Soc. Med.,* **70,** 149

Asscher, A.W. and Brumfitt, W. (1975). Urinary tract infection symposium. *Kidney Int.,* **8,** S1-149

Badenoch, A.W. Infections and inflamations of the urinary tract. In *Manual of Urology*. (London: Heinemann) *1974*

Beeson, P.B. (1968). The case against the catheter. *A.J. Med.,* **24,** 1

Cotran, R.S. (1969). The renal lesion in chronic pyelonephritis. *J. Infect. Dis.,* **120,** 109

Cox, C.E. (1968). Urethral flora of the female and recurrent UTI. *J. Urol.,* **99,** 632

Domingue, J. (1970). Microbial L-forms in pyelonephritis. *J. Urol.,* **104,** 790

Hallett, R.J. (1967). Urine infection in children. *Lancet,* **ii,** 1107

Hand, W.L. (1971). Antibacterial effect of the urinary bladder. *J. Lab. Clin. Med.,* **77,** 605

Heptinstall, R.H. (1962). Epidemiology of non-enteric *E. coli* infections. *J. Clin. Invest.*, **41**, 1760

Hodson, C.J. (1965). The natural history of chronic pyelonephritic scarring. *Br. Med. J.*, **2**, 191

Holmgren, J. and Smith, J.W. (1975). Immunological aspects of urinary tract infection. *Prog. Allergy*, **18**, 289

Kleeman, C.R. (1960). Pyelonephritis. *Medicine (Baltimore)*, **39**, 3

Kraft, J.K., Stamey, T.A. (1977). Natural history of symptomatic recurrent bacteriuria in women. *Medicine (Baltimore)*, **56**, 55

Kunin, C.M. (1970). Natural history of recurrent bacteruria in schoolgirls. *N. Engl. J. Med.*, **282**, 1443

MacGregor, M.E. (1975). Childhood urinary tract infection with uretero-vesical reflux. *Q. J. Med.*, **44**, 481

Montgomerie, J.Z. (1968). Renal failure and infection. *Medicine*, **47**, 1

Rolleston, G.L. (1974). Intrarenal reflux and the scarred kidney. *Arch. Dis. Child*, **49**, 531

Schwartz, M.M. and Cotran, R.S. (1973). Common enterobacterial antigen in pyelonephritis. *N. Engl. J. Med.*, **289**, 830

Smellie, J. (1964). Urine infection in childhood. *Br. Med. J.*, **2**, 1222

Smellie, J. (1975). Vesico-uretero reflux and renal scarring. *Kidney Int.*, **8**, S65

Stamey, T.A., Wehner, N., Mihara, G., and Condy, M. (1978). Immunological basis of recurrent bacteruria. *Medicine*, **57**, 47

Turck, M. (1966). Relapse and infection in chronic bacteruria. *N. Engl. J. Med.*, **275**, 70

White, R. (1977). Urine infection in children. *Br. Med. J.*, **1**, 1650

Bacteruria and pregnancy

Gower, P.E. (1968). *Lancet*, **1**, 990

Norden, C.W., Kass, E.H. (1968). *Ann. Rev. Med.*, **19**, 431

Savage, W.E. (1967). *Medicine*, **46**, 385

E. coli antibodies

Anderson, H.J. (1967), *Acta Paediatr. Scand.*, **56**, 637

Antibiotic sensitivity tests

Bell, S.M. (1975). *Pathology (Australia)*, **7**, 1

Ryan, K.J. (1976). *Human Pathol.*, **7**, 277

Sabath, L.D. (1976). *Human Pathol.*, **7**, 287

Treatment of UTI

Asscher, A.W. (1977). Therapy of UTI. *Br. Med. J.*, **1**, 1332

Kass, E.H. (1955). Chemotherapeutic and antibiotic drugs in management of UTI. *Am. J. Med.*, **18**, 764

Winterborn, M.H. (1977). Management of urinary tract infections in children. *Br. J. Hosp. Med.*, **17**, 453

Perinephric abscess

Thorley, J.B. (1974). *Medicine (Baltimore)*, **53**, 441

Salvatierra, O. (1967). *J. Urol.*, **98**, 296

Analgesic nephropathy

Abel, J.A. (1971). *Clin. Pharmacol. Ther.*, **12**, 583

Bangtsson, U. (1974). *Clin. Nephrol.*, **2**, 123

Clausen, H. and Jensen, K. (1968). Renal biopsies from patients with high analgesic intake. *Acta Pathol. Microbiol. Scand.*, **72**, 219

Gault, M.H. (1968). *Ann. Intern. Med.*, **68**, 906

Goldberg, M. (1975). *Ann. Rev. Med.*, **26**, 537 and *N. Engl. J. Med.*, 1978, **299**, 716

Grimlund, K. (1974). *Acta Med. Scand.*, (suppl. 405) 3

Harvald, B. (1963). Renal papillary necrosis. *Am. J. Med.*, **35**, 481

Kincaid-Smith, P. (1968). Lesions of the blood supply of the papilla in analgesic nephropathy. *Med. J. Aust.*, **1**, 203. Lesions of the blood supply of the papilla in analgesic nephropathy. *Lancet*, 1967, **1**, 859

Murray, T. (1975). *Ann. Intern. Med.*, **82**, 453

Retroperitoneal fibrosis

Ormond, J.K. (1960). *J. Am. Med. Assoc.*, **174**, 1561

Renal tuberculosis

Borthwick, W.M. (1970). *Br. J. Urol.*, **42**, 642

Christensen, W.I. (1974). *Medicine (Baltimore)*, **53**, 377

Kerr, W.K. (1970). Prognosis in reconstructive surgery for urinary tuberculosis. *Br. J. Urol.*, **42**, 672

8
Kidney stones and congenital diseases of the kidney

Calcium

The normal serum calcium is 2.5 mmol/l (or 10 mg%); of this, half is ionized, some 40% is bound to the serum proteins, and 10% is complexed with citrate or other organic anions. So the normal ionized calcium is 1.25 mmol/l and the concentration in the extracellular fluids is just below this at 1.0 mmol/l (10^{-3}M). In the actual cytoplasm of cells the calcium concentration is only 10^{-5}M, for cells have both the ability to actively extrude calcium, and alternatively to regulate the level in the cytosol by an energy-dependent uptake into the mitochondria. Phosphate moves likewise. Conversely, if calcium is taken up by mitochondria independently of phosphate, hydrogen ions are then secreted into the cytosol.

It is a fundamental point that the calcium content of the cytosol and intracellular membranes regulates the activity of many enzymes. Calcium is known to inhibit adenylcyclase, and high concentrations interfere with enzymes, bind nucleic acids and uncouple oxidative phosphorylation. Even a modest rise of calcium in the cytosol inhibits the normal intercellular coupling between cell surfaces.

Absorption

Both 24,25- and 1,25-dihydroxy-*vitamin* D promote the intestinal absorption of calcium. There is a calcium-activated ATPase in the intestinal mucosa which may aid the absorption process. Parathormone has no direct action on gut absorption but acts indirectly by promoting 1,25-dihydroxy-cholecalciferol formation. In sarcoidosis there is an excessive absorption of calcium which appears to be vitamin D-mediated and this is inhibited by cortisone, whose administration is the basis of a therapeutic test.

Losses

Of the 10 g/day calcium that are filtered by the kidneys, 98% is reabsorbed, most in the proximal tubules, some 25% in the loops of Henle and 10% in the distal tubules. Normally calcium excretion follows sodium excretion, possibly because a calcium transport ATPase parallels the distribution of Na–K ATPase—which is essentially an enzyme that activates a proton pump into the interior of a cell.

The following points are of direct clinical interest:

(1)   Extracellular fluid *volume expansion* with saline reduces calcium as well as sodium reabsorption.

(2)   Administration of most *diuretics* causes a loss of calcium with sodium. However in the long term thiazides result in calcium retention and even hypercalcaemia.

(3)   *Parathormone* enhances reabsorption of calcium; but when hyperparathyroidism causes hypercalcaemia, hypercalcuria will follow.

(4)   Under the influence of mineralo*corticoids* there is mobilization of calcium from bone and a marked urinary loss leading in the long term to osteoporosis.

Hypercalcaemia and hypocalcaemia

In hypercalcaemia *metastatic deposition* of calcium with phosphate occurs in various areas. In the cornea a band keratopathy develops, because egress of carbon dioxide from the exposed parts of the cornea leaves an alkaline interstitium. Other alkaline areas occur on the opposite side of acid secreting epithelia, as in the gastric mucosa and renal tubules. It is here that calcium deposits occur.

In hypocalcaemia one expects *tetany,* but this is lessened by the acidosis of chronic renal failure. Calcium is of course very critical to neuromuscular function: (a) it controls sodium fluxes (action potentials) across nerve cell membranes. This is now understandable since calcium ions are known to cross-link the negative phosphate groups of acidic phospholipids such as phosphatidyl-serine. The following diagram shows the binding of calcium to acidic phospholipids. Note that aluminium will displace both Mg^{2+} and Ca^{2+}; (b) release of calcium within heart or muscle fibres initiates contraction by joining actin with myosin. This process is energized by a calcium-dependent ATPase.

$$
\begin{array}{ll}
& O \\
& \parallel \\
O \qquad CH_2-O-C-R \qquad\qquad R-C-O-CH_2 \qquad O \\
\parallel \quad\qquad | \qquad\qquad\qquad\qquad\qquad\qquad\quad | \qquad \parallel \\
R-C-O\!-\!-\!-CH \qquad O \qquad\qquad P \quad CH-O-C-R \\
\qquad\qquad\quad | \qquad\qquad \parallel \qquad\qquad\qquad \parallel \quad | \\
\qquad\qquad CH_2-O-P-X \qquad\qquad X-O-CH_2 \\
\qquad\qquad\qquad\qquad | \qquad\qquad\qquad\qquad\qquad | \\
\qquad\qquad\qquad\qquad O^- \qquad\qquad\qquad\qquad\quad O^- \\
\qquad\qquad\qquad\qquad\qquad\qquad \boxed{Ca^{2+}}
\end{array}
$$

Magnesium

The serum magnesium is 0.7–0.9 mmol/l of which 25% is bound to protein and the remainder is complexed to anions such as citrate, phosphate and sulphate. It is a major intracellular cation that is essential for the function of many enzymes: muscles contain some 10 mmol/l. Of the 1800 mg/day of magnesium that is filtered by the kidneys, only 3–5% is lost in the urine. In the proximal tubules reabsorption of magnesium, like that of calcium, is closely linked to sodium reabsorption, and parathormone enhances tubular reabsorption of magnesium. The following factors lead to increased *urinary loss* of magnesium:

(1) ECF expansion and diuretics;
(1) alcoholism, glucose loading (as in diabetes);
(3) hypercalcaemia;
(4) glucocorticoids and mineralocorticoids (aldosteronism).

Although intracellular levels of magnesium are well maintained, in deficiency there is a vacuolation of the distal tubules. This might be seen in a alcoholism or after diabetic ketosis.

A low magnesium may result in tremors and convulsions; this is seen in alcoholism. Conversely, the nephrologist will see hypermagnesaemia as part of chronic renal failure. There is somnolence, peripheral vasodilatation with hypotension and defective function in the cardiac conducting system.

Phosphate

The serum phosphate is 1.0–1.5 mmol/l (3.0–4.5 mg%) but is higher in growing children. Phosphate is vital to intracellular metabolism and a recent meal, glucose, insulin, muscle activity and increased glycolysis induced by alkalosis (as with hyperventilation) all lead to phosphate uptake by cells. The 2:3 DPG of erythrocytes is increased in alkalosis; 2:3 DPG retards the release of oxygen from haemoglobin and this is one reason why bicarbonate therapy in diabetic ketosis has to be used with caution.

Low levels of serum phosphate lead to muscle weakness and to osteomalacia. High levels of serum phosphate may depress the serum calcium to the point at which tetany and convulsions occur, since there is precipitation with calcium in extracellular sites.

In hyperparathyroidism the serum phosphate is depressed. PTH inhibits proximal tubule reabsorption of phosphate (via stimulation of adenylate cyclase). However as the GFR falls, the renal clearance of phosphate falls, so that a raised serum phosphate is still the feature of the secondary hyperparathyroidism of chronic renal failure.

Damage to the proximal tubules as in Fanconi syndrome (p. 51) results in phosphaturia, and bone mineralization is impaired.

KIDNEY STONES AND THEIR FORMATION

Kidney stones are important, for one-third of patients will lose one kidney either from unavoidable operation or as the result of infection. A stone may pass down the ureter causing colic and when impacted produce obstruction to the urine flow; long-term irritation by a stone can produce cancerous changes in the renal pelvis; and once a stone has occurred, there is a 25% recurrence rate on the same side and 15% chance on the opposite side.

Two-thirds of all kidney stones are made of calcium oxalate or of calcium oxalate mixed with the hydroxyapatite form of calcium phosphate. When there is recurrent urinary tract infection, magnesium ammonium phosphate stones are formed. Other stones form for precise metabolic causes as is the case with uric acid stones, xanthine stones, cystine stones, silica stones and those calcium stones which occur as a result of prolonged hypercalcaemia or excessive urinary excretion of calcium.

The stone-forming situations are summarized in Table 23.

Calcium is filtered in the renal glomeruli and is reabsorbed along with sodium in the proximal tubule and, under the influence of parathormone, in the ascending loop of Henle. In general, therefore, calcium losses tend to parallel sodium losses. More important still there is a steep calcium concentration gradient within the renal substance:

Table 23

Types of stone	Predisposing situations
Calcium phosphate (hydroxyapatite)	Hypercalcaemia or hypercalcuria
Calcium phosphate/Calcium oxalate	Immobilization
	Hot climate
	Alkalinuria/obstruction/ medullary sponge kidney
Calcium oxalate	Oxaluria/pyridoxine deficiency
Magnesium ammonium phosphate (struvite)	Infection or obstruction
Uric acid	Gout/acid urine due to diarrhoea/ blood dyscrasia
Xanthine	Inborn error/allopurinol administration
Cystine stones	COAL transport defect

Calcium content: renal cortex	8.9 mmol/kg wet tissue
outer medulla	10.1
inner medulla	16.9
renal papilla	23–38

and this explains why Randall noted small calcified areas beneath the epithelium of the renal papillae in as many as 17% autopsies. One has to know then how calcium precipitation is prevented in the face of such a high ionic concentration. Very likely it is kept in solution by citrate anions that are produced and excreted by the renal tubules; indeed there is often a low citrate/calcium ratio when there is stone formation. Other inhibitor substances include pyrophosphates, diphosphonates and certain mucopolysaccharides.

In considering the generation of stones discussion centres on three mechanisms:

(1) *Absence of an inhibitor of calcium precipitation*—citrate, pyrophosphate or certain mucopolysaccharides.

(2) *Causes of supersaturation of the crystalloids*—or why the calcium:phosphate solubility product is so easily exceeded in calcium formers, and the fact that uric acid is so insoluble in an acid urine.

(3) *How an initiation centre* may be formed by bacterial debris, by Boyce mucoprotein or by brushite (calcium phosphate monohydrate) acting as a precipitation nucleus for oxalate.

Simple physicochemical principles no doubt explain the supersaturation of crystalloids, so if one studies solute precipitation in urine in relation to the pH, it is found that below pH 6.5 brushite crystals form, between 6.5 and 7.0 apatite crystals, and above pH 7.1 struvite (Figure 88). Brushite, hydroxy-apatite or monosodium urate monohydrate serve as seeds for the crystalliza-tion of calcium oxalate. The activity: product ratio (APR) expresses the state of saturation: the value 1 represents saturation, values greater than 1 indicate supersaturation, and values less than 1 indicate undersaturation. Calcium oxalate comes nearer to the precipitation limit than any other compound in normal urine. Some 40% of day urines and 70% of night urines actually become supersaturated with calcium oxalate.

The theories of stone formation outlined above may be integrated with the clinical realities in a classification as shown in Table 24.

Table 24   Factors predisposing to stone formation

   I. Absence of a crystallization inhibitor in the urine:
       lack of citrate, magnesium, pyrophosphate etc.
   II. Increased crystalloid concentration of the urine, as in:
       dehydration
       hypercalcuria, hyperoxaluria, uricaciduria, cystinuria
       acid pH causing uric acid precipitation
       alkaline pH 'initiation centres' in patients with renal tubular defects
   III. Urinary tract abnormalities predisposing to stone formation:
       congenital abnormalities and recurrent infection
       medullary sponge kidneys (MSK)
       polycystic kidneys

We can now consider the predisposing metabolic defects in further detail and derive a rational approach to the management.

Hypercalcuria

This is known to be associated with the supersaturated state for brushite and oxalate. If the calcium excretion in the female exceeds 300 mg% (0.75 mmol/l), or 250 mg/day, or in the male 350 mg% (0.87 mmol/l), or 300 mg/day, then calcium stone formation is quite possible. In reality 'idiopathic hypercalcuria' is a common cause of stone formation, but one also has to look

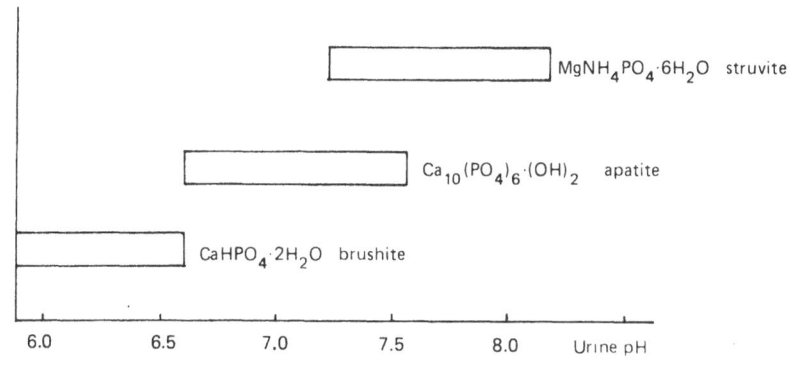

Figure 88. Crystallization in urine

closely for the various forms of hypercalcaemia. A serum calcium which exceeds 11.0 mg% (2.75 mmol/l) on several occasions, in venous blood taken without stasis, is abnormally high. It is often helpful to adjust the total plasma calcium to a protein of 70 g/l using the formula 10 g/l = 0.75 mg% (0.1875 mmol/l) of calcium.

Causes of hypercalcuria (and nephrocalcinosis in the long term)

(1) *Hypercalcuria with normal serum calcium*
idiopathic hypercalcuria ? due to increased intestinal absorption;
normocalcaemic hyperparathyroidism;
renal tubular acidosis.

(2) *Hypercalcuria with raised serum calcium*
Primary hyperparathyroidism (some 4% of all stone formers). At first site the hypercalcuria seems paradoxical for the action of parathormone is to stimulate renal tubular reabsorption of calcium. In fact the hypercalcuria occurs because the filtered load of calcium is so great that total reabsorption is impossible.

(3) *Hypercalcuria with a normal or raised calcium*
vitamin D intoxication or hypersensitivity (sarcoid);
malignant tumours and myeloma involving the skeleton;
milk-alkali syndrome due to sodium bicarbonate ingestion;
Paget's disease;
hyperthyroidism;
immobilization.

Idiopathic hypercalcuria is a common cause of recurrent stone formation. This condition can now be subdivided into:

227

type   I: patients with absorptive hypercalcuria;
type IIa: those with a renal calcium leak and secondary hyper-
                        parathyroidism;
     IIb: those with a renal calcium leak and non-suppressible hyper-
                        parathyroids;
type III: patients who have a primary renal phosphate leak.

In type I the urinary calcium can be lowered by a low calcium diet, or by means of oral sodium cellulose phosphate binding resin. In type II thiazides will reduce the calcium leak. In IIb they and 25-hydroxy-vitamin D will raise the serum calcium and yet not reduce the serum PTH.

Hyperoxaluria

Oxalate metabolism is dealt with on page 247. The normal urinary oxalate is 15–60 mg/day. The various forms of hyperoxaluria are:

(1)   *Primary inherited hyperoxaluria*
           Type I: oxaluria with glycolic aciduria (Figure 92).
           Type II: oxaluria with glyceric aciduria
(2)   *Secondary causes*
           (a) excess dietary oxalate, derived from tea, rhubarb, spinach, nuts,
               ascorbic acid; pyridoxine deficiency;
           (b) ethylene glycol poisoning or methoxyfluorane anaesthesia on
               account of conversion to oxalate;
           (c) ileal impairment; when there is interruption of bile acid absorp-
               tion, there is excess absorption of oxalate from the colon.

Magnesium ammonium phosphate stones (struvite)

When there is urinary tract obstruction and infection by urea-splitting organisms, a combination of increased concentrations of ammonia with alkali leads to triple phosphate crystallization.

Uric acid stones

Uric acid excretion should not exceed 600 mg/day (36 mM) on a low purine diet. Since uric acid is insoluble in an acid urine, the causes are simply divided into:

(1)   *Increased production of uric acid:*
           gout;
           polycythaemia, leukaemias and lymphomata
           psoriasis

(2)   *Increased urine acidity*
reduced ammonia excretion;
loss of alkaline gut fluids—as in chronic diarrhoea or ileostomy.

Cystinuria

This is discussed on page 246. Cystine is insoluble in an acid urine. The definitive test is to add 5% sodium cyanide to urine to convert cysteine to cystine and then to detect the latter by sodium nitroprusside which forms a magenta colour.

The calculi tend to form at night when there is a poor urine flow and an acid urine (the postprandial acid tide), and it is therefore important to maintain an alkaline diuresis. Penicillamine converts cystine to more soluble cysteine and mixed disulphides but in view of its toxicity, enthusiasm for its use is waning.

THE APPROACH TO KIDNEY STONE INVESTIGATION

The following screening procedures are required when stone formation is being investigated:

(1)   urea and electrolytes;
(2)   serum calcium, phosphate and alkaline phosphatase;
(3)   endogenous creatinine clearance with 24 h urinary calcium (not greater than 300 mg);
endogenous creatinine clearance and 24 h urinary uric acid (not greater than 600 mg);
(4)   random urinary pH and possibly an ammonium chloride-loading test (0.1 gram per kilo);
(5)   cystine screening test;
(6)   routine urine bacteriology.

In primary hyperparathyroidism the serum calcium is elevated in all but 15% of cases, and there is hypercalcuria in 70%. Such patients are best investigated while on a fixed dietary intake of 400 mg/day calcium. The serum phosphate is only low in about 20% of cases. Urinary cyclic AMP is elevated in 70% of cases.

The urinary calcium in the fasting state is a measure of the mobilization of calcium from bone. It is high in any renal hypercalcuria and in primary hyperparathyroidism, in which case it bears a relation to the decrease in bone density, as measured by photon absorption in the distal end of the radius.

The absorption of a 1.0 g load of oral calcium is elevated in primary hyperparathyroidism. A routine absorption test should consist of a 2 h fasting urine, following overnight fast, and thereafter a 4 h urine collection following

229

the 1 g calcium load. This test is used to diagnose renal hypercalcuria. It also divides absorptive hypercalcuria into those with excessive renal excretion of calcium at all levels of calcium intake, and those who only show hypercalcuria after a load.

THE APPROACH TO TREATMENT

This can be summarized as a series of rules.

(1)   Maintain a high urinary output; this means drinking 500 ml of fluid 4 hourly even through the night. Relieve any stasis in the urinary tract.

(2)   Acidify the urine (with hexamine or mandelamine) for magnesium ammonium phosphate stones, but alkalinize the urine for uric acid and cystine stones or for renal tubular acidosis.

(3)   Consider the use of a special diet:
(a) low calcium diet for idiopathic hypercalcuria;
(b) low purine diet for gout or uric acid stones, with allopurinol;
(c) low methionine diet for cystinuria (not very practical) and ? penicillamine;
(d) low oxalate intake; high pyridoxine intake for type I oxaluria.

(4)   For idiopathic hypercalcuria administer oral cellulose phosphate and use the thiazide diuretics to reduce the urinary calcium. Consider the use of diphosphonates.

(5)   In hypercalcaemia try a therapeutic trial of hydrocortisone 40 mg t.i.d. to reduce intestinal calcium absorption after the routine investigations for hyperparathyroidism.

Sodium cellulose phosphate is an ion-exchange resin that binds calcium in the gut. In patients with absorptive hypercalcuria who are on a low calcium intake (400 mg Ca diet), sodium cellulose phosphate decreases urine calcium by 200 mg/day and increases urinary phosphate by up to 400 mg.

Orthophosphates are useful because they promote the excretion of pyrophosphates that are inhibitors of crystallization, but they can lead to soft tissue calcification and deterioration in renal function.

Diphosphonates, such as EHDP are synthetic analogues of pyrophosphate that are resistant to pyrophosphatases; they inhibit nucleation and crystal growth.

CALCIUM NEPHROPATHY

Hypercalcaemia impairs the renal concentrating ability and results in polyuria and sodium depletion. In fact high concentrations of calcium inhibit

Na–K ATPase, as well as enzymes vital to energy metabolism, and thus the medullary interstitium loses its hypertonicity. With the hypercalcuria there is deposition of calcium in the medulla and collecting ducts. The tubular epithelium and the renal interstitium is damaged and fibrosis ensues with distortion which creates a liability to infection. This scarring determines the degree of reversibility. Although the whole renal substance may become more radio-opaque, the calcium deposits are typically seen only by the microscope.

Hypercalcaemia

'Hypercalcaemic crisis' occurs when the serum calcium is over 15 mg% (2.75 mmol/l). There is polyuria leading to dehydration, vomiting and ensuing shock and acute renal failure. Death may occur from cardiac arrhythmias.

The approaches to treatment are as follows:

(1) Give large amounts of intravenous saline and then supplement this with frusemide therapy in order to cause body depletion of calcium.

(2) In emergency hypercalcaemia resort to renal dialysis.

(3) Intravenous sodium sulphate at 122 mmol/l is an osmotic diuretic and causes the loss of large amounts of calcium in the urine.

(4) Intravenous disodium hydrogen phosphate with potassium dihydrogen phosphate, given as 100 mmol/l of 5% dextrose in 6–8 h, lowers the calcium by precipitation in extracellular sites. It is, however, potentially dangerous since some intravascular precipitation might occur (so causing pancreatitis).

(5) Large oral doses of corticosteroids counteract the enhancing effect of vitamin D on gut absorption. Paradoxically, parenteral steroids do not work.

(6) Calcitonin therapy (160 MCR units in 2 ml i/m) causes a rapid decrease in the numbers and activity of osteoclasts.

(7) Chelation of calcium with sodium versanate (trisodium edetate) is now rarely used.

(8) For the hypercalcaemia of malignancy the cytotoxic antibiotic from *Streptomyces*, known as mithramycin C, is recognized to be extremely useful. (25 μg per kilo by slow infusion daily x 10).

URIC ACID AND THE KIDNEY

The normal serum urate is less than 7.0 mg% in men (0.4 mmol/l) and less than 6.0 mg% (0.36 mmol/l) in women. Average serum urates are 5.0 mg% for men and 4.0 mg% for women. In fact, the normal male synthesizes 500–700 mg/day (30–42 mmol/day) of uric acid and 75% of this is excreted in the urine. It is relatively insoluble. Some uric acid is lost into the gut and a little is degraded by leucocytes.

The average uric acid pool in the body is 1 g. Dietary intake contributes less than 20% to this pool, and the major part is derived from the endogenous breakdown of cell nucleic acids. There is considerable recycling of purines and pyrimidines.

For *de novo* synthesis entry of ribose-5-phosphate to the pathway requires an amido-transferase which uses ATP to form the key compound PRPP (phosphoribosylpyrophosphate). There is then utilization of glutamine to form phosphoribosylamine and thereafter the sequence is: $\rightarrow$ inosinic acid $\rightarrow$ hypoxanthine + PRPP (recycled $\xrightarrow{X.O}$ xanthine $\xrightarrow{X.O}$ uric acid (Figure 89)).

The final conversion to uric acid involves the enzyme xanthine oxidase, which is inhibited by allopurinol.

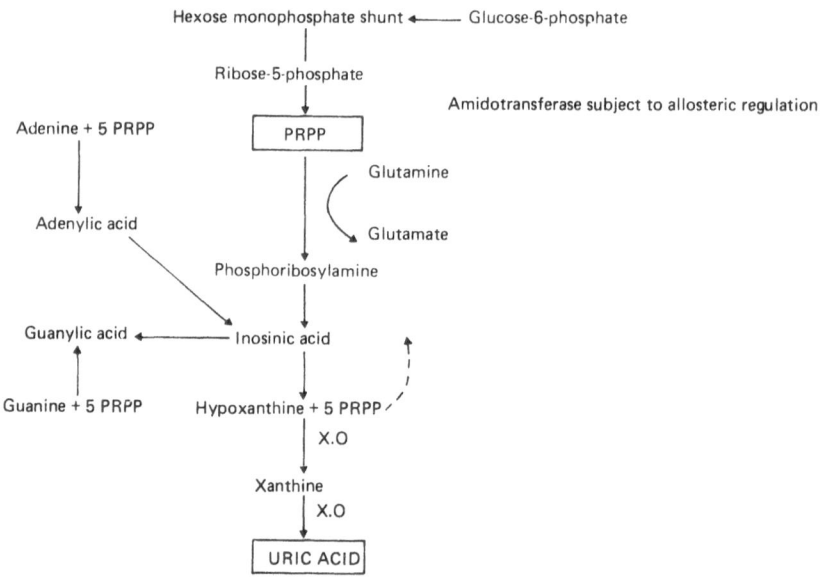

Figure 89. PRPP regulation and uric acid biosynthesis

Details of the system are found in standard biochemical texts. The rate of purine synthesis is undoubtedly determined by the availability of PRPP. In turn this depends on the activity of the hexose monophosphate shunt, for example when uric acid synthesis is increased by fructose infusion. PRPP synthetase (amidotransferase) activity is increased in some forms of gout.

Reutilization of purine bases is more efficient than *de novo* synthesis which is energy requiring. In the brain enzymes for purine synthesis are lacking and it achieves major importance.

Causes of a raised serum urate

These can be categorized as follows:

(1) *Increased uric acid production*
gout (several enzyme defects which increase PRPP availability);
lymphoproliferative diseases and psoriasis causing increased nucleic acid turnover;
Lesch–Nyan syndrome (HGPRT deficiency).

(2) *Decreased renal clearance*
intrinsic renal disease;
gout;
hypertension, hyperparathyroid, idiopathic hypercalcuria;
hypothyroidism.

(3) *Competitive inhibition of renal tubular secretion*
by organic acids such as diuretics, low dose salicylate, pyrazinamide;
by lactate or ketones (as caused by ethanol consumption or by pre-eclampsia, starvation);
in glycogen storage disease.

(4) *Decrease of extra-renal disposal* is not of significance.

It is apparent that a raised blood urate may come to the attention of the nephrologist in any patient with chronic renal failure or hypertension, as part of the investigation of renal stone formation, and when he is called upon to determine whether gout is primary or secondary. Assay of enzymes in red cells or fibroblasts will be of use in the rare congenital anomalies of uric acid overproduction.

Secondary hyperuricaemia due to congestive heart failure, cirrhosis, hypertension, diuretics, alcohol or pregnancy toxaemia should always be sought and identified because it is quite possible for it to accentuate any renal deterioration.

The renal clearance of urate rises progressively with impaired renal function, so the clearance rate per nephron rises. In fact this is due to an increase of tubular secretion. However when the GFR is less than 10 ml/min, tubular secretion becomes less than anticipated, but there is then a decrease in reabsorption to account for increased urine loss. (See below).

Uric acid excretion

700 mg uric acid are produced daily. 500 mg are excreted in the urine and 200 mg are eliminated via the gastrointestinal tract. A urinary excretion of more than 600 mg/day is considered abnormal (36 mmol/l). Patients under assessment should be on a purine-free diet and give three daily urine collections to assess uric acid clearance in comparison with that for creatinine.

Uric acid has a pK_a of 5.7 and so if the urine pH is low, the acid will be insoluble. There are three problems as far as the kidney is concerned: (a) the high serum urate results in high filtered loads to the kidneys; so that (b) uric acid may precipitate in the distal tubules as water is reabsorbed; and (c) because acidification occurs at this level.

There are three distinct components to uric acid excretion: (a) the serum urate is *filtered* at the glomerulus; (b) there is *reabsorption* in the proximal tubule; and then (c) there is *secretion* in the distal tubule. Almost all urate is filtered, yet not quite all because there is loose binding to albumin and to $a\text{-}_1\text{-}_2$ urate-binding globulins. 98% of the urate is then reabsorbed, and the 2% that escapes reabsorption eventually accounts for 20% of that which appears in the urine, the other 80% being derived from distal tubular secretion. The overall result is a urate–inulin clearance of 0.1, so indicating the considerable degree of reabsorption.

Animals such as the rabbit, chicken and dalmatian dog have a urate clearance exceeding that of inulin and indicating a net secretion. The dalmatian dog defect is only found in man very rarely; there is hypouricaemia and a urate–inulin clearance exceeding 0.1. Other animals such as the rat, monkey and mongrel dog have like man a urate clearance that is only 10–20% that of inulin. Clearances can always be increased by infusions of glucose, saline or mannitol.

The *pyrazinamide* (or like pyrazinoic acid—PZA) test produces complete suppression of urate secretion and has been used to elucidate the clearance mechanism. After three study periods of a standard inulin clearance 3g of pyrazinamide is given by mouth, or pyrazinoic acid is given intravenously. After 1h delay three more clearances are determined. Tubular secretion of urate is quantitated from the maximum decrement in uric acid excretion per ml of glomerular filtration rate.

Probenicid is known for its ability to increase urate loss by suppression of tubular reabsorption. Interesting results are obtained if probenicid is given before or after pyrazinamide. When the pyrazinamide is given after probenicid, it actually counteracts its uricosuric effect and causes urate retention. It seems, therefore, that under these peculiar circumstances pyrazinamide stimulates the reabsorption that has been blocked by probenicid. When probenicid is given after pyrazinamide there is no change in excretion. Uric acid studies in animals and man are still somewhat controversial. No drug has been found to increase urate reabsorption; glycine stimulates secretion.

As uric acid is an organic acid it is secreted by the *organic acid secretory mechanism,* so there is competition by a number of natural substances, which accounts for the raised serum urate that occurs in lactic acidosis or ketoacidosis. Salicylates and phenylbutazone show an interesting biphasic effect. The secretory mechanism is sensitive and is blocked by low doses of salicylate, but the reabsorption mechanism is blocked at higher salicylate dosages so that there is then uricosuria.

The extracellular fluid volume influences the proximal tubule reabsorption of both sodium and uric acid. So saline infusion or other form of *volume expansion* will increase uric acid clearances. Although in heart failure there is increased proximal sodium reabsorption and serum urate is raised, in general in sodium-retaining states hyperuricaemia is only provoked by the use of diuretics.

Renal damage due to uric acid

Renal stones

In this country 5% of stones are caused by urates. About 20% of patients with such stones actually have hyperuricaemia and 10% have gout.

Stones may form on account of increased urinary *uric acid excretion* as in gout or in those syndromes in which there is uric acid overproduction, namely myeloproliferative and lymphoproliferative diseases or psoriasis. They also form when there is increased *acidity* of the urine due (a) to reduced ammonia secretion, or (b) loss of alkaline gut fluids with dehydration as in any chronic diarrhoea, or when there are ileostomy problems.

Uric acid damage to the kidney

This causes interstitial nephritis and nephrosclerosis. In addition acute or chronic sodium urate nephropathy is due to uric acid precipitation in the distal tubules and the collecting ducts within the renal papillae. Then there is segmental damage to papillae with tophus formation and interstitial fibrosis. A sclerosing process is induced and the result is vascular sclerosis, glomerulosclerosis and interstitial nephritis with papillary damage which may appear to be a pyelonephritis. In fact about 25% patients with gout have proteinuria, 25% have hypertension, and all have autopsy evidence of renal damage.

In asymptomatic hyperuricaemia or mild gout there can be minimal albuminuria and occasional haematuria, attacks of ureteric colic or loin pain presumably due to crystalluria, and in 25% of symptom-free patients an impairment of renal concentrating ability.

Patients with clinical gout have many vascular problems. Certainly increased atherogenesis is associated with hypertriglyceridaemia and hypercholesteraemia. The type A aggressive striving coronary-prone individual, who has excessive secretion of catecholamines and hyperlipaemia with hyperinsulinaemia, has an elevated blood urate. Indeed there is a triangle of interactions between elevated uric acid–lipaemia–glucose intolerance that accompanies atherosclerosis and to which genetic factors clearly contribute.

Acute uric acid nephropathy

This is most likely to be a consequence of the treatment of reticuloses with cytotoxic drugs or irradiation, so that a sudden catabolism of nuclear material results in uric acid precipitation in the collecting tubules of the kidneys. The result is oliguric renal failure. If this has already happened, it is necessary to insert ureteric catheters and to promote a diuresis of alkaline urine. Clearly prophylaxis is desirable (a) by giving allopurinol (so that xanthine and not uric acid is excreted), (b) by drinking large volumes of fluid, and (c) by taking sodium bicarbonate to alkalinize the urine. Additionally, the chemotherapy should be given as spaced doses rather than as a single massive dose.

CYSTIC DISEASE OF THE KIDNEYS

Cysts in the kidney can pose problems for both the clinician and the radiologist. Classification of the possible types of cysts is as follows:

(1)   renal dysplasia—familial cystic dysplasia;
(2)   polycystic disease—infantile or adult forms;
(3)   renal cysts in hereditary syndromes:
    (a) chromosome disorders;
    (b) phakomatoses;
    (c) tuberose sclerosis;
    (d) Lindau's disease;
    (e) Zellweger's cerebrohepatorenal syndrome;
(4)   diffuse cortical cystic disease;
(5)   renal medullary cysts:
    (a) medullary sponge kidneys (MSK);
    (b) medullary cystic disease complex;
    (c) medullary cystic disease (same as juvenile nephronophthisis) associated with pigmentary retinal degeneration;
(6)   miscellaneous renal cysts:
    (a) hydrocalicosis, associated with stone and with TB;
    (b) hydatid;
    (c) cystic degeneration of carcinoma;
    (d) dermoid;
    (e) intrarenal haematoma.

It will be apparent that most of these conditions are subtle. Enlargement of a kidney is not very common. When a renal swelling is present it moves downwards and slightly forwards on inspiration and is felt bimanually. It has therefore to be distinguished from a spleen on the left and a Riedel's lobe of the liver on the right.

The *usual causes of renal enlargement* are:

236

(1) malignancy—renal carcinoma; Wilm's tumour in a child (embryonic adenosarcoma);
(2) hydronephrosis or pyonephrosis: a tuberculous abscess;
(3) polycystic disease, usually bilateral;
(4) single unilocular or hydatid cyst.

Ultrasonography and CAT scans are now invaluable in differentiation.

Polycystic disease

Infantile form
This is due to an autosomal recessive gene which accounts for a failure of union between the primitive collecting ductules and the nephrons. The kidneys are therefore enlarged at birth owing to cyst formation in the proximal tubules. Other cysts are found in the lungs and liver, and there can be neurological and skeletal deformities. It is a rare condition. Death occurs shortly after birth or within a year.

Adult polycystic disease
The autopsy incidence is 1/500. However 75% cases may not be detected in life since the milder forms may not cause clinical illness. The inheritance is as a Mendelian dominant, so that the progeny have a 50% chance of acquiring the condition. Cysts appear in the collecting tubules of both kidneys, although one organ may be larger than the other. There may also be cysts in the liver and pancreas. Renal failure often does not occur until the age of 40–50. In fact when symptoms appear at the age of 20, chronic renal failure may be anticipated at 40; when symptoms do not appear until 50, then renal failure may appear by 55 years.

The clinical presentation is as:

(a) a *loin mass;*
(b) loin pain, urinary infection or haematuria from the *cysts;*
(c) nocturia as an early symptom of *chronic renal failure.*

Accidental discovery might be early due to *hypertension* or hypertension in pregnancy, or of course during surgery.

The IVU shows cysts of all shapes and sizes and the distortion causes a spidery stretched-out arrangement of the calyces (Figure 77). A high dosage urogram with nephrotomography is essential in order to make out the correct differential features. Diagnostic ultrasound is very useful and isotope scintigraphy might also be used.

The differential diagnosis of polycystic disease is therefore:

(1) multiple cortical cysts, or simple solitary cysts;
(2) bilateral hydronephrosis;

(3)   tuberose sclerosis with hamartomas and cysts;
(4)   bilateral renal carcinomata or adenomata;
(5)   tumour of one kidney and hypertrophy of the other.

Tuberose sclerosis is very rare and consists of a triad of adenoma sebaceum, epilepsy and mental deficiency. In fact not all patients have mental deficiency or epilepsy but intracranial calcification may be found. Hamartomatous 'tubers' occur in the lungs, bone and kidneys, so differentiation from polycystic disease may be necessary.

When the patient with polycystic kidneys reaches the stage of dialysis or transplantation it may be considered advisable to remove the kidneys if there is recurrent renal infection, haematuria or stone formation. There are however compelling reasons for avoiding this if possible, namely (a) the need to preserve a urine output giving the patient flexibility in fluid intake; (b) a higher haemoglobin level, which is a blessing derived from ERP production; and (c) preservation of the metabolism of vitamin D so that there is less renal bone disease.

Simple solitary cysts

These may be cortical and lie just under the renal capsule, or they may lie in a peripelvic situation. Although they might on occasion account for a dull ache or dragging pain, they are more likely to be discovered accidentally. This can occur during the course of an IVU retrograde pyelogram or renal arteriogram, and the above-mentioned investigatory procedures will be required to clarify the diagnosis—it is essential that a renal carcinoma is not missed. If the cyst appears benign, aspiration of the contents with a renal biopsy needle with a view to cytological examination, and also further X-ray after injection of contrast medium will be very helpful.

Medullary sponge kidneys (MSK)

This condition is associated with a normal lifespan and may be asymptomatic, but on the other hand it can present in early adult life on account of urinary tract infections or calculus formation. It does not cause hypertension for salt wasting can be prominent. It occurs in about 1/1000 people.

There is dilatation of the renal collecting tubules so that cysts form in the medullary pyramids. The resulting urinary stagnation leads to (a) hypercalcuria and stone formation, (b) impaired urinary acidification, and (c) infections. Since parathormone-mediated calcium reabsorption takes place principally in the ascending loop of Henle, it appears that a diminished sodium reabsorption at this site accounts for the concurrent hypercalcuria.

The IVU appearance is diagnostic (Figure 90). The kidneys are normal in size or even enlarged, and typically there is a blush at the base of

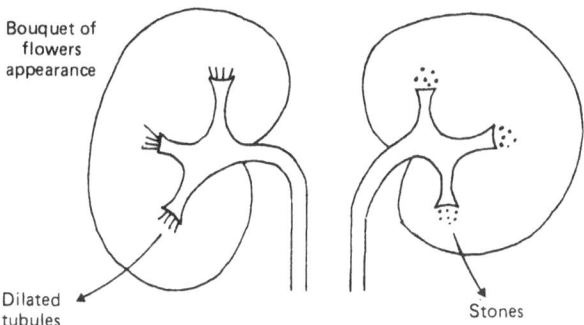

Figure 90.   Appearances of medullary sponge kidneys (MSK)

each renal papilla due to ectasia of the collecting tubules. This may be only unilateral and it may involve only some of the papillae. It is seen best when ureteral compression is applied. Additionally there may be a nephrocalcinosis caused by small calculi in the ectatic ducts and these will be visible on the plain control radiograph.

Juvenile nephronophthisis

This is a cause of small kidneys and renal failure early in life. Children or young adults present with polyuria, enuresis and polydipsia which all indicate a urinary concentrating defect and also salt wasting. Additionally they often have weakness and pallor due to their uraemia, and short stature due to bone disease.

This condition shows genetic heterogeneity since it can be inherited either as a dominant or as a recessive trait. It can be associated with retinitis pigmentosa or other ocular defects.

The nephrons are altered by cyst and diverticular formation along the distal and collecting tubules. Electron microscopy shows intracytoplasmic vesicles and widely dilated intercellular spaces. Thus each suggests that there is active fluid transport involved in the distortion.

This entity therefore, has only a superficial resemblance to medullary sponge kidney. The differential diagnosis between this and polycystic disease is shown in Table 25 below.

Syndromes of renal cystic dysplasia

These are mixed syndromes of chromosomal or single gene disorders associated with neuromuscular dysfunction and obstructive uropathy and renal cysts.

The following syndromes may have to be considered systematically.

Table 25   Points in differential diagnosis

Criteria	Polycystic disease	Medullary sponge kidney MSK	Juvenile nephronophthisis
Loin pain/ haematuria	Present	Occasional	—
Hypertension	Frequent (+ berry aneurysm)	—	—
Impaired GFR	Frequent	—	Usual
X-ray	Large kidneys with cysts; can have calculi	Normal to large Papillary blush Medullary calcification	Small kidneys No calculi
Family	+	Only 20%	+
Lifespan	40–50 years	Normal	10–40 years

Chromosomal anomalies
Trisomy 18 and 13.

Single gene disorders
(1) Zellweger: cerebrohepatorenal syndrome with hypotonia and glaucoma, biliary dysgenesis and renal cortical microcysts;
(2) Ivemark: renal cysts with congenital hepatic fibrosis;
(3) Meckel: encephalocoele, cleft lip, polydactyly;
(4) Jeune syndrome: asphyxiating thoracic dystrophy with constriction of the thorax and renal cystic dysplasia;
(5) Beckwith–Wiedemann syndrome: gigantism, visceromegaly and renal cysts;
(6) Lawrence–Biedl–Moon: renal failure is a frequent cause of death;
(7) Ehlers–Danlos: associated with renal cysts due to the connective tissue defect;
(8) Phakomatoses: An ocular defect associated with neurological visceral or connective tissue abnormality;
    (a) tuberous sclerosis: adenoma sebaceum, mental deficiency with fits and renal hamartomata;
    (b) von Hippel–Lindau disease: angiomata and renal cell carcinoma.

Malignancy in renal cystic disease

Malignancy in polycystic kidneys or the von Hippel–Lindau syndrome is quite possible. Warning signs include an episode of haematuria, discrepancy in renal size, a solid mass on tomography and intrarenal calcification. A renal arteriogram and urinary cytology are essential.

Renal carcinoma (hypernephroma)

This was described in 1883 by von Grawitz who considered that it arises from a 'rest' of adrenal cortex embedded within the kidney. Certainly hypernephroma cells resemble those of the z.fasciculata of the adrenal cortex, since both contain lipoid and glycogen, and 'rests' of adrenal cortex occur on the surface of the kidney. The tumour forms a spherical golden yellow mass which accounts for some 2% of all cancers and 85% renal neoplasms. Typically there is a mass in the loin which results in pain and haematuria, but this only occurs in 15% cases. Some 50% of patients, however, have painless haematuria at some time. Distant metastases tend to occur late but meantime the tumour may spread along the renal vein to cause thrombosis of the vena cava, whilst on the left side renal vein thrombosis may cause a left varicocoele and there may be metastases in the genitals. In the silent phase the patient may be under investigation for weight loss, fever, anaemia, a raised ESR, thrombophlebitis or hypertension.

The urinary lactic dehydrogenase and the urinary alkaline phosphatase will be elevated.

Unusual aspects of renal carcinoma
  (1)   *The pyrexia of unknown origin (PUO)* is accompanied by the refractory anaemia of infection, with a low serum iron and iron-binding capacity, and one or more features of *Stauffer's syndrome*. This refers to the finding of Kupffer cell hyperplasia with mild BSP retention, increased alkaline phosphatase activity, increased alpha-2 globulins with a decreased serum albumin, and possibly a prolonged thrombin time (which is accounted for by raised serum FDP). All these features are reversed by successful removal of the tumour. The alkaline phosphatase originates from the tumour. Indeed note that a rise in serum alkaline phosphatase is useful for confirmation of renal infarction, since the enzyme originates in renal tubules.
  (2)   *Hypercalcaemia* is another possibility and is due either to bony metastases or to parathormone production. As mentioned metastases are late but can occur in many sites. 'Cannonball' secondaries in the lung are characteristic, as also is a predilection for the bronchial mucosa; secondaries commonly occur in the liver and bones.

241

(3)   *Polycythaemia* occurs in some 5% of cases and is due to erythropoietin production. There can also be an impressive leukemoid reaction.

(4)   *Hypertension*. Investigations may lead to the discovery of a hypernephroma; in some cases the tumour might cause renal artery obstruction.

(5)   Coincidental amyloid, polymyositis or dermatomyositis are known to occur.

Summary of the presentations of renal carcinoma

(1)   Loin mass/pain/haematuria;
(2)   unexplained fever and weight loss;
(3)   abnormal liver function tests—Stauffer's syndrome;
(4)   hypertension or proteinuria or haematuria;
(5)   hypercalcaemia;
(6)   polycythaemia or leucocytosis;
(7)   secondary amyloid;
(8)   neuropathy or myositis;
(9)   anaemia, high output heart failure and raised gammaglobulins.

It is clear that as part of the investigations an IVU will be performed and that there are several possible appearances as shown in Figure 91 below.

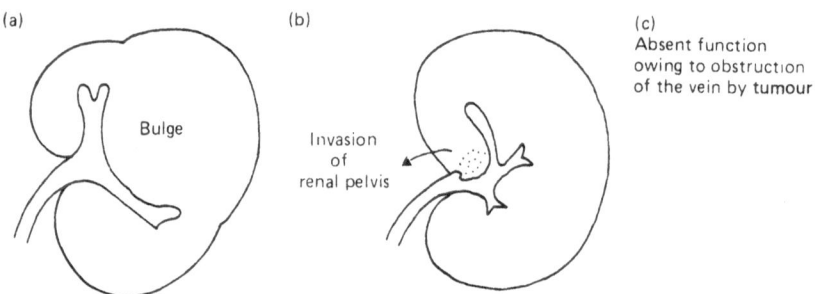

Figure 91.   Hypernephroma appearances

The problem lies in the differentiation of benign cysts, abscesses or secondary malignant growths. If there is calcification in a renal mass, this indicates malignancy. It may be patchy, diffuse or form part of the wall of a cystic tumour.

Isotope scanning, cyst puncture for aspiration of cells and outline of the contents by dye injection, and ultrasonography all play a part in the investigations. Selective renal arteriography is useful to reveal small lesions and also to make the distinction from a benign cyst. A cyst forms only a radiolucent mass, whereas the neoplasm is a vascular structure in which areas of irregular opacification indicate abnormal tumour vessels. Normal vessels can be constricted by adrenaline but not those of a tumour. Then later in the nephrogram phase one should be able to see a benign cyst as a sharply demarcated structure with a thin wall, while a neoplasm has a thick irregular wall and merges with the renal parenchyma.

As part of the further assessment bone, liver and brain scans, a chest radiograph and lymphangiograms are required, since radical surgery is the treatment of choice. Even bilateral nephrectomy followed by dialysis may be a reasonable approach.

Two further points of interest concerning this interesting tumour are (a) its ability to produce a variety of ectopic hormones including parathormone, prolactin, prostaglandins, gonadotrophins, and steroids such as aetio-cholanalone that is known to induce fever, and (b) the occasional occurrence of immune complex glomerulonephritis.

Urine cytology

There is no doubt that this requires expert attention. Although renal adeno-carcinoma cells can occur in urine and are characteristic, exfoliation into the urine is more likely with urothelial transitional cell carcinomata.

CONGENITAL SMALL KIDNEYS

The causes can be briefly summarized as follows:

(1) bilateral symmetrical hypoplasia—causes renal insufficiency and hypertension (page 200);
(2) bilateral asymmetrical hypoplasia ... due to previous pyelo-nephritis;
(3) bilateral oligomeganephronic hypoplasia;
(4) renal dysplasia and other malformation syndromes (such as Ivemark/Jeune/Meckel);
(5) the result of renal artery or renal vein thrombosis very early in life.

Categories (1), (2) and (5) have no certain genetic aetiology and the small kidney is likely to be the result of postnatal inflammatory or ischaemic contraction.

Most cases of renal vein thrombosis are associated with perinatal asphyxia, especially in infants of diabetic mothers. The thrombosis is consequent upon hypercoagulability within the kidneys and progresses from the smaller to the larger renal veins. In some cases there is papillary necrosis. Endotoxinaemia should be considered as a causative factor.

243

Other congenital malformations

As many as 3% of all births might have some congenital anomaly of the urinary tract. Presentation may be early with vomiting and failure to thrive, or as daytime wetting or enuresis leading to the discovery of urinary tract obstruction or malformation. Other cases may only be revealed in early adult life in the course of routine investigation of a urinary tract infection.

These other congenital anomalies may be thought of briefly in terms of of renal location, number of kidneys and amount of tissue.

Renal location
 (1) *Ectopia* refers to a kidney located at the level of the pelvic brim, where it derives its blood supply from the lower aorta or iliac arteries.
 (2) *Horseshoe kidney* when the lower poles are fused.
 (3) *Malrotation* when the pelvis instead of being medial is facing either anteriorly or posteriorly.

Number of kidneys
 (1) Bilateral renal agenesis (Potter's syndrome) which is incompatible with life and which in any case is associated with hypoplastic lungs.
 (2) Unilateral agenesis occurs in 1/1500 cases. Care must be taken not to damage the remaining enlarged kidney.
 (3) Duplication of the renal pelvis or ureters.

Amount of tissue
 (1) Unilateral hypoplasia, as referred to above.
 (2) Foetal lobulation persisting in 3–4% of individuals. It may be necessary to differentiate the projections on the surface of the kidney from cystic change.

CONGENITAL AND FAMILIAL NEPHROTIC SYNDROME

Infant nephrotic syndrome

The nephrotic syndrome in infancy can be due to congenital or acquired causes:

 (1) idiopathic 'congenital' nephrotic syndrome;
 (2) microcystic disease;
 (3) congenital syphilis;
 (4) renal vein thrombosis;
 (5) nail-patella syndrome.

Familial nephrotic syndrome

This may not become fully developed until later. The following conditions should be considered.

(1) *Congenital nephrotic syndrome.*
(a) *Finnish type.* This is inherited as an autosomal recessive. It may be a cause of intrauterine death. Electron microscopy shows only fusion of the foot processes of the epithelial cells. The alpha-fetoprotein of the amniotic fluid is markedly elevated.
(b) A focal glomerulosclerosis or mesangial hypercellularity.
(c) Minimal change nephrosis associated with HLA-B12 (see page 140).
(2) *Amyloid* due to familial Mediterranean fever.
(3) *Alport's syndrome* (page 162).
(4) *Nail-patella syndrome.* This is a skeletal abnormality which after a long period of asymptomatic proteinuria may present as progressive renal failure. The glomerular basement membrane shows thickening and wrinkling and even the appearance in the membrane of collagen fibrils. The associated abnormalities include patella aplasia or hypoplasia, iliac horns, elbow deformities due to hypoplasia of the proximal head of the radii, and also fingernail dysplasia.

INHERITED RENAL TRANSPORT DEFECTS

These can be discussed briefly.

Renal glycosuria and renal phosphaturia

Renal glycosuria is due to reduction of Tm in the proximal tubule leading to impaired reabsorption of glucose. Renal phosphaturia or vitamin D-resistant rickets is due to a proximal tubule and gut phosphate transport defect.

Bartter's syndrome

Sodium loss in Bartter's syndrome accompanies hypokalaemic alkalosis due to renal potassium wasting, increased plasma renin and aldosterone and yet a normal blood pressure on account of insensitivity to angiotensin. Since PGAi infusions lead to facilitation of the aldosterone-stimulating effects of angiotensin, yet abrogation of its pressor response, and indomethacin inhibition of PGA synthesis causes sodium retention, attention was drawn to the role of prostaglandins in Bartter's syndrome. It appears that overproduction of vasodepressor and natriuretic prostaglandins explains the situation. There is hyperplasia of the renal medullary interstitial cells. Prostaglandins will account for proximal tubular rejection of sodium and thereby distal Na–K exchange. Indomethacin with spironolactone therapy is now recommended.

Aminoaciduriasis

There are common transport mechanisms for gut absorption and proximal renal tubular reabsorption of amino acids:

(1) Anion transport system for aspartic and glutamic acid.
(2) Cation carrier system for COAL amino acids: cystine, ornithine, arginine, lysine. This defect accounts for cystinuria.
(3) Neutral amino acid carrier system. Thus in Hartnup disease which presents as skin photosensitivity, cerebellar ataxia, pellagra and mental retardation there is a transport defect of neutral A (alanine type) and L (leucine) amino acids and of the system which transports the ring amino acids, namely phenylalanine, tyrosine and tryptophan.

Bicarbonate wasting (proximal tubular renal acidosis) and *Hydrogen ion wasting* (distal renal tubular acidosis) are discussed on page 50.

BIOCHEMICAL DEFECTS WITH RENAL IMPLICATIONS
Cystinuria

This comes on at the age of 20–30 with staghorn calculi or multiple large smooth renal stones leading to obstructive uropathy, urinary infections and failure. Hexagonal crystals are found in the urine. The cyanide–nitroprusside test confirms the excretion of cystine, and chromatography of urine will reveal COAL.

Cystinosis (Lignac–Fanconi syndrome)

This is a syndrome of renal tubular acidosis with aminoaciduria caused by deposition of cystine crystals in the kidneys, cornea, bone marrow, liver, spleen and lymph nodes. Cystine deposits occur especially in the lysosomes of reticuloendothelial cells. In cystinosis the first part of the proximal tubule is damaged by the high concentration of cystine. The result is that cells grow down from the glomerulus to produce the 'swan-neck' abnormality.

Fabry's syndrome

This is a recessive condition consequent on deficiency of the enzyme trihexosyl-ceramide-galactosyl-hydrolase. Since circulating and urinary levels of ceramide trihexoside are increased and there is deposition of the abnormal lipid in the small blood vessels, even from early childhood patients may have pain in the fingers and toes. Tiny painless angiomatous punctae occur on the skin of male patients, who are affected more than females. By early adult life accumulation of the lipid is beginning to cause more severe problems and eventually there are corneal opacities, retinal vein abnormalities, intracranial haemorrhages and renal failure. The accumulation of trihexosyl-ceramide (Gal-Gal-Glc-ceramide) in the glomerular epithelial cells and tubules creates a characteristic appearance for the epithelial cells are expanded by whorled myelin figures. There are also glomerular foam cells.

Familial gout

Hypoxanthine-guanine-phosphoribosyl-transferase deficiency is one ex-plantation. (HGPRT deficiency—page 232).

Xanthinuria

In xanthine oxidase deficiency the excretion of large amounts of urinary xanthine can lead to stone formation.

Oroticaciduria

Orotic acid is an intermediate in pyrimidine biosynthesis. Accumulation is due to lack of orotidylate pyrophosphorylase and orotidylate decarboxylase. There is a failure of growth, a megaloblastic anaemia which responds only to uridine and excretion of orotic acid crystals in the urine.

Oxalosis

The normal urinary oxalate excretion is less than 40 mg/day, but in primary hyperoxaluria it increases to 100–400 mg/day. Most cases (type I) are due to α-ketoglutarate-glyoxylate-carboxylase deficiency, so that glyoxalate ac-cumulates and is oxidized to oxalic acid. A second type (II) is due to deficiency of the enzyme that would divert some glyoxylate to glycolic acid (Figure 92).

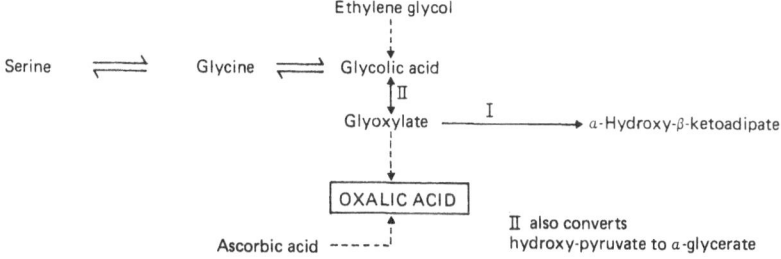

Figure 92. Oxalic acid formation

247

Patients form calcium oxalate calculi so that they have pyelonephritis, hypertension and end-stage renal failure. Oxalate crystals are found in the arteries and myocardium and in the long bones. The crystals lie in the renal tubules where they show a radial or fan-shaped orientation. They remain yellow-brown with haematoxylin and eosin strains but are turned black by von Kossa. Crystals in the urine have the 'coffin lid' appearance.

Familial LCAT deficiency (lecithin-cholesterol acyl-transferase deficiency)

Patients with LCAT deficiency are unable to form cholesterol ester in the usual reaction—cholesterol + lecithin $\longrightarrow$ cholesterol ester + lysolecithin. They develop a normochromic anaemia, proteinuria and lipid deposits in the cornea. Examination of the kidneys reveals a stripping of the endothelium off the basement membrane of the glomerular capillaries. Renal failure ultimately occurs after 15–30 years of symptomless proteinuria.

DIABETES INSIPIDUS

There are three main types:

(1) *Primary idiopathic type* (which may be familial), with a failure to produce ADH. It occurs in both sexes and may appear at any age after infancy. There is reduction of the number of neurones in the supraoptic and paraventricular hypothalamic nuclei.

(2) *Nephrogenic diabetes insipidus,* due to failure of the renal tubules to respond to ADH. Hence there is a defective receptor that should trigger the cyclic AMP 'second messenger', that actually mediates the increase in permeability to water of the collecting tubules.

(3) *Secondary to pituitary disease,* so resulting in a gradual failure of ADH production. Causes include pituitary tumours, trauma, birth injury, postpartum collapse (Sheehan's syndrome) or granulomata e.g. sarcoid, eosinophilic granuloma, tuberculosis or syphilis.

Presentation and investigation

The patient has polyuria and polydipsia so that it is necessary to think in particular of intrinsic renal disease, diabetes mellitus and compulsive water drinking. Therefore the approach will be as follows.

(1) *Measure daily fluid intake and output* and the early morning urine and plasma osmolality. One will expect the urine osmolality to be very low and the plasma osmolality raised.

(2)   *Six-hour water deprivation test.* Start in the early morning and allow no fluids for 6 h. A normal subject is expected to reduce his urine flow to less than 0.5 ml/h, and so urine osmolality will rise to above 800 mosmol/kg.

In the Miller test the same procedure is adopted. The urine is collected hourly until its osmolality is constant. At this stage the plasma osmolality is measured and then an injection of 5 units aqueous vasopressin is given subcutis; urine and plasma osmolalities are measured again after 60 min. In diabetes insipidus the urine osmolality will never rise to that of the plasma but will increase by some 50% after the injection of vasopressin. In normal persons the urine osmolality at the end of water deprivation is very much greater than that of plasma but, being maximally concentrated, it cannot rise more than a further 5% after vasopressin.

(3)   *Partial diabetes insipidus* can pose a real problem for which a strict analytical regime must be followed. The same Miller test is used. Water is deprived until the urine osmolality reaches its maximum, and any rise after the injection of vasopressin is carefully monitored.

Table 26   Expected results in the dehydration/vasopressin test (mosmol/kg)

	U_{osm} *with dehydration*	U_{osm} *after vasopressin*	*Trend*	P_{osm}	*Weight loss*
Normal	1100 ± 200	980 ± 250	—	290 mosmol	3%
Diabetes insipidus	160	460	↑ ↑	305	5%(care)
Partial diabetes insipidus	440	540	↑	295	3%
Compulsive drinking	700	800*	↑	290	4%

* Excessive consumption of water blunts the response of the kidney to administered vasopressin.

Diabetes insipidus used to be treated by the injection of vasopressin and later by use of a snuff, but allergic reactions occurred. Currently the most convenient method is a twice-daily inhalation intranasally of 2.5 ml DDAVP snuff. This 1-deamino-8-D-arginine-vasopressin is a long-acting derivative.

The drugs chlorpropamide, carbamazepine and clofibrate all have some effect in potentiating the action of small quantities ADH. Conversely the thiazide diuretics help by inducing depletion of extracellular fluid, and so increase the fraction of the glomerular filtrate that is reabsorbed in the proximal tubules.

REFERENCES

Calcium, magnesium and phosphate

Bank, N. (1965). Impaired renal concentration–hypercalcaemia. *J. Clin. Invest.*, **44,** 681

Epstein, F.H. (1968). Calcium and the kidney. *Am. J. Med.*, **45,** 700

Gitelman, H.J. (1962). Magnesium deficiency. *Ann. Rev. Med.*, **20,** 233

Knapp, E.L. (1946). Urinary excretion of calcium. *J. Clin. Invest.*, **26,** 182

Krane, S.M. (1956). Urinary excretion of calcium. *J. Clin. Invest.*, **35,** 874

Lemann, J. (1967). Urinary excretion of calcium. *J. Clin. Invest.*, **46,** 1318

Lennon, E.J. (1970). Urinary excretion of calcium. *J. Clin. Invest.*, **49,** 1458

Lim, P. (1972). Magnesium deficiency due to diuretics. *Br. Med. J.*, **3,** 620

Manitius, A. (1960). Impaired renal concentration in hypercalcaemia. *J. Clin. Invest.*, **39,** 693

Massry, S.G. (1967). Steroids and the excretion of sodium, calcium and magnesium. *J. Lan. Clin. Med.*, **70,** 563

Massry, S.G. (1977). Magnesium deficiency. *Ann. Rev. Pharmacol.*,

Vallee, B.L. (1960). Magnesium deficiency. *N. Engl. J. Med.*, **262,** 155

Walser, M. (1962). Ion balance in plasma. *J. Clin. Invest.*, **41,** 1454

Uric acid

Danovitch, G.M. (1972). Uric acid transport in renal failure. *Nephron,* **9,** 291

Gutman, A.B. (1969). Renal function in gout: use of pyrazinamide. *Am. J. Medicine,* **47,** 575

Rastegar, A. and Thier, S. (1972). The physiological approach to hyperuricaemia. *N. Engl. J. Med.*, **286,** 470

Steele, T.H. (1969). Altered renal urate reabsorption during changes in ECF volume. *J. Lab. Clin. Med.*, **74,** 288

Steele, T.H. (1971). Control of uric acid secretion. *N. Engl. J. Med.*, **284,** 1193

Pathogenesis of gouty kidney

Cameron, J.S. (1976). Uric acid and the kidney. *Roy. Coll. Phys. Adv. Med.*, **12,** 378

Emmerson, B.T. and Row, P.G. (1975). *Kidney Int.*, **8,** 65

Nuki, G. (1975). Significance of hyperuricaemia. *Roy. Coll. Phys. Adv. Med.*, **11,** 334

Uses of allopurinol (1971). *Br. Med. J.*, **4,** 185

Renal stone formation

Badenoch, A.W. (1974). *Calculous Disease of the Urinary Tract.* (London: Heinemann.)

Boyce, W.H. (1956). Mucoprotein matrix of calculi. *J. Clinical Invest.*, **35,** 1067

Boyce, W.H. and King, J.S. (1959). Crystal-matrix inter-relations in calculi. *J. of Urol.*, **81,** 351

Chaplin, A.J. (1977). Occurrence and characterisation of calcium oxalate. *J. Clin. Pathol.*, **30,** 800

Coe, F.L. and Raisen, L. (1973). Allopurinol treatment of uric acid disorders in calcium stone formers. *Lancet,* **i,** 129

Crawhall, J.C. *et al.* (1967). Cystine stones dissolved by d-penicillamine. *Br. Med. J.*, **2,** 216

Dent, C.E., Watson, L. (1965). Metabolic studies in idiopathic hypercalcuria. *Br. Med. J.*, **2,** 449

Fleisch, H. (1964). Orthophosphate in the prevention of lithiasis. *Lancet,* **i,** 1065

Fleisch, H., Bisaz, S. and Case, A.D. (1964). Effect of orthophosphate in the prevention of urolithiasis. *Lancet,* **i,** 1065

Harrison, A.R. (1959). Metabolic investigation of stone. *Br. J. Urol.*, **31,** 398

Hodgkinson, A. and Nordin, B.E.C. (1969). *Renal Stone Research Symposium.* (J.A. Churchill Ltd.)

Howard, J.E. and Thomas, W.C. (1968). Control of crystallisation in urine. *Am. J. Med.*, **45,** 693

Kimbrough, J.C. *et al.* (1950). Calculi in recumbent patients. *J. Am. Med. Assoc.*, **142,** 787

Kleeberg, J. (1976). Analysis of calculi. *J. Clin. Pathol.*, **29,** 1038

Leonard, R.H. (1961). Quantitative composition of kidney stones. *Clin. Chem.*, **7,** 546

Modlin, M. (1967). Aetiology of stone: a new concept. *Ann. Roy. Coll. Surg.*, **40,** 155

Nordin, B.E.C. (1973). *Metabolic Bone and Stone Disease.* (Churchill Livingstone.)

Pak, C. (1973). Hydrochlorothiazide therapy for renal stones. *Clin. Pharmacol. Ther.*, **14,** 209

Pak, C. (1976). Management of calculi. *New Concepts in Endocrinology and Metabolism.* Ed. L. Rose and R. Lavine. (New York: Grune and Stratton)

Pak, C., Kaplan, R. and Bone, H. (1975). Simple test for absorptive, resorptive and renal hypercalcurias. *N. Engl. J. Med.*, **292,** 497

Paterson, C.R. (1974). *Metabolic Disorders of Bone.* (Oxford: Blackwell) p. 129

Prien, E.L. (1971). Riddle of urinary stone disease. *J. Am. Med. Assoc.*, **215,** 503

Steele, T.H. (1977). Pharmacology of renal lithiasis. *Ann. Rev. Pharmacol. Toxicol.,* **17,** 11-25

Williams, H.E. (1974). Nephrolithiasis. *N. Engl. J. Med.,* **290,** 33

Wrong, O., Feest, T.M. (1976). Nephrocalcinosis. *Roy. Coll. Phys. Adv. Med.,* **12,** 394

Yendt, E.R. *et al.* (1970). Thiazides in the prevention of renal calculi. *Can. Med. Assoc.,* **102,** 614

Symposium on Renal Stones. (Ed.) L.H. Smith. *Am. J. Med.* **November** 1968

Cystic disease of the kidneys

Boichis, H. (1973). Nephronophthisis with hepatic fibrosis. *Q. J. Med.,* **42,** 221 *Cystic disease of the Kidneys.* Ed. K.D. Gardner. (New York: John Wiley and Sons) 1976

MacDougall, J.A. (1968). Medullary sponge kidneys. *Br. J. Surg.,* **55,** 130

Mitcheson, H.D. (1977). Polycystic disease. *Br. Med. J.,* **1,** 1196

Mongeay, J.G. (1967). Nephronophthisis. *Am. J. Med.,* **43,** 345

Malformations

Kissane, J.M. Malformations in *Pathology of the Kidney.* R.H. Heptinstall ed. Churchill. Ltd.

Williams, D.I. (1961). Congenital anomalies. *Practitioner,* **186,** 467

Tumours

Badenoch, A.W. (1974). Tumours of the upper urinary tract. *Manual of Urology.* (London: Heinemann)

Kiely, J.M. (1966). Hypernephroma. *Med. Clin. N. Am.,* **50,** 1067

Ochsner, M.G. (1965). Hypernephroma. *J. Urol.,* **93,** 361

Riches, E.W. (1951). New growths of the kidney and ureter. *Br. J. of Urol.,* **23,** 297

Trott, P.A. (1977). Ureteric urine examination. *Br. J. Hosp. Med.,* **17,** 493

Biochemical anomalies

Crawhall, J.C. (1964). Cystinuria. *Br. Med. J.,* **1,** 1411

Dent, C.E., Senior, B. (1955). Cystinuria. *Br. J. Urol.,* **27,** 317

Eberlein, W.R. (1953). Aminoaciduria in childhood. *Am. J. Med. Sci.,* **225,** 677

Fichman, M.P. (1976). Prostaglandins in Bartter's syndrome. *Am. J. Med.,* **60,** 785

Gjone, E. and Norum, K.R. (1968). LCAT as a familial deficiency. *Acta Med. Scand.*, **183,** 107

Hunt, D.D. (1966). Fanconi syndrome. *Am. J. Med.*, **40,** 492

Kjessler, B. (1975). Congenital nephrotic syndrome. *Lancet*, **i,** 432

Milne, M.D. Renal transport defects. In Thompson and Wootton, eds. *Chemical Pathology*, 3rd Edition. p. 553 (Churchill.)

Morris, R.C. (1969). Renal tubular acidosis. *N. Engl. J. Med.*, **281,** 1405

Myhre, E. and Gjone, E. (1977). LCAT as a familial deficiency. *Nephron*, **18,** 239

Robinson, M.G. (1960). Nephrogenic diabetes insipidus. *Am. J. Dis. Child.*, **99,** 164

Scriver, C.R. and Rosenberg, L.E. (1973). *Amino acid Metabolism and its Disorders.* W.B. Saunders Co.

Wade, D.N. (1969). Renal tubular disorders. *Br. J. Hosp.*, **2,** 820

Williams, T.F. (1968). Vitamin D resistant rickets. *Ann. Intern. Med.*, **68,** 706

9
Acute renal failure

If the blood urea rises and urine output falls, one has to consider the following categories of acute renal failure:

(1) *Prerenal failure*, when there is impairment of the renal circulation either due to blood loss or dehydration, or due to a poor cardiac output.

(2) *Acute intrinsic renal failure*, which signifies ischaemic or nephrotoxic damage resulting in focal acute tubular necrosis. Recovery of function may then take 2–3 weeks.

(3) *Postrenal failure*, when there is obstruction to the outflow of urine, as by stone or pelvic neoplasm. In this latter situation one clue may be total anuria which can alternate with periods of normal flow.

Acute intrinsic renal failure was fully documented in the Second World War as 'crush syndrome'. After an episode of traumatic *shock*, particularly when complicated by muscle damage and supervening sepsis, there developed a period of *oliguria*, with associated uraemia and hypertension. This would last for a few days during which the mortality was high. Then in the recovery phase there would be *polyuria* prior to restoration of normal function. In the final event the GFR might be permanently reduced by 20%.

255

This situation is not due to haemorrhagic shock *per se,* for this is a form of prerenal failure that is easily reversible by transfusion. It rarely leads on to acute tubular necrosis. Superimposed trauma or sepsis makes all the difference.

Tubular poisoning affects the proximal tubules, since a nephrotoxin arriving by the bloodstream will reach these first. On the other hand renal ischaemia causes 'tubulorrhexis' in which there is widespread and random necrosis with an associated disruption of the basement membrane. The actual necrosis can be quite elusive, but the lower segments of the nephrons often show foci of epithelial necrosis and associated casts block the tubular lumina. There is an accompanying interstitial inflammatory reaction with thrombosis of small venules. With late histology this phase will be missed and instead the distal tubules are seen to be lined by flattened non-necrotic epithelium, and there is patchy interstitial oedema and cellular infiltration. The glomeruli almost always look normal by light microscopy. Rarely there may be some evidence of focal glomerular thrombosis. The proximal tubules show only some minimal degeneration or cloudy swelling.

Of course the problem is that biopsy or autopsy material is always obtained some days after the initial shock-event that led to the establishment of the ischaemic lesion. Some clue as to the nature of the initial insult comes from the recognition that there is, in both animals and man, a spectrum of disease ranging from the extreme situation of renal cortical necrosis, to situations in which there is some minimal glomerular thrombosis, to acute tubular necrosis, and finally to that more common situation in which there is only some focal tubular degeneration (Figure 93).

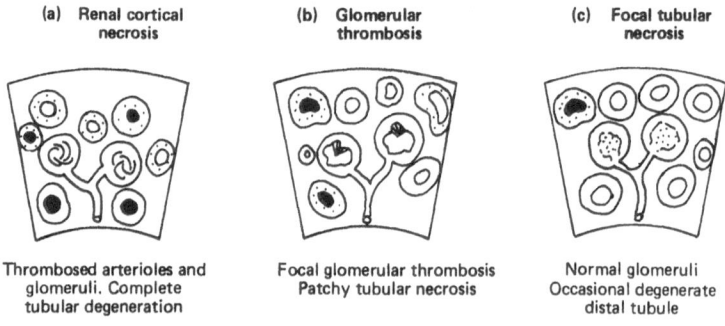

(a) Renal cortical necrosis

(b) Glomerular thrombosis

(c) Focal tubular necrosis

Thrombosed arterioles and glomeruli. Complete tubular degeneration

Focal glomerular thrombosis Patchy tubular necrosis

Normal glomeruli Occasional degenerate distal tubule

Figure 93.   The histological spectrum in acute intrinsic renal failure

PATHOGENESIS

The events in Figure 93 suggest that the *vasoconstriction* of shock causes a profound reduction in renal cortical blood flow and plays an important role in determining ischaemic tubular damage, but that there is in addition a liability to *thrombosis* within the renal circulation. This thrombosis is manifest when the lining endothelium of the arterioles and glomeruli has been completely damaged, as in renal cortical necrosis, but often it is so evanescent that evidence will later be lacking in biopsy material.

Therefore apart from those types of acute renal failure that are due to recognized nephrotoxic chemicals and drugs, the pathogenetic factors which lead to acute ischaemic renal failure are as shown in Table 27.

Table 27 Pathogenetic factors leading to acute ischaemic renal failure

Factors causing the initial increase of renal vascular resistance	Factors mitigating against re-establishment of the circulation
Sympathetic nervous vasoconstriction	Endothelial cell swelling
Catecholamine vasoconstriction	Sludging of red cells
Angiotensin II generation (local?)	Clumping of platelets and leucocytes
Disseminated intravascular coagulation (DIC)	Fibrin thrombi
Endotoxinaemia	Interstitial oedema

Sympathetic nervous vasoconstriction

In traumatic shock the pain and loss of blood each cause sympathetic nervous vasoconstriction of peripheral arterioles which help to maintain the central circulation to the most vital organs. The renal cortex is not privileged and like the skin and muscles is the site of intense vasoconstriction. Clearly such a mechanism helps to reduce fluid losses.

Initial renal vasoconstriction acts at the postglomerular level and can thus decrease renal blood flow from 1250 to 800 ml/min, while still maintaining a normal GFR. This means that an extra 400 ml/min blood is available for distribution in the main circulation. Then hypovolaemia causes renal vasoconstriction at both the afferent and efferent arterioles producing a reduction in renal blood flow to 500 ml/min so that 700 ml/min is available for redistribution, but the GFR now falls to 80 or even 50 ml/min. When trauma is so severe as to produce such low filtration rates, the superadded coagulation may cause acute renal failure.

Assessment of renal blood flow by the ^{133}Xe washout technique shows that preferential renal ischaemia of the outer renal cortex is the cause of the suppression of glomerular filtration. Once established renal vaso-constriction may persist from a few hours to several days, depending on the renal insult. However, by the time that patients are fit for study total renal blood flow may be back to 30–40% of normal, even though they remain oliguric.

Catecholamine release from the adrenals

This plays an important supportive role. Most nervous reflexes are easily fatigued and the humoral factor, noradrenaline, is a most important accessory to the vasoconstrictive process.

It is also not so widely known that stimulation of the alpha-adrenergic receptors of blood vessels leads to activation of clotting via Hageman factor XII. In this way sympathetic activation is linked to the genesis of local intra-arteriolar and capillary thrombosis.

The renin–angiotensin system

Renal ischaemia leads inevitably to release of renin by the juxtaglomerular apparatus so that there are high levels of plasma renin activity in both shock and acute renal failure, and local angiotensin II generation could be a cause of continued renal cortical ischaemia. Indeed Thurau has made the important point that when sodium-rich fluid reaches the macula densa owing to failure of proximal reabsorption, local angiotensin II generation causes a reduction in glomerular filtration until such time as the tubular epithelium is healing! Otherwise there would be massive fluid losses.

Disseminated intravascular coagulation (DIC)

As Hardaway has pointed out there comes a phase in all types of shock when there is stasis of blood in dilated capillaries, where the pH is very acid owing to the accumulation of local metabolites such as lactate. This blood clots so that there is no chance of intermittent blood flow through the capillaries, as is normally the case, and the result is focal tissue necrosis.

Additionally in those situations in which there is tissue trauma, thrombo-plastins enter the circulation and cause disseminated intravascular coagula-tion. This is particularly evident as the formation of platelet aggregates and fibrin microthrombi in the main venous stream; they result in the picture of 'shock lung'. That process is also accompanied by the formation of activated coagulation factors which in passing to the arterial system can give rise to microthrombi, especially in those arteriolar beds in which there is vasoconstriction. Thus muscle damage may in theory give rise to fibrin microthrombi in the kidneys; in reality this is not so common because active fibrinolysis dissolves away the microthrombi. However, it is known that there can be a profound post-traumatic inhibition of fibrinolysis. Clearly this will result in the persistence of platelet aggregates and thrombi in the arterioles and capillaries.

It is an interesting fact that the causes of acute renal failure are identical with the many situations in which disseminated intravascular coagulation is known to occur (Table 28). Animal experiments demonstrate that local intrarenal coagulation is associated with impairment of renal blood flow not only on account of mechanical obstruction, but also because aggregating platelets release serotonin, which is a powerful vasoconstrictor, and fibrino-peptides and fibrin degradation products have weak vasoconstrictor effects that work in synergism with angiotensin.

Endotoxinaemia

The factors which account for acute renal failure can be summarized as follows:

(1)	Infection	40%
(2)	Trauma	12%
(3)	Obstetric	11%
(4)	Primary renal disease	15%
(5)	Obstruction	7%
(5)	Nephrotoxins	10%
(6)	Carcinomata	5%

It can, therefore, be seen at a glance that endotoxinaemia could complicate as many as 50% of cases of acute renal failure. Since Gram-negative bacteraemia is increasing, endotoxin is now (and probably was in the various wars) the major cause of acute renal failure. This is another way of saying that the spectrum of acute renal failure outlined above is, in fact, a modified Shwartzman reaction. In its classical form the Shwartzman reaction means that when a rabbit is given two spaced doses of endotoxin by intravenous injection, the end result will be renal cortical necrosis. Endotoxin is a powerful vasoconstrictor agent, which also damages vascular endothelium causing coagulation and inhibition of fibrinolysis. Additionally it triggers disseminated intravascular coagulation by causing platelet damage. Thus after the first injection there is a minor episode of DIC (Figure 94) and the products of that coagulation and the endotoxin itself lead to blockade of the reticuloendothelial phagocytic system, (represented principally by the Kupffer cells of the liver) so that when a second dose is given there is

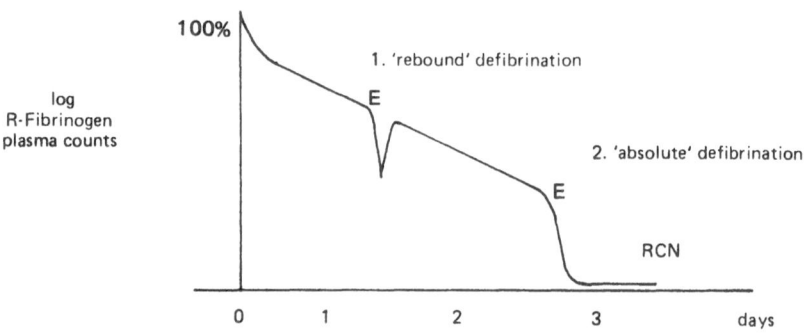

Figure 94.   DIC initiated by the first and second doses of endotoxin

widespread intravascular coagulation and the result is renal cortical necrosis. Initial contact with endotoxin in fact damages Kupffer cells, but if liver blood flow is restored, recovery is rapid.

The Shwartzman reaction need no longer be defined by the histological finding of renal cortical necrosis, since a variety of more subtle tests applicable to dynamic situations are available:

(1)   the study of coagulation factors;
(2)   labelled platelet studies;
(3)   the radiofibrinogen catabolism study;
(4)   the detection of endotoxin by the Limulus lysate assay and radio-immunoassay.

Knowledge accumulated in this way has led to the conclusion that endotoxin does indeed account for the majority of cases of acute renal failure and also for the adult post-traumatic respiratory distress syndrome (shock lung) from which many of these patients die.

Moreover, animal studies have made it clear that endotoxin itself is capable of causing (a) sympathetic nervous vasoconstriction, (b) catecholamine release, (c) renin–angiotensin activation in the whole animal, and (d) disseminated intravascular coagulation. It is thus a deadly and destructive agent. Studies also show that, by manipulation of the dose, the same spectrum as is seen in acute renal failure can be produced by means of endotoxin given either intermittently or as a continuous infusion.

Cell swelling and sludging of the blood cells

Although we can accept that continued activation of the renin–angiotensin system is a cause of prolonged renal vasoconstriction, since the macula densa is stimulated by the high sodium content of the tubules owing to depression of proximal tubular resorption, there are other important local causes. Often the vascular endothelium has been damaged and is swollen, as also are the tubular cells, and restoration of blood flow is impaired. The process can be facilitated by means of a hyperosmolar agent such as mannitol. One knows in addition that the microscopist is used to seeing sludged red cells and platelet aggregates, which signify that there is a local increase in blood viscosity.

Functional cause of the oliguria

Endotoxin damage is widespread and has numerous modes of action, but the physiologists have always sought to define a single mechanism that will explain oliguria. The following are to be considered:

(1) Afferent arteriolar constriction; this will explain cessation of filtration.
(2) Necrosis of tubular epithelium allowing passive backflow of fluid; clearly such necrosis has to be extensive.
(3) Intrarenal renin release at the macula due to sodium that has not been reabsorbed proximally. So intrarenal renin depletion by chronic sodium loading is known to confer some resistance to experimental acute renal failure.
(4) An increase in renal vascular resistance due to depletion of the vasodilator prostaglandins, in particular endothelial prostacyclin.

THE DIAGNOSIS OF ACUTE RENAL FAILURE

Patients with acute intrinsic renal failure pass less than 400 ml/day urine, or less than 50 ml/day in the case of a child. Their blood urea, therefore, rises at 6–8 mM/l per day if they have moderate protein catabolism, but at 10 mM/l per day when there is post-operative or post-traumatic catabolism. Infection, or bleeding into the gut causing a protein load, also worsen the position.

It is useful to consider those factors which affect the rate of urea accumulation, because they are relevant to the management of renal failure.

(1) *Urea production* is increased by high protein diets, tissue catabolism, steroid-induced protein catabolism, and tetracycline-induced protein catabolism. It is reduced by a low protein diet or by a high calorie diet.
(2) *Urea excretion* is reduced by any form of renal failure. A transient rise of urea due to prerenal uraemia is to be expected after major surgery, but there is concern when the level continues to rise. Such patients have to be followed by daily estimations of the blood urea and electrolytes.

The specific features of acute renal failure, as opposed to prerenal uraemia, are:

(1)   a urine SG<1014;
(2)   a urinary sodium above 20 mmol/l;
(3)   a urinary urea below 133 mmol/l (and thus urine osmolality<360 mosmol/kg);
(4)   a urine/plasma urea ratio of less than 10;
(5)   a urine/plasma osmolality ratio of less than 1.1.

It is very important to confirm acute intrinsic renal failure by measuring these indices.

When cardiac insufficiency is causing prerenal failure and a rising urea, a high central venous pressure (CVP 20 cmH$_2$O) will indicate an urgent need for digoxin and frusemide therapy and, the use of a short-acting vasodilator such as dopamine or chlorpromazine in order to encourage the kidneys to secrete urine and reduce the hypervolaemia.

Table 28   Causes of acute renal failure

Shock	Obstetric	Haemolysis with DIC	Hyper sensitivity	Other DIC	Liver disease	Direct nephrotoxins
Haemor-rhagic.	Septic abortion	Malaria	Due to anaphyl-axis:	Haemorrhagic pancreatitis	Acute hepatic with renal failure	Chemicals: mercury, arsenic, ethylene
Septic.	Detached placenta.	Incom-patible trans-fusion	serum sickness:	Carcinomata Extracorporeal circulation	Obstructive jaundice	glycol, paraquat
Trau-matic	Amniotic fluid		acute nephritis	Proteolytic enzymes.		Antibiotics:
Heat stroke.	embolism.		IVP or chole-cystogram			kanamycin: colomycin: gentamycin
Burns.	Eclamptic		collapse			amphotericin
Fat em-bolism.						methicillin polymyxin B sulphonamide
Pan-creatitis.						cephaloridine
Muscle injury						

One must also be aware that in burns, sepsis and acute pancreatitis a *polyuric type* of acute renal failure may occur. Urinary urea concentrations and urine osmolality do not have the same predictive value in these circumstances, but the blood urea and serum creatinine still rise. In fact it is important to stress that when renal failure is induced in animals by endotoxin, there is a phase of polyuria which precedes the oliguria. Polyuric renal failure is discussed (page 274).

Knowing the situation in which acute renal failure has developed is often sufficient to establish the diagnosis. An episode of shock and a fall of the urine output are the usual clinical clues, but it has been emphasized that urine volumes can remain high.

DEFENCES AGAINST DIC AND ENDOTOXINAEMIA

As emphasized above, apart from those situations in which there is some toxin acting on the tubular epithelium, all the other conditions known to cause acute renal failure are also recognized to be situations in which DIC can occur. The outcome of these syndromes depends very much on the patient's defences against intravascular coagulation. There are two main lines of defence (Figure 95): (a) the plasma fibrinolytic system, which may or may not be inhibited by the level of plasma protein fibrinolytic inhibitors, and (b) the activity of the reticuloendothelial system, which is represented principally by the Kupffer cells of the liver.

Whether or not microthrombi persist in the microcirculation, so as to give rise to foci of tissue necrosis, is crucial to the outcome of these shock syndromes.

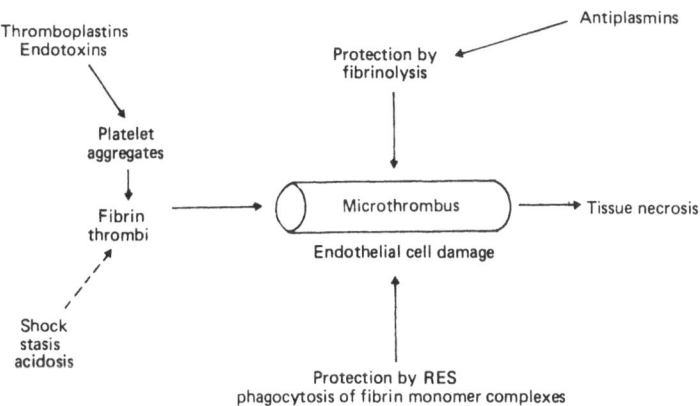

Figure 95. The principle of DIC and the defences against it

Since Gram-negative sepsis is so often linked to the onset of acute renal failure that it can be said with confidence that most cases of renal failure in the context of trauma or shock are 'Shwartzman equivalents' (Hjort and Rapaport, 1965), the body defences against endotoxin and how they can be supported are of increasing interest.

The normal defences against endotoxins and Gram-negative bacterial are as follows.

Action by the Kupffer cells

First, there is phagocytosis of bacteria by polymorphs and the Kupffer cells in a complement-dependent interaction.

Second, there is clearance and inactivation of endotoxin by the Kupffer cells. Exactly how endotoxin is cleared by the Kupffer cells is under intensive investigation. However, it is certain that esterases are capable of inactivating endotoxin in those Kupffer cells that have acquired 'resistance' to membrane lysis by endotoxin. This situation presents a paradox whose explanation appears quite simple: Kupffer cells may be inactivated and even destroyed by their first contact with endotoxin, but thereafter they become resistant and capable of neutralizing the toxic lipid-A end of the molecule.

The endotoxin may be circulating freely in the systemic or portal blood or it may be bound as an antigen–antibody complex according to the nature of the antibodies that the patient already has. All patients have some antibodies to the O-antigens of *E. coli* and other organisms but because the other antigens are relatively inaccessible, there are many patients who do not have adequate antibodies to the CEA (common enterobacterial antigen) and lipid-A antigens. Since lipid-A is the toxic part of the endotoxin molecule which actually destroys cell membranes, this is indeed an alarming situation. Reference to Figure 76 shows that the toxic lipid-A is a concealed antigen. Indeed few normal persons have raised titres of antitoxin (antilipid-A antibody).

Inactivation by non-specific esterase

It has been shown by Skarnes that endotoxin in the blood becomes bound to an a_1-lipoprotein and that final inactivation is achieved by an alpha-l-globulin, which acts as an esterase of the organophosphate-resistant type. This makes sense since the lipid-A end of the molecule is rich in long-chain fatty acids such as myristic acid.

These esterases function more efficiently when the serum calcium is low and, in fact, this is a common feature in endotoxinaemia.

Inactivation by polymyxins

Polymyxins will bind to the endotoxin binding site of cell membranes and thus prevent the noxious effects of the lipid-A. They are thus endotoxin-neutralizing agents, as also is colistin but the action of the latter is weaker.

Other means of combating endotoxins

The commonest organism in the bowel is *Bacteroides fragilis,* which is an anaerobe. It is a common cause of endotoxinaemia, although it may not be grown if the appropriate cultures are not requested. It can be controlled by Flagyl (metronidazole) which is given either orally to sterilize the bowel or intravenously.

Charcoal and various resins will also bind endotoxins and haemoperfusion (p. 381) is likely to come into greater use in the future.

Once a diagnosis of endotoxinaemia is established, it is normally wise to give that patient methylprednisolone (Solumedrone). This has the following beneficial actions, although on account of its long-term immunosuppressive effects therapy should be restricted to one or two pulse doses (15 mg/kg):

(1)   It reduces the powerful vasoconstrictor responses to endotoxin.
(2)   It protects cells against the damaging effects of endotoxins and thus against lysosomal enzyme release.
(3)   Although in large dosage steroids will paralyse the Kupffer cells, smaller dosages appear to facilitate endotoxin inactivation.
(4)   Renal blood flow is more likely to be maintained.

THE MANAGEMENT OF ACUTE RENAL FAILURE

The shock phase

Maintenance of blood volume and blood pressure
If the perfusion of the kidneys and also of the liver (so that there is Kupffer cell protection) can be maintained in a patient with haemorrhage, trauma or septicaemic shock, there is little risk of acute renal failure. Once endotoxinaemia is established it is difficult to combat. Such patients develop oliguric or polyuric renal failure. Fluid deficits should be replaced using central venous pressure monitoring. Blood, plasma or saline should not be spared.

Mannitol, dextran and frusemide therapy
Mannitol, an osmotic diuretic and anti-sludging agent which maintains renal cortical blood flow, is a safe means of establishing urine flow. 25 g is given intravenously within 3 min and within 2 h the urine output should increase to 40 ml/h. In such a case the patient only has prerenal uraemia. A like dose is given intravenously in the early stage of high-risk operations such as those for obstructive jaundice, cardiac bypass surgery and burns.

Dextran is also known for its ability to prevent circulatory sludging. It should, however, be used with care for if too much is filtered into the tubules when there is a poor urine flow, it will be reabsorbed by the proximal tubules and so cause swelling of the epithelium, known as an 'osmotic nephrosis'. A reduced urine output is a contraindication to dextran. More than 500 ml should not be given if the urine output is less than 1½ l/day, if the specific gravity of the urine exceeds 1045, of if the blood urea is above 10 mmol/l (60 mg%). Even normally no more than 1 litre day dextran should be given; in fact each year one sees several patients whose acute renal failure has been precipitated after surgery by misuse of dextran.

Frusemide therapy is justified if the patient is overhydrated and is indeed capable of passing urine. But if the patient is already volume depleted, its use may worsen acute renal failure. Frusemide, in any case, does not alter the course of established acute intrinsic renal failure, but only increases the free water clearance.

Summary of vital measures
The following measures are therefore mandatory:

(1) Treat causative factors including volume depletion.
(2) Flush the renal circulation with mannitol.
(3) Treat sepsis vigorously. This will mean the use of antibiotics and metronidazole for anaerobes, as well as possible surgery for evacuation of pus. Consider more specific antiendotoxin measures such as the use of steroids, isoprenaline infusion, and whether heparinization for septic (non-traumatic) shock is justified. Polymyxin infusion and charcoal perfusion might also be used.
(4) At the same time any nephrotoxic aminoglycosides should be stopped.

Intravenous dopamine is currently being advocated for support of the circulation in various types of shock and heart failure. The infusion is started at 0.5–1.0 µg/kg per min and is carefully increased to 10 or even 20 µg/kg per min. It can cause nausea and vomiting, but it has the triple advantage that:

(1) It is a potent renal vasodilator by reason of stimulation of dopamine receptors.
(2) It increases cardiac output by stimulation of cardiac beta-receptors.
(3) It causes peripheral vasoconstriction and a rise of arterial blood pressure.

Intravenous isoprenaline is slightly more dangerous as it can precipitate cardiac arrhythmias. Nevertheless it is a pure beta-stimulant that is very good at increasing myocardial contractility and output. An infusion is started at 2 µg/kg per min and is gradually increased to 6–8 µg/kg per min.

Heparin at a dosage as low as 5000 units intravenously every 6 h will help to prevent DIC in endotoxin shock. Larger dosages should only be used if there are facilities for accurate monitoring of coagulation. A Dale and Laidlaw coagulometer can be used at the bedside for a simple measurement of clotting time. (Lancet 1970, ii, 1006.) One can then give 10 000 units of heparin stat followed by an infusion of 1000–2000 units/h. Figure 96 summarizes the phases through which the patient with acute oliguria will pass. The phases are discussed in detail below; they are self-explanatory if the characteristics detailed above are considered.

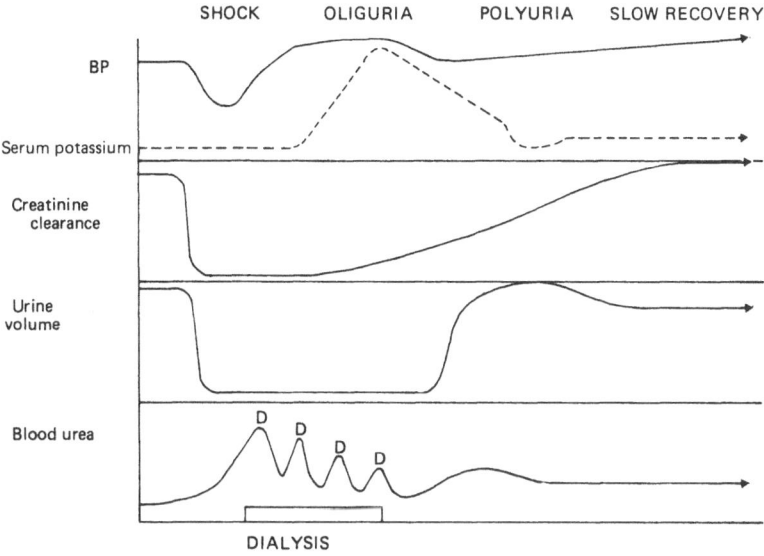

Figure 96. The phases of acute tubular necrosis

The oliguric phase

In special centres confused uraemic oliguric patients sometimes turn up from nowhere with muddled stories which have been inadequately documented. The first task therefore is to ensure that one is truly dealing with acute intrinsic renal failure. Many patients in fact turn out to have insidious chronic renal failure that has undergone a sudden deterioration.

In pre-existing chronic renal failure, there is evidence of:

(1)   anaemia, so that the haemoglobin is less than 10 g/100 ml;
(2)   a systemic acidosis;
(3)   pigmentation and scratch marks indicative of pruritis;

(4)　possible loin masses signifying polycystic kidneys or hydronephrosis;

(5)　evidence of retarded growth or renal bone disease;

(6)　small size of the kidneys on plain abdominal X-ray, if the cause is either chronic glomerulonephritis or chronic pyelonephritis.

At this stage renal biopsy is not practical because the patient is too ill and heparinization for dialysis may follow. There are, however, accessory aids to diagnosis. If a patient has complete anuria one should suspect urological obstruction and a story of anuria alternating with episodes of polyuria also suggests obstruction. In that case a high dose IVP using 150 ml of Conroy 280 might be tried. The possibilities are:

(1)　Chronic glomerular disease—there is a faint nephrogram owing to poor concentration of the contrast medium but often a reasonable pyelogram.

(2)　Acute tubular necrosis—there is a good nephrogram that persists for hours or even days and yet since there is no urine secretion, there is no pyelogram.

(3)　Acute renal vein thrombosis—there is a good nephrogram on the unaffected side.

(4)　Acute obstruction—there is usually sufficient contrast excreted to show up a dilated calyceal system, a stone, or an asymmetrical obstructive pattern.

A word of warning is appropriate here. An intravenous urogram in the oliguric patient can be dangerous as the high viscosity of the contrast medium, precipitation of proteins in the renal tubules and a uricosuric effect of some dyes can all lead to anuria. It is well known that this can happen in myeloma, but it is less well recognized that it may happen in any oliguric patient and particularly in patients who have hypertensive renovascular disease or shrunken kidneys due to chronic nephritis or diabetes.

If the story of acute tubular necrosis due to shock is clearcut and the patient is oliguric but not in need of urgent dialysis, it is still standard practice to try the effect of either 500 mg frusemide given intravenously or 50 ml/25% mannitol. It must be realized that these drugs can cause an increase of 'free water' excretion without having any effect on established tubular necrosis. They are meant to select any missed cases of prerenal failure.

When using mannitol it must be remembered that it can provoke pulmonary oedema. Moreover since mannitol shifts water from the intracellular to the extracellular compartment it leads to a decrease of the serum sodium concentration. This can be interpreted as dilutional hyponatraemia, which is in any case common in this situation.

The priorities in established oliguria are to:

(1) Assess fluid balance and the electrolytes.
(2) Attend to nutrition and the minimization of protein catabolism.
(3) Institute dialysis to correct uraemia, hyperkalaemia, and fluid overload.
(4) Try to prevent superimposed infection.

It is important that the following are avoided.

(1) Catheterization, since this introduces infection.
(2) Intravenous infusions, which load the patient with fluid and ruin the veins.
(3) Immobilization, since this predisposes to deep venous thrombosis.
(4) Display of unnecessary and nephrotoxic antibiotics.

Fluid balance and electrolytes
Many patients arrive with signs of fluid overload; they have a raised jugular venous pressure, pulmonary oedema, and ankle and sacral oedema. In any case it is essential to *restrict fluid intake* to 400 ml/day (the amount that the patient can lose by perspiration) and only later to allow in addition an amount equal to the volume of urine that is being passed. Remember that metabolic water that is produced by oxidation amounts to 300 ml/day.

The patient's urea and electrolytes will naturally be estimated immediately on admission. *Hyperkalaemia* can cause cardiac arrest and arrhythmias. It is easily corrected by dialysis and emergency treatment is seldom needed, but the choices are:

(1) To give 50 g dextrose (100 ml/50%) with 20 units of soluble insulin i/v, so that glucose with potassium moves temporarily into the body cells.
(2) To give 40–80 mEq (40–80 ml) 8.4% sodium bicarbonate i/v.
(3) If there is minimal acidosis, to give 50–100 ml 10% calcium gluconate i/v.
(4) To use a rectal enema of 20–60 g of resonium-A polystyrene sulphonate ion-exchange resin. This, however, releases 3 mEq sodium/g resin which is absorbed by the gut and leads to sodium loading. Calcium phase resin is preferable.

If there is very severe *hypertension,* this requires treatment using intravenous diazoxide, methyldopa or sodium nitroprusside infusion. This applies particularly to patients who have become oliguric on account of acute nephritis or accelerated hypertension. Otherwise hydralazine is used.

It is also very important, since uraemic *gastric atony* produces nausea and vomiting and potential aspiration pneumonia, to pass a nasogastric tube and to aspirate the contents of the stomach. At the same time this procedure may reveal whether there is any *gastrointestinal bleeding*. Nausea and vomiting are now best controlled by the use of Maxolon (10 mg orally or i.m.) or by Torecan (thiethylperazine 10 mg orally or i.m. or as a suppository).

Diet and nutrition

In the oliguric phase one must give a diet of 20–30 g protein only, with no more than 30 mEq each of sodium and potassium (0.5 g of sodium chloride is 22 mEq), and in order to limit protein catabolism it is vital to ensure a high carbohydrate and calorie intake. The patient may be able to tolerate dextrose drinks, but with fluids such as Hycal the problem is that the high glucose content may lead to delayed gastric emptying and nausea; it should therefore be diluted. Protein catabolism can be reduced by giving injections or tablets of an anabolic steroid, such as Deca-durabolin 50 mg/2 weeks or 25–50 mg/day norethandralone orally.

So, therefore, the immediate prescription for the oliguric phase will read:

(1) fluids: 400 ml/day;
(2) diet: 20 g protein; 100 g CHO 20 mEq/day of Na^+ (all food must be cooked without salt) and only two helpings of fruit and vegetables — and the latter must be cooked in water for 30 min; K 30 mEq/day;
(3) daily dialysis;
(4) resonium (calcium phase) 15 g q.i.d.;
(5) Vitamins: Albee with C 1 g/day; norethandralone 10 mg t.i.d. Epanutin 100 mg t.i.d. to prevent any convulsions.

Doctors have to understand how to translate a dietary prescription into practice. A basic diet could be:

(1) *20 g protein* comprising 75% first class protein, i.e. one egg/one-third pint milk, together with 25% second class protein, i.e. 180 g potatoes, fruit and vegetables; and this is made up to
(2) *3000 calories in toto* by use of high carbohydrate additives such as 56 g salt-free butter/jam/sugar/double cream, 1 bottle Hycal, and low protein bread and low protein pasta.

Dialysis

One great advantage of dialysis is that fluid balance is easily corrected, so the patient can be fed on an intravenous nutrition regime using dextrose, fructose or sorbital with amino acids and some added insulin, and by the use of Intralipid. Indeed the need to provide adequate calories may be the most important reason for daily dialysis. Additionally in hypercatabolic patients (in whom the blood urea is rising more than 10 mmol/l per day) daily dialysis is necessary to control the uraemia.

Dialysis should be instituted as soon as is possible. The rule is always to dialyse early so as to keep the blood urea below 200 mg% (33 mmol/l); the only discussion centres around the method. Peritoneal dialysis is available in all institutions and can be used as an interim measure. Haemodialysis, however, is a much more efficient way of rapidly removing excess fluid and potassium. It requires the insertion of a silastic arteriovenous shunt, but this can be done under local anaesthesia in about half an hour.

As an alternative, a Seldinger puncture in the femoral vein may be utilised, so as to insert a large bore catheter into the vena cava that is then used as the 'arterial line', with the venous return line running into an arm vein. In small children it is possible to dialyse by means of fine catheters passed up the long saphenous veins.

At the onset of dialysis one has to be very much aware of the 'dialysis dis-equilibrium syndrome'; which is due to a delay in the equilibrium of urea across the blood-brain barrier (Figure 97). Rapid dialysis can result in osmotic swelling of the brain. (See also Figure 131.)

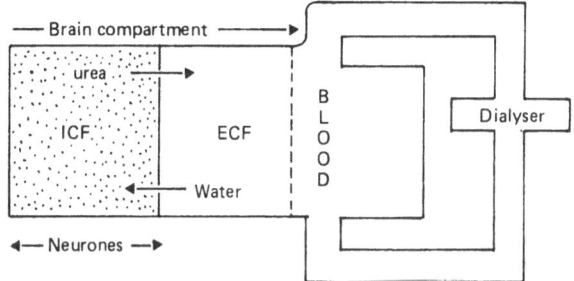

Figure 97. Explanation of dialysis dis-equilibrium

At first dialysis has to be restricted to 2–4 h per session, although by the end of the first week 6 h dialyses are possible. During this time there is a risk of convulsions and the patients should be given prophylactic injections of Epanutin 100 mg three times daily; if a fit does occur, it can be controlled by giving i/v diazepam (Valium). It must be remembered that uraemic patients are much more liable to respiratory depression from sedative drugs, particularly as hyperkalaemia itself can induce muscle weakness.

Prevention of infection
The mortality of acute renal failure following trauma is at least 50% in spite of good intensive care and dialysis. Deaths in the early phase are undoubtedly due to the original endotoxinaemia which was consequent on the traumatic shock. This probably causes the acute renal failure and most certainly contributes to the 'shock lung' which is the explanation for these early deaths.

271

A patient who has an intravenous drip regime, a nasogastric tube, a urinary drainage, who is being dialysed by means of a shunt or catheters and who may even have a tracheostomy and be on a mechanical ventilator, is at considerable risk from secondary infection. Uraemia *per se* impairs the phagocytic defence mechanisms, and wound infections occur in some 50% persons with acute renal failure.

Attention to the following points of detail are essential:

(1) The patient should be barrier-nursed in a closed ventilation cubicle.
(2) All effluents and septic sites should be cultured and appropriate antibiotics used.
(3) Regular mouth toilet, and aseptic handling of tracheostomies should be used.
(4) Early mobilization and chest physiotherapy should be instituted; catheterize only when necessary.
(5) Closed-system peritoneal dialysis should be used.

Antibiotics in renal failure

When antibiotics are used, they must be bactericidal and be prescribed in accordance with the sensitivities of the infecting organisms. Additionally since antibiotics themselves can be nephrotoxic, attention must be paid to a dosage schedule which is adjusted to the patient's glomerular filtration rate (see Chapter 12).

It is clear that the half-life of drugs normally excreted by the kidneys will be prolonged in renal insufficiency, even though alternate pathways of metabolism might become important. Additionally one has to allow for dialysis losses, so it is normal to give a drug such as *gentamycin post-dialysis*. In a patient with acute renal failure and Gram-negative infection the MIC for the pathogen might be $4\mu g/ml$, so the policy is to give 1 mg/kg body weight post-dialysis, producing a peak serum level'of $8.8\mu g/ml$ which after some 22 h is down to $4.0\mu g/ml$. A serum level of $10\mu g/ml$ is regarded as toxic and is to be avoided, while therapeutic levels ought to be in the range $5-7\,\mu g/ml$.

Gentamicin is liable to cause ototoxicity and nephrotoxicity. In fact, if its elimination constant $k\,(= \log 2/\,T\frac{1}{2})$ is plotted against the creatinine clearance, it will be found that it rises with GFR up to a clearance of 70 ml/min when the drug has a normal half-time of elimination of 2.5 h (Figure 98).

With a normal urine clearance one would give the standard loading dose of 1.7 mg/kg every 8 h. As the GFR falls so does the dose of the drug that can be given, in logarithmic fashion, so that at a GFR of 10 ml/min this loading dose will be reduced to 0.3 mg/kg. Such nomograms are available for many drugs (see Chapter 12).

However, this is a complicated system and where possible some rule of

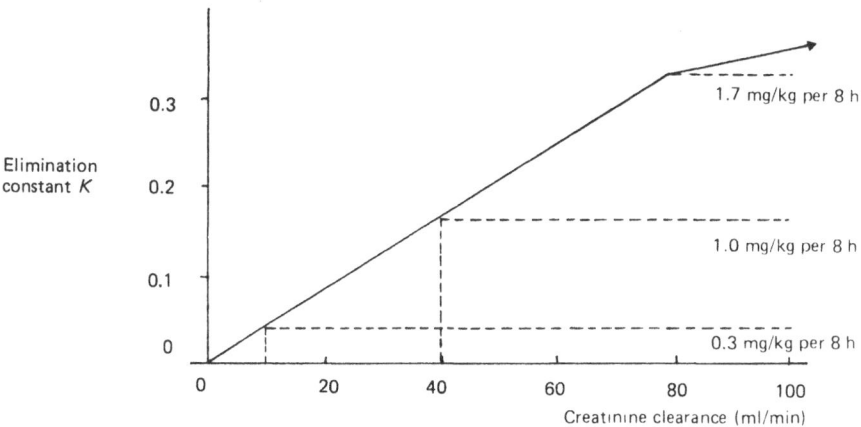

Figure 98.   Gentamicin elimination and creatinine clearance

thumb has to be adopted. Simply to reduce the drug dosage according to a scheme is a reasonable approach. The *rule of eight* is that a normal gentamicin dosage is 1 mg/kg every 8 h, and that this time interval is prolonged according to the level of the serum creatinine, so if it is 200 *u*mol/l the dosage schedule could be 80 mg every 16 h. Other antibiotics are administered as shown in Table 29.

Table 29   Antibiotic administration

12 h	*24 h*	*48 h*	*72 h*
Carbenicillin	cephalosporins	gentamicin*	streptomycin
Penicillin G	minocycline	ethambutol	kanamycin
Methicillin	isoniazid	colistin	
Ampicillin	cotrimoxazole		
Nalidixic acid	allopurinol		
Phenothiazines	azathioprine		
Aspirin			
Phenobarbitone			

* when the serum creatinine is 600 *μ*mol/l, according to the rule of eight.

273

The polyuric phase

When urine output starts to improve (say 750 ml/day), the patient may be allowed freedom from strict fluid restriction. Even so the blood urea may not begin to fall until the urine output is 2l/day.

At first the tubules do not concentrate the urine, so the patient may go through a phase in which he passes 3–4l/day. He then runs the risk of sodium, potassium and water depletion, and this has to be treated with intravenous crystalloid infusions.

At this stage also the patient will be anaemic, and remain so for weeks.

Histological evidence of tubular regeneration can be seen within 48 h of the initial injury. The tubules show large cells with basophil cytoplasm and dense nuclei, and an occasional mitosis. However, the actual regeneration takes some weeks, as it includes the reconstitution of brush borders and intracellular organelles; this explains the prolonged phase of impaired urine concentration that can last at least 3 weeks and sometimes for months.

Renal function will return to normal within 1–2 years but many patients show some evidence of glomerular filtration reduction, indicating glomerular loss, and there is an accompanying interstitial fibrosis.

POLYURIC ACUTE RENAL FAILURE

From the outset these patients have urine volumes greater than 600 ml/day and yet a serum creatinine in excess of 200 μmol/l. Whereas in oliguric renal failure the urinary sodium is usually over 60 mmol/l, in the polyuric type it can be in the range 20–60 mmol/l. The urine/plasma urea ratios are higher (for example, oliguric 3.3: non-oliguric 7.0). Many cases occur in association with sepsis, pancreatitis or burns. With a urine osmolality of 340 mosmol/kg (which is average for a polyuric case) if the patient excretes 1250 ml urine, he will lose only 400 mosmol of solute. In sepsis, however, the solute loads may be 600–1000 mosmol so there will be a positive solute accumulation and progressive nitrogen retention.

The possible causes of the polyuria are briefly as follows:

(1)   There is hyperosmolaemia in septic patients which facilitates renal vasodilation and diuresis.

(2)   Although there is cortical ischaemia, there may be juxtamedullary washout secondary to increased medullary blood flow.

(3)   Low-grade endotoxinaemia is causing pyrogenic activation of renal prostaglandin synthesis and thereby renal vasodilatation, especially in the inner renal cortex and medulla.

274

HAEMOLYTIC—URAEMIA SYNDROME (HUS)

In 1955 Gasser described a syndrome of young children who have oliguric renal failure in association with purpura and a haemolytic anaemia, with evident red cell fragmentation. In the florid case there are thrombi in the glomerular capillaries and in the renal arterioles, so that there is a gradation from patchy tubular damage to areas of cortical necrosis. By the light microscope there may only appear to be thickening of the glomerular capillary walls, but electron microscopy shows that there is really a separation of the endothelium from the basement membrane by accumulation in the subendothelial space of granular material, which gives a positive immunofluorescence for fibrin. At a later stage the subendothelium is invaded by the phagocytic mesangial cells, so that ultimately the appearance will resemble mesangiocapillary glomerulonephritis. In the arteries the thrombi become organized into the walls which therefore show intimal fibrosis, hyalinization and fibrinoid necrosis. Narrowing of the arterioles can then be the cause of persistent hypertension.

The red cell fragmentation has been shown by Brain and Regoeczi to be due to tearing of erythrocytes on fibrin strands in the small vessels. The red cells have the appearance of 'tear cells', 'helmet cells' or 'schistocytes' or they can simply be referred to as fragmented cells; they are distinct from those 'burr cells' or spiny cells which merely represent the sick cells of the uraemic state. Cell tearing explains the haemolysis. The thrombocytopenia is likewise caused by fibrin deposition in small vessels and seems to reflect a Shwartzman reaction to endotoxin. Certainly some agent has caused damage to vascular endothelium, just as in the analogous syndrome of thrombotic thrombocytopenic purpura, which is a variant of SLE in which antibodies to vascular endothelium are found. There is endothelial prostacyclin deficiency.

HUS commonly occurs between 3 and 10 months of age. It is often preceded by a gastrointestinal upset or urinary tract infection, giving credence to the endotoxin theory. Indeed many children have *E. coli* or Shigella diarrhoea. Moreover hypogammaglobulinaemia has been described as a predisposing factor in such young infants and there can be transient depression of C3 and partial conversion of factor B (properdin) to Ba and Bb products. However, many other precipitating factors have been noted. There are reports of the syndrome in South and Central America due to an haemorrhagic virus infection. Coxsackie A virus enteritis, Echo, influenza and infectious mononucleosis have all preceded the syndrome, as also have inoculations with live measles vaccine. Certain drugs such as the oral contraceptives, pyran copolymer, and ergometrine as given for post-partum haemorrhage have also been implicated.

Although there is a spectrum of disease, clinical forms can be identified:

(1) *Mild cases* without anuria but with oliguria, hypertension or convulsions.

(2) *Anuric cases* accompanied by neorological symptoms such as convulsions, stupor, aphasia or hemiparesis, and also hypertension.

(3) *Progressive oliguria and hypertension.*

(4) *Recurrent* haemolytic–uraemic syndrome in which the first episode is mild but months or years later there is a further episode.

The characteristic red cell picture enables a prompt diagnosis but the prognosis is closely correlated with the extent of the renal vascular damage. The half-life of infused platelets is shortened and fibrinogen catabolism can also be accelerated. Whether DIC is diffuse, as would be expected in endotoxinaemia, or whether it is localized to the kidneys is not really clear for in fact the endotoxaemia probably occurs in the early phase of the illness. There are anecdotal reports of the efficacy of heparin. However, it is also certain that some cases may show spontaneous recovery, while others may have prolonged anuria which necessitates dialysis. Even in children who recover there is a high incidence of renal dysfunction, and for this reason fibrinolytic therapy has been advocated. Systemic streptokinase infusion is dangerous but encouraging results have been claimed for combined heparin–streptokinase infusion by means of a catheter in the aorta at the level of the renal arteries. In fact, the amassed data from several centres does suggest a better outcome with heparin therapy (78% survival for treated patients and only 43% otherwise).

Steroid therapy is of no value. There is no serious argument in favour of platelet-inhibitory drugs unless an ongoing immunological process can be demonstrated as in TTP. In this latter situation plasma exchange should be considered; it may hasten endothelial recovery.

THE LIVER AND THE KIDNEYS

The functional renal failure of cirrhosis

Long after the initial diagnosis of cirrhosis the patient develops a 'functional renal failure' in which there is oliguria leading on to uraemia and terminal hyperkalaemia. The kidney, however, is histologically normal and it can be transplanted successfully into a suitable recipient. It is for this reason that the main problem is thought to be renal hypoperfusion due to a reduction of the 'effective plasma volume'. Such patients have reached an advanced stage of liver disease in which they have a high serum bilirubin, a low serum albumin and a prolonged prothrombin time, and also an elevated blood urea. In general such patients also have a low arteriolar resistance and a high cardiac output. Yet the renal cortical hypoperfusion, which can be readily demonstrated by xenon washout studies, raises the question as to whether (a) the cardiac output is actually high enough; or (b) is the vasoconstriction due to a pooling of the blood volume in the veins of the splanchnic bed entirely caused by 'functional hypovolaemia'? In this case powerful diuretics should be avoided.

That the latter is indeed the case is suggested by the fact that volume expansion by ascites reinfusion or a peritoneojugular shunt causes a rise of blood pressure, and an increase in renal blood flow, and hence a diuresis in most of these patients. Added to this there is certainly a suspicion in some patients of impaired myocardial function, since although the left ventricle appears to behave normally and may even be in a high output state in relation to the low arteriolar resistance, cardiac failure can easily be precipitated. The majority of patients have alcoholic cirrhosis, so some degree of cardiomyopathy or coronary artery disease is to be anticipated.

The typical *clinical features* of this state are:

(1)   Increased plasma and extracellular fluid volume seen as *oedema and ascites,* due to continuing sodium retention which is related to increased renin and aldosterone generation, due in turn to decreased renal plasma flow.

(2)   A decreased diuresis after water loading, in other words an *inability to excrete free water.*

The possible *pathogenetic factors* are therefore:

(1)   Diversion of blood from the kidneys due to effective volume depletion and thus active renal vasoconstriction.

(2)   Potential cardiac insufficiency owing to
        (a) functional hypovolaemia due to splanchnic pooling;
        (b) superadded myocardial dysfunction.

The actual mechanism of hepatic ascites can be viewed as in Figure 99.

The features of the cirrhotic renal performance of physiological interest are:

(1)   the active vasoconstriction;
(2)   the inability to excrete free water;
(3)   the relevance of renin;
(4)   the role of aldosterone in causing sodium retention;
(5)   enhanced proximal sodium reabsorption.

Active vasoconstriction
Studies by means of the ^{133}Xe washout technique and by renal

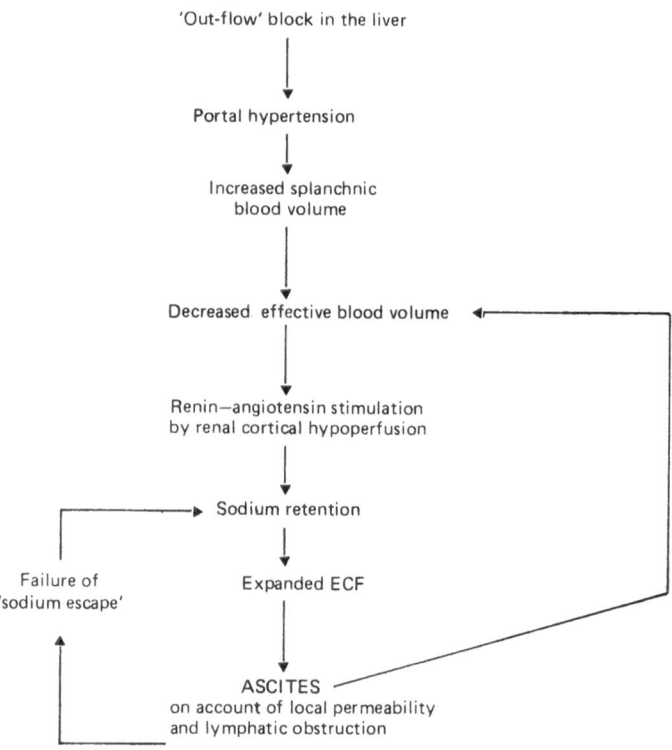

'Out-flow' block in the liver

Portal hypertension

Increased splanchnic
blood volume

Decreased effective blood volume

Renin—angiotensin stimulation
by renal cortical hypoperfusion

Sodium retention

Failure of   Expanded ECF
'sodium escape'

ASCITES
on account of local permeability
and lymphatic obstruction

Figure 99. Genesis of hepatic ascites

arteriography confirm that there is a marked reduction in renal cortical perfusion in cirrhosis. They also show that the active vasoconstriction is marked by haemodynamic instability. Together a low cardiac output and reduction of the effective plasma volume could be the whole answer. Also vasoconstriction as a result of endotoxinaemia seems to be quite a possibility, even though such patients have high *E. coli* antibody titres and the mechanism has to involve endotoxin—antibody complexes.

The renal cortical vasoconstriction actually means a diversion of blood flow from the glomeruli of those cortical nephrons that have short loops of Henle and are thus 'salt losers', and instead a greater perfusion of the juxtamedullary nephrons that are known to be 'salt-retaining'. This difference can be shown up by deconvolutional analysis of the clearance curve of an intravenous bolus of radioiodohippurate as measured by a detector over each kidney. Normally there is a first peak at 2½ min followed by a second at 5 min; the former is the highest, but when there is redistribution of flow from the outer cortex, the second peak is the larger. Thus it is possible that the redistribution itself causes salt retention.

The inability to excrete free water
This might also be due to increased plasma flow to the juxtamedullary nephrons, for then there could be an increased hydrostatic pressure in the capillaries around the loops of Henle of a magnitude sufficient to reduce sodium reabsorption. Hence free water excretion would be diminished.

Plasma renin levels
These are high in the patient with cirrhosis and especially so when there is renal failure. This occurs even though renin substrate, which is synthesized by the liver, is low, and in some cases is quite a limiting factor in angiotensin generation. Without doubt any factor that reduces renal perfusion is a strong stimulus to renin release and it is often difficult to separate cause and effect. However the increased plasma renin falls when renal blood flow is increased by volume expansion or dopamine, so it seems that renin release is secondary factor. All the same the combination of a low bradykinin (a vasodilator) and elevated renin will lead to vasoconstriction.

The role of aldosterone
There is compelling evidence that distal tubular sodium reabsorption as mediated by aldosterone has to be increased in cirrhosis. The renal handling of sodium, osmols and water can be expressed as sodium clearance (C_{Na}), osmolar clearance (C_{osm}) and free water clearance ($UV-C_{osm}$). With normal water and salt intake both the C_{Na} and the C_{osm} average 1–3% of the glomerular filtration rate. Yet the clearance of free water (C_{H_2O}) is usually negative, reflecting the excretion of concentrated urine. A decrease in either renal blood flow or effective circulating blood volume causes C_{Na} and the C_{osm} to fall indicating sodium conservation. Conversely damage to the juxtamedullary nephrons causes C_{Na} and the C_{osm} to increase. The actual distal tubular aldosterone effect for those patients with a positive C_{H_2O} is estimated by dividing the free water clearance by the clearance of free water plus sodium. Hence the formula

$$\frac{C_{H_2O}}{C_{H_2O} + C_{Na}} \times 100$$

gives the percentage of distal tubule sodium reabsorption. In general when cirrhotic subjects are compared with normal control patients during hypotonic *saline* infusion, it is found that they have a reduced delivery of sodium from the proximal tubule to the distal reabsorbing site. Aldosterone-mediated sodium reabsorption is also taking place in those with cirrhosis.

279

Undoubtedly the patient with ascites and hyperaldosteronism fails to 'escape' from the sodium-retaining effect. Although, in theory, this might be due to impaired production of the natriuretic hormone, in fact it is more simply explained by leakage of ascitic fluid into the peritoneum.

Proximal sodium reabsorption
There are some cirrhotic patients who produce a low volume of hypotonic urine during water diuresis which suggests that they have excessive proximal as well as distal sodium reabsorption. Moreover the fact that the urine can be hypotonic excludes antidiuretic hormone as the cause of the low urine volume. In fact all patients with cirrhosis have an increase in sodium reabsorption in their proximal tubules, which is based on the sequence:

   (1)   vasoconstriction causes decreased glomerular filtration and a low hydrostatic pressure in the peritubular vessels;
   (2)   so there is increased sodium reabsorption in the proximal tubules;
   (3)   in turn there is less sodium available for reabsorption in the loops of Henle, and this causes a lowered medullary interstitial pressure;
   (4)   but this is counteracted in part through increased sodium reabsorption by aldosterone acting on the distal tubules.

Thus at all levels of GFR the cirrhotic patient produces a lower urine volume/min than normal persons. As mentioned their free water clearance is reduced, whereas it would be increased if distal tubular sodium reabsorption were the only problem. GFR values are always reduced and proximal tubular reabsorption of fluid amounts to 80% of the filtered fluid, while normally it is 65%.

In practice many patients with cirrhosis have GFRs in the range 20–90 ml/min so that sodium retention is due to a combination of reduced renal perfusion and hyperaldosteronism. In the later stages of cirrhosis the GFR is reduced from 20 down to 3 ml/min and even lower. These patients have a low urinary sodium of less than 10 mmol/l, and yet a hyperosmolar urine with a high urea (U/P > 10/l). This indicates that there is intact tubular function and confirms the functional basis for the defect. Additionally the reduction of free water clearance explains the development of water overload and the frequent occurrence of hyponatraemia.

When the GFR is less than 3 ml/min the urine becomes virtually iso-mosmolar, and the urine sodium is then high at more than 15 mmol/l. These findings indicate the occurrence of renal tubular necrosis at such poor levels of perfusion. Indeed it has been shown that under these circumstances there is a proximal tubular dysfunction, as shown by lysozymuria.

Quite early on in cirrhosis radiofibrinogen catabolism studies and a lowering of the platelet count will prove that there is a continuing intravascular coagulation. Unlike those conditions that lead to acute renal failure, there is a marked increase of fibrinolysis in cirrhosis so no permanent fibrin deposition. However since fibrin degradation products can act synergistically with other peptides to cause contraction of smooth muscle, a role for this process in the renal failure of cirrhosis is yet possible.

The management of ascites

It has already been emphasized how easy it is to induce prerenal uraemia in the patient with cirrhosis and ascites. The advice now given is to treat ascites with spironolactone alone for as long as possible, and to avoid the powerful loop diuretics. Patients need not be subjected to sodium restriction, which always leads to hyponatraemia. Instead paracentesis can be used to remove no more than 2 l of fluid at a time in order to make the abdomen comfortable. In refractory cases a Le Veen shunt can be inserted.

As for the practical diuretic therapy of ascites, it does follow from what has been said that there are probably three categories of patient.

(1)   There are patients who can still excrete adequate salt and water so that they can be treated by a low sodium intake only.

(2)   There are many who have a poor capacity to excrete sodium, but who still have a high free water excretion. Ideally they are treated with a low salt intake together with distal tubule inhibitory diuretics such as spironolactone or triamterene; frusemide is best avoided.

(3)   There are those patients with such a low GFR that they can neither excrete salt nor water, and few of these will respond to diuretics. Ascites reinfusion at this stage is too late but insertion of a peritoneovenous Le Veen shunt may help. Haemodialysis is of no help to such patients.

Renal azotaemia induced by diuretics

Unfortunately prerenal failure which has been induced by diuretics is common in the cirrhotic patient. It is characterized by an increased blood urea and a decreased GFR, yet there is a high urinary flow and high urinary sodium concentration. The patient actually looks dehydrated, although there may be ascites. It is less likely to occur in the cirrhotic patient who has peripheral oedema. The treatment is simply to stop the diuretics.

Intrinsic renal failure in association with cirrhosis

Occasionally a patient who has chronic nephritis as well as cirrhosis will be found. There is likely to be significant proteinuria with casts, a low urinary urea and a low urine/plasma osmolality ratio (less than 1.3). This could indicate acute tubular necrosis except that in this latter there is an acute oliguria, while the patient with chronic renal failure passes a good volume of poor quality urine.

Hepatic failure with renal failure

In this context one is concerned with patients with acute hepatic necrosis due to infectious or serum hepatitis, paracetamol overdose or multiple halothane exposure who develop a progressive or sudden terminal renal failure. The patients have oliguria with a urine volume of less than 400 ml/day, a low GFR and, of course, azotaemia. In fact there seems to be a spectrum of change from a functional renal failure as in cirrhosis (in which it is known that the kidneys have normal histology) to definite acute tubular necrosis. Very often the situation seems to be precipitated by a gastrointestinal haemorrhage, abdominal paracentesis or by an infection. In these situations the Limulus lysate assay for endotoxin is almost always positive, indicating a Gram-negative bacterial cause. Since these patients are usually being nursed under intensive therapy conditions with a nasogastric tube, urinary catheter and intravenous fluid regime a source of entry can often be found. Failing this one has to assume that the endotoxin has gained entry to the portal bloodstream from the bowel and that because of shunting or Kupffer cell dysfunction, there has been a failure of the normal inactivation mechanisms. The escape of endotoxin into the general circulation will undoubtedly cause renal vasoconstriction and possibly the renal tubular necrosis (see page 260).

At this point, therefore, it is useful to summarize the tests which help with the differential diagnosis of these various types of renal failure (Table 30).

Table 30   Tests for differential diagnosis of renal failure in liver disease

Type	24 h urine volume	U/P osmolality	Urine sodium
Functional renal failure	600 ml	1.2–1.8	<15 mmol/l
(cirrhosis or hepatic failure)			
ATN (with liver disease)	<400 ml	1.0	>15 mmol/l
Chronic renal failure	>600 ml	1.1	>40 mmol/l

Acute tubular necrosis with obstructive jaundice

If the term 'hepatorenal syndrome' is used at all, it is best reserved for the patient with obstructive jaundice who gets acute tubular necrosis. Often it is precipitated by acute ascending cholangitis or by operation on the biliary tract or pancreas. Moreover, it is known that the longer a patient has obstruction before operation is attempted, the more likely is it that the patient will develop renal ischaemic damage. Therefore Dawson has advocated the preoperative administration of 1.5 litres of glucose-saline and an infusion of 5% mannitol prior to and for 48 h after operation.

All this suggests that obstructive jaundice sensitizes the renal parenchyma to ischaemic damage. In fact conjugated bilirubin, although albumin-bound, will filter into the urine in free form and in being reabsorbed will cause degenerative mitochondrial changes in the renal tubules, indicative of its effect in causing uncoupling of oxidative phosphorylation. Additionally the elevated serum bile acids tend to damage the renal vascular endothelium and may cause a loss of the protective fibrinolysis (see Figure 95 page 263).

The real blow comes, however, when there is endotoxinaemia from the biliary tract. The effect can be particularly devastating because the Kupffer cells of the liver are not well perfused and are unable to detoxify the endotoxin molecule with their usual avidity.

REFERENCES

Clinical acute renal failure

Alexander, R.D., Berkes, S.L. and Abuelo, J.G. (1978). Contrast media-induced oliguric renal failure. *Arch. Intern Med.*, **138**, 381

Anderson, R.J. (1977). Non-oliguric renal failure. *N. Engl. J. Med.*, **296**, 1134

Bates, C.P. (1970). Post-operative renal function. *Br. J. Surg.*, **57**, 361

Cameron, J.S. (1967). Renal function due to burns. *Br. J. Surg.*, **54**, 132

Clarkson, A.R. (1969). Post-partum renal failure: the generalised Shwartzman reaction. *Aust. Ann. Med.*, **18**, 209

Fletcher, J.R. (1971). Renal function after sepsis in combat casualties. *Surg., Gynecol. and Obstet.*, **33**, 237

Hermreck, A.S. (1972). Polyuria of sepsis. *Surg. Forum*, **23**, 53

Lindsay, R.M. (1965). Post-operative renal function. *Lancet*, **i**, 978

Lucas, C.E. (1973). Altered renal homeostasis with sepsis. *Arch. Surg.*, **106**, 444

Maddox, D.A. (1977). Glomerular filtration in response to injury. *Ann. Rev. Med.*, **28**, 91

Maher, J.F. and Schreiner, G.E. (1962). Cause of death in acute renal failure. *Arch. Intern. Med.*, **110**, 493

McEvoy, J., McGowen, M.G. and Kumar, R. (1970). Contrast media-induced oliguric renal failure. *Br. Med. J.*, **4,** 717

Muehrck, R.C. (1969). *Acute Renal Failure: Diagnosis and Management.* (St. Louis: C.V. Mosby)

Ray, J.F. (1974). Post-operative renal failure. *Arch. Surg.*, **103,** 175

Rosenberg, I.K. (1971). Renal insufficiency after trauma and sepsis. *Arch. Surg.*, **103,** 175

Selmonosky, C.A. (1969). Renal failure after cardio-pulmonary bypass. *Arch. Surg.*, **99,** 64

Stone, W.J. (1974). Post-traumatic renal insufficiency in Vietnam. *Clin. Nephrol.*, **2,** 186

Swan, R.C. and Merrill, J.P. (1953). Clinical course of acute renal failure. *Medicine*, **32,** 215

Teschan, P.E. (1955). Post-traumatic renal insufficiency. *Am. J. Med.*, **18,** 172

Vertel, R.M. (1967). Non-oliguric renal failure. *J. Am. Med. Assoc.*, **200,** 598

Whelton, A. (1969). Vietnam experience compared with Korea. *Johns Hopkins Med. J.*, **124,** 95

Pathogenesis—circulatory

Brun, C. and Munck, O. (1957). Lesions of the kidney following shock. *Lancet*, **i,** 603

Finn, W.F. (1975). Pathogenesis of oliguria in acute renal failure. *Circ. Res.*, **36,** 675

Henry, L.N. (1968). Micropuncture studies of the pathophysiology of acute renal failure. *Lab. Invest.*, **19,** 309

Hollenberg, N.K. (1968). Evidence for preferential renal cortical ischaemia. *Medicine*, **47,** 455

Lauson, H.D. (1944). The renal circulation in shock. *J. Clin. Invest.*, **23,** 381

Logan, A. (1971). Distribution of renal blood flow in haemorrhagic shock. *Circ. Res.*, **29,** 257

Oliver, J., MacDowell, M., Tracy, A. (1951). ARF associated with traumatic and toxic injury. *J. Clin. Invest.*, **30,** 1307

Phillips, R.A. (1946). Effects of acute haemorrhagic and traumatic shock. *Am. J. Physiol.*, **145,** 314

Priano, L.L. (1971). Cell membrane changes in haemorrhagic shock. *Am. J. Physiol.*, **220,** 705

Sevitt, S. (1959). Pathogenesis of traumatic uraemia. *Lancet*, **2,** 135

Wells, J.D. (1960). Renal cortical necrosis. *Am. J. of Med.*, **29,** 257

Pathogenesis—endotoxin

Donnell, O. (1976). Experimental endotoxinaemia. *Surg. Forum,* **26,** 25

Hjort, P.F. and Rapaport, S.I. (1965). The generalised Shwarztman reaction. *Ann. Rev. Med.,* **16,** 135

Wardle, E.N. (1975a). Endotoxin and acute renal failure. *Nephron,* **14,** 321

Wardle, E.N. (1975b). Endotoxin and acute renal failure. *Q. J. Med.,* **44,** 389

Wardle, E.N. (1976). Functional role of intravascular coagulation in renal disease. *Scot. Med. J.,* **21,** 83

Treatment

Holloway, E.L. (1975). Dopamine compared with isoprenaline. *Am. J. Cardiol.,* **35,** 656

Tallex, R.C. (1969). Dopamine compared with isoprenaline. *Circulation,* **39,** 361

Post-obstructive nephropathy

Jaenicke, J.R. (1972). *J. Clin. Invest.,* **51,** 2999

Wilson, D.R. (1977). *Ann. Rev. Med.,* **28,** 329

Haemolytic—uraemia syndrome

Berman, W. (1972). Haemolytic—uraemia syndrome mimicking ulcerative colitis. *J. Paediatr.,* **81,** 275

Brown, C.B. *et al.* (1973). Oral contraceptives in haemolytic—uraemia syndrome. *Lancet,* **1,** 1479

Finkelstein, F.O. *et al.* (1974). Post-partum haemolytic—uraemia syndrome. *Am. J. Med.,* **57,** 649

Giantantonio. *et al.* (1973). Nephron, **11,** 174

Habib, R. *et al.* (1967). *Nephron,* **4,** 139-172

Kaplan, B.S. (1971). *J. Paediatr.,* **78,** 420

Kaplan, B.S. and Koornhof, H.J. (1969). *Lancet,* **2,** 1424

Katz, J. (1973). *J. Paediatr.,* **83,** 379

Koster, F., Levin, J. *et al.* (1978). *N. Engl. J. Med.,* **298,** 927

Moncrieff, W.M., Glasgow, E.F. (1970). *Br. Med. J.,* **1,** 188

O'Regan, S. (1975). Decreased serum tocopherol levels in haemolytic—uraemia syndrome. *Paediatr. Res.,* **9,** 377

Piel, C.F. and Phibbs, R.H. (1966). *Paediatr. Clin. N. Am.,* **13,** 295

Remuzzi, G. (1978). Deficiency of plasma factors regulating prostacyclins? *Lancet,* **ii,** 871

Vitacco, M. (1973). *J. Paediatr.,* **83,** 271

Cirrhosis

Auld, R.B. *et al.* (1971). Proximal tubular function in dogs with thoracic caval constriction. *J. Clin. Invest.*, **50,** 2150

Baldus, W.P. *et al.* (1964). The kidney in cirrhosis. *Ann. Intern. Med.*, **60,** 366

Chaimouitz, C. *et al.* (1972). Increased renal tubular sodium malabsorption in cirrhosis. *Am. J. Med.*, **52,** 198

Eggert, R.C. (1970). Spironolactone diuresis in cirrhosis with ascites. *Br. Med. J.*, **4,** 401

Epstein, M. *et al.* (1970a). Renal failure in cirrhosis: active vasoconstriction. *Am. J. Med.*, **49,** 175

Epstein, M. *et al.* (1970b). Active renal vasoconstriction in cirrhosis. *Am. J. Med.*, **49,** 175

Kew, M. (1972). Progress report: renal changes in cirrhosis. *Gut,* **13,** 748

Lieberman, F.L. (1970). Plasma volume, portal hypertension and ascites. *Ann. N.Y. Acad. Sci.,* **170,** 202

Papper, S. and Saxon, L. (1959). Diuretic response to water in liver disease. *Arch. Pathol.,* **103,** 7501

Reynolds, T.B. (1967). Functional renal failure: plasma expansion therapy. *Medicine,* **46,** 191

Schroeder, E.T. *et al.* (1970). Plasma renin in cirrhosis. *Am. J. Med.,* **49,** 187

Stein, J.H. *et al.* (1973). Alterations in renal blood flow distribution. *Circ.Res.,* **32,** (suppl. 1.) 61

Wilkinson, S.P. *et al.* (1976). Endotoxinaemia and renal failure in cirrhosis. *Br. Med. J.,* **4,**

Wilkinson, S.P. and Williams, R. (1975). Renal and electrolyte disorders in liver disease. *Postgrad. Med. J.,* **51,** 481

Hepatic with renal failure

Wilkinson, S.P. *et al.* (1974a). Renal and electrolyte disorders in hepatic failure. *Br. Med. J.,* **1,** 186

Wilkinson, S.P. *et al.* (1974b). Renal impairment and endotoxin in fulminant hepatic failure. *Lancet,* **i,** 521

Wilkinson, S.P. *et al.* (1976). Sodium excretion in fulminant hepatic failure. *Gut,* **17,** 501

Obstructive jaundice and acute renal failure

Dawson, J.L. (1965). Post-operative renal failure in obstructive jaundice. *Br. J. Surg.,* **52,** 663

Gollan, J.L. *et al.* (1976). Changes in the kidney by conjugated bilirubin and bile acids. *Br. J. Exp., Pathol.,* **57,** 571

Wardle, E.N. (1975). Renal failure in obstructive jaundice–pathogenic factors. *Postg. Med. J.,* **51,** 512

10
Renal problems in pregnancy

The problems that may arise in pregnancy are:

(1) bacteruria or pyelonephritis;
(2) complications due to previous nephritis or hypertension;
(3) hypertension of pregnancy, so-called 'pre-eclamptic toxaemia';
(4) acute renal failure. .

URINARY TRACT INFECTION IN PREGNANCY

The kidney in pregnancy leaks amino acids and glucose making the urine an excellent culture medium for bacteria. In addition, since there is stasis of urine flow in the ureters and renal pelves, particularly on the right side in primiparous women, from the second trimester onwards there is a liability to pyelonephritis. The stasis is due to obstruction caused directly by the pressure of the gravid uterus or as a result of venous congestion.

Symptoms of dysuria and nocturia are unhelpful in pregnancy, so all women should have routine clinical cultures because symptomatic bacteruria will occur in at least 4%, and of these almost one-half will go on to develop overt pyelonephritis. Not only does this carry the risk of some permanent renal damage and hypertension, but it can lead to premature delivery, fetal loss and superimposed pre-eclamptic toxaemia. Post-natal follow-up has shown that infection may persist in one or other kidney for as long as 5 years unless effective therapy is given. Indeed pyelonephritis of pregnancy has contributed significantly in the past to the development of chronic renal failure in women.

For the treatment of asymptomatic bacteruria a 2 week course of sulphonamide should suffice, but recurrences are common and occur just as much in those who have only cystitis as those who have pyelitis. Prolonged therapy is required for renal infection. Sulphonamides may still be the choice, but one has to be aware that they should be stopped near to term because they displace bilirubin from its binding site on the albumin and can thereby precipitate kernicterus in the neonate.

PRE-EXISTING RENAL DISEASE AND PREGNANCY

Evaluation of renal function in pregnancy

Allowances have to be made for the important physiological changes that occur in normal pregnancy.

Renal plasma flow

Since the cardiac output increases up to the 32nd week of pregnancy, so also does the renal plasma flow which shows an overall increase of 200 ml/min (550–750 ml/min), though there is a fall in the month prior to delivery.

The renal plasma flow is also reduced quite markedly whenever the patient lies on her back, allowing pressure of the gravid uterus on the vena cava. The result is a fall of both urine flow and sodium excretion. Even in the upright position there is some pressure on the vena cava and it will be seen shortly that this may explain why oedema as part of toxaemia is only seen in man, and not in other animals.

Glomerular filtration rate

The creatinine clearance is increased in pregnancy by some 30–50% above normal non-pregnant values, so that results of 150–200 ml/min are usual. In turn this is probably due to the abrupt fall of the plasma albumin and hence of colloid osmotic pressure occurring in the first weeks of pregnancy. Therefore, a creatinine clearance of 120 ml/min in the patient with PET represents a significant reduction; likewise a serum creatinine value above 0.8 mg% (70 μmol/l) should be regarded with suspicion.

Proximal tubular function

The normal daily leak of protein in the urine is less than 40 mg; in pregnancy it may be of the order of 300–400 mg.

Additionally some 50% of women show a benign glycosuria on account of a lowered proximal tubular reabsorption (a low T_{mG}). There are also marked increases in the excretion of amino acids.

Sodium excretion

Plasma renin activity is increased greatly in pregnancy and so is the secretion of aldosterone. On the other hand the normal pregnant woman has a reduced sensitivity to angiotensin probably on account of increased angiotensinases.

Both the total body sodium and body water are increased (but separately), so there is expansion of the extracellular fluids and a normal (in pregnancy) tendency to oedema. In fact it seems that there is an active binding of free water to connective tissue ground substances that is mediated by the oestrogens.

Since the GFR is increased, it follows that the tubular reabsorption must also be increased; this cannot be mediated by aldosterone alone and presumably 'third factor' is switched off.

Distal tubule function: water excretion

In pregnancy the plasma osmolality is reduced by 10 mosmol/kg from 290 to 280 mosmol/kg. Yet in the mid-trimester the ability to excrete a water load is actually increased. However this falls off in the last trimester, and especially so if there is impending toxaemia.

Nephritis in pregnancy

It can be difficult to diagnose renal disease late in pregnancy because proteinuria with some oedema and hypertension add up to 'toxaemia'. Indeed toxaemia is a recognized risk when there is any pre-existing hypertension or renal disease.

As a general rule the more severe the renal insufficiency or the hypertension, whatever its cause, the less likely is the pregnancy to succeed. If deterioration occurs in the first half of pregnancy, then termination must be performed in order to save the mother.

However, in the absence of hypertension, patients with polycystic kidneys are expected to do well, as also can patients with present or past nephrotic syndrome. This can also be the case for the woman with diabetic nephropathy. Proteinuria *per se* is not an indication for termination but increasing red cells in the urine, a rising blood urea and an increasing blood pressure all demand action.

Any patient with active nephritis, in particular lupus nephritis, can be expected to show deterioration in pregnancy but case reports show that this is not always the case. In general the incidence of pre-eclampsia is increased and there is a high fetal loss. The marked reduction in fibrinolysis during pregnancy with a tendency to intraglomerular coagulation may play a part in this. Certainly the hypertensive changes with stasis of flow in the placental circulation all lead on to placental degeneration, which plays an important part in the toxaemia process (see **Figure 100**).

HYPERTENSION OF PREGNANCY (PRE-ECLAMPTIC TOXAEMIA)

When Lever first recognized albumin in the urine in eclampsia, it was natural that he should attribute it to a nephritis, for 50 years earlier Richard Bright had described the finding in renal disease. About 1900, however, the eclamptic syndrome was recognized as consisting of fits with hypertension and a typical peripheral necrosis of the lobules of the liver. Indeed eclampsia is the end-stage of untreated hypertension of pregnancy, in which epilepsy develops due to the hypertensive encephalopathy with its associated spasm of cerebral vessels and petechial haemorrhages throughout the brain. *Pre-eclampsia* itself does not occur before the 26th week unless due to hydatidiform mole or when associated with pre-existing renal disease. When it appears the normal physiological oedema of pregnancy is exaggerated and there is proteinuria and a blood pressure exceeding 140/90 mmHg.

Thus the 'pre-eclamptic triad' is hypertension/proteinuria/oedema. Simple hypertension of pregnancy indicates that there is a persistent diastolic blood pressure of 90 mmHg or more and yet no proteinuria, which merely means that the renal lesion is not so advanced. The underlying pathology is the same, namely, uteroplacental ischaemia with degeneration.

The histology of pre-eclampsia can be unimpressive but the discerning eye will note that the glomeruli are bloodless as a reflection of the vasoconstriction. Moreover the typical lesion of 'endotheliosis' is caused by swelling of the endothelium of the glomerular capillaries and a proliferation of the mesangium. Immunofluorescence shows fibrin-reactive material within and beneath the endothelial cells (see **Figure 101**).

Serum urate levels have been found to correlate with the severity of the illness. In part this is the result of an elevation of blood lactate which is known to cause decreased urate secretion. Lactate levels are elevated in proportion to the degree of vasoconstriction that occurs in any severe hypertension. It is also recognized that angiotension or noradrenaline-induced vasoconstriction leads to decreased urate secretion. *Eclampsia* means that after a period of mounting blood pressure and headache, there is encephalopathy with convulsions. Those patients who come to autopsy have manifest fibrin thrombi in their glomeruli and on occasion there can be acute renal failure.

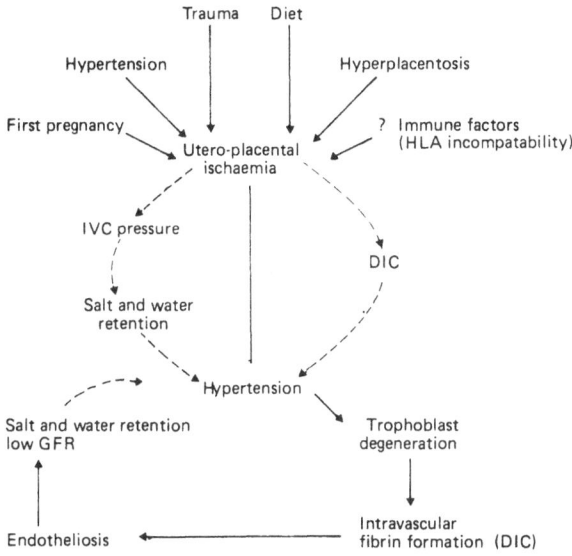

Figure 100. View of pre-eclampsia

Aetiology of pre-eclampsia

The syndrome is based on poor uteroplacental blood flow, that results in:

(1)   sludging of the placental circulation leading to placental degeneration and infarcts;
(2)   release of thromboplastin causing disseminated intravascular coagulation;
(3)   release of renin from the chorion adding to the hypertension.

Pre-eclampsia is more common in the first pregnancy and Sophian has attributed this to lack of elasticity of the uterine muscle producing a uterorenal vasoconstrictive reflex. It is also more likely when there is pre-existing hypertension, trauma to the placenta as by rough journeying, and when there is a poor diet lacking in vitamin E, which in animals is definitely known to cause placental degeneration. A very bulky placenta occurs in diabetes, twin pregnancy, rhesus incompatibility, etc., and since this leaves less room there will be restriction of the blood supply. The prime cause is therefore hypertensive vascular degeneration with accompanying DIC in the placental bed leading to trophoblast degeneration. The secondary effects are (a) release of chorionic renin, and (b) release of thromboplastins.

Origin of the hypertension

As indicated above Sophian has proposed that the generalized arteriolar constriction of pre-eclampsia arises as a reflex response to uterine distension. This may be so, but it does not account for those cases of 'toxaemia' which occur actually after delivery or those due to hydatidiform mole. Salt and water retention is quite physiological in pregnancy and seems to be due to the salt-retaining effect of progesterone. Of particular importance is the fact that release of renin from a degenerating chorion is expected to generate angiotensin and aldosteronism. Indeed there is evidence that women who later develop pre-eclampsia have supranormal plasma renin levels in the mid-trimester, but as salt accumulates under the influence of aldosterone, renin levels fall below the values to be expected; they are thus low in the last trimester.

Additionally one has to note that the upright posture in man means that the gravid uterus presses against the vena cava and that in turn this will cause renal vasoconstriction and salt retention.

Relevance of intravascular coagulation

There are interesting changes in the coagulation system in pregnancy which taken together account for the histological finding of fibrin in the pulmonary circulation, in the Kupffer cells of the liver, and in the mesangial cells and swollen endothelial cells of the renal glomeruli, whose overall appearance is referred to as 'endotheliosis'.

The sequence of these changes is shown in Figure 101.

Hypertensive vasoconstriction *per se,* as in essential hypertension, gives the appearance of bloodless glomeruli in which no red cells are seen, but it does not give rise to fibrin deposition. The fibrin-like material of pre-eclampsia is shown by immunofluorescence to lie either in a subendothelial position or within the swollen endothelial and mesangial cells. In fact it represents circulating high-molecular weight fibrin complexes which have been previously referred to in the literature as 'cryofibrinogen', that is a fibrin-like material which precipitates in the cold.

Three factors explain the deposition of this material within the glomeruli.

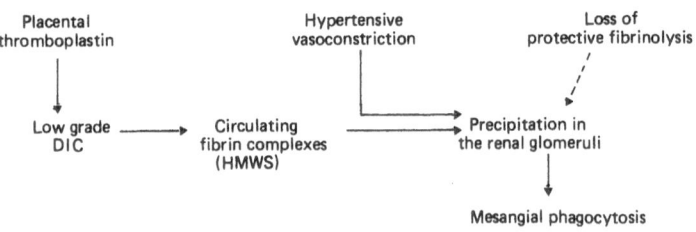

Figure 101. Explanation of the origin of fibrin in the renal glomeruli

(1)   The physiological inhibition of fibrinolysis of middle and late pregnancy. This is due to hormonal changes, principally the high secretion of lactogen from the placenta.

(2)   Release of thromboplastin into the circulation from degenerate placenta. It is this process which is so marked in pre-eclampsia as to account for a low-grade intravascular coagulation syndrome; so there can be lowered platelets, an increased turnover of radiofibrinogen, and the appearance of HMWS (high-molecular weight substances) which are demonstrable either as 'cryofibrinogen' or as a high-molecular weight peak on a plasma fibrinogen chromatogram.

(3)   Increased activity of the reticuloendothelial cells such as the Kupffer cells of the liver and the mesangial cells of the renal glomeruli; this is caused by high oestrogen levels. The phagocytic cells are, therefore, primed to deal with fibrin debris that is trapped in the renal filters.

Treatment of hypertension in pregnancy

The old idea of strict bed rest and sedation has been discarded; both approaches make the patient feel worse and anxious. Methyldopa is a most trustworthy hypotensive agent for this situation, and propranolol has also been shown to be safe. Certainly a diastolic blood pressure of 110 mmHg is an indication for hospitalization, as the fetus can be in jeopardy. Currently both salt restriction and diuretics are condemned. When patients lie down they are asked to rest on one or other side in order to avoid vena caval compression. There is a rise of blood pressure that results from aortic compression by a gravid uterus, when the patient changes from the lateral to the supine position. This is actually used as a 'supine pressor response' test.

The maternal blood pressure must be monitored and a record is kept of premonitory symptoms of eclampsia such as epigastric pain and vomiting, and of course headache or visual disturbance. Proteinuria is highly significant. Measurements of the serum urate can be made.

A reduction in fetal activity (kick-counting) has to be taken seriously. Monitoring facilities are now available and in addition ultrasound can be used to measure the size of the fetal head, amnioscopy performed to assess the volume of the liquor and to look for meconium staining, and measurements made of urinary oestriol output, and of serum placental lactogen.

ACUTE RENAL FAILURE IN PREGNANCY

The above comment on physiological changes in the coagulation system in pregnancy is also relevant to the occurrence of acute renal failure, either as tubular necrosis or as renal cortical necrosis. As explained above in Chapter 9 on acute renal failure, DIC is part of all shock syndromes and the occurrence of fibrinolytic inhibition in this situation can set the scene for renal cortical necrosis.

Although glomerulonephritis, hepatorenal syndrome and sepsis might all cause acute renal failure in pregnancy, in practice the vast majority of cases occur in association with toxaemia among women who have not attended for regular antenatal care. In the early weeks of pregnancy attempted criminal abortion with septicaemia, hydatidiform mole or hyperemesis gravidarum all have to be considered.

One of the interesting facts about obstetric (non-septic) acute renal failure is that its prognosis with dialysis is very good. The likely explanation is that with the delivery of the placenta the elevated blood pressure of toxaemia and the predisposition to intravascular coagulation are each removed. Moreover normal fibrinolysis is restored within a few hours of separation of the placenta.

REFERENCES

Physiological renal changes in pregnancy

Hytten, F.E. *et al.* (1966). Body water. *J. Obstet. Gynecol. Br. Common.*, **73**, 533

Hytten, F.W. and Leitch, I. (1971). Other functional changes. *The Physiology of Human Pregnancy*. (Oxford: Blackwell)

Langgard, H. (1967). *Dan. Med. Bull.*, **14**, 533

Lauritsen, O.S. (1969). Fibrinolysis. *Scand. J. Clin. Lab. Invest.*, **23**, 191

Kidney disease and pregnancy

Lindheimer, M.D., Katz, A.I. (1977). Kidney function and Disease in Pregnancy. (Lea & Febiger)

Kincaid-Smith, P. *et al.* (1967). *Med. J. Aust.*, **11**, 1155

Strauch, B.S. and Hayslett, J.P. (1974). *Br. Med. J.*, **4**, 578

Studd, J.W. and Blainey, J.D. (1969). *Br. Med. J.*, **1**, 276

Pregnancy toxaemia

Birmingham Eclampsia Study Group, (1971). *Lancet,* **ii**, 889

McKay, D.G. (1964). *Circulation.* suppl. 2, 66

Page, E.W. (1972). *J. Obstet. Gynecol. Br. Common.*, **79**, 883

Schneider, C.L. (1951). *J. Obstet. Gynceol. Br. Common.*, **58**, 538

Wardle, E.N. (1974). *Clin. Nephrol.*, **2**, 85

11
Chronic renal failure (CRF)

PRESENTATION

Only one-half of patients with CRF are known beforehand to have disease, and most present insidiously in the following ways:

(1)   with *polyuria and nocturia,* which are indicative of tubular damage. The time of onset of these symptoms will give an indication of the duration;

(2)   with *loss of energy and weakness,* which are indicative of uraemia and anaemia;

(3)   with uraemic *nausea and vomiting,* or skin itching and paraesthesiae;

(4)   with *headache, blurred vision and breathlessness* indicative of hypertension.

The blood urea is the normal screening test and guide to renal insufficiency, although clearly it can be influenced by the amount of protein in the diet and it is not as reliable as the serum creatinine (Figure 102). Uraemic symptoms appear when the urea exceeds 25 mmol/l (150 mg%) and this may correspond to a creatinine clearance of 7–8 ml/min.

So it appears that at a serum creatinine of 1.5 mg% there is only half normal renal function, at a creatinine of 3.0 mg% one-fifth of renal function, and at 6 mg% serum creatinine only one-tenth of normal renal function. It is useful to

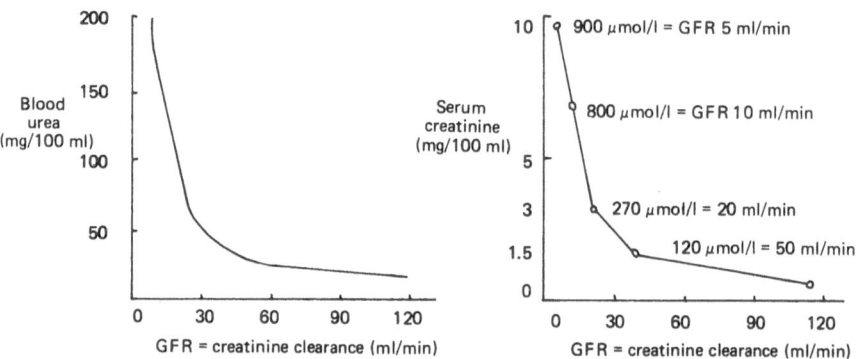

Figure 102. **Relation of the blood urea and serum creatinine to renal insufficiency.**

have a simple nomogram so as to relate a serum creatinine (which can be available in 1 h) with the patient's creatinine clearance (which is delayed owing to requirement for urine collection):

For men

creatinine clearance ml/min = 100/serum creatinine mg%   − 12

for women

creatinine clearance ml/min = 80/serum creatinine mg%   − 7

A slightly more complex formula which is still more accurate is:

$$\frac{\text{creatinine}}{\text{clearance}} = \frac{(140 - \text{age})\,(\text{weight in kg})}{\cdot 72 \times \text{serum creatinine (mg\%)}}$$

or for children

$$\frac{\text{creatinine}}{\text{clearance}} = \frac{0.55 \text{ length in cm}}{\text{serum creatinine}} \times \frac{\text{SArea}}{1.73}$$

Although the creatinine clearance comes to exceed the inulin clearance by as much as 50% at low glomerular filtration rates, because creatinine is actually secreted by the tubules, for practical purposes a serum creatinine or the 24 h endogenous creatinine clearance is the most useful guide to renal malfunction. The patient can be regarded as having *renal insufficiency* as the glomerular filtration rate falls from 20 →5 ml/min (serum creatinine rising 1.5 → 7.0 mg% or 140 →620 μmol/l) and established *renal failure*; requiring dietary measures and haemodialysis with clearances below this (serum creatinine →7 mg%) (blood urea →35 mmol/l or 200 mg%).

Furthermore the reciprocal of the serum creatinine (which as the above nomograms suggest is the equivalent of the creatinine clearance) can be shown to decline linearly with time as chronic renal failure progresses. This means that a few serial estimates predict the time at which dialysis becomes necessary.

ASSESSMENT OF THE CRF PATIENT

In the first instance it is necessary to arrive at a definitive diagnosis, although, since supportive therapy may have to take precedence, this can often be difficult or impossible.

The *causes of chronic renal failure* must be borne in mind:

(1)   chronic glomerulonephritis—small granular kidneys;
(2)   chronic pyelonephritis or analgesic nephropathy;
(3)   urinary tract obstruction, stones, or renal tuberculosis;
(4)   polycystic kidneys, medullary cystic disease or hereditary nephritis with deafness;
(5)   systemic disease—gout, diabetes, amyloid, myeloma, polyarteritis, scleroderma, SLE;
(6)   hypertensive disease, arteriosclerotic or senile nephrosclerosis.

Therefore, as soon as possible an *IVU with tomography* will be required. The hope is not only to make a diagnosis but to find a potentially reversible

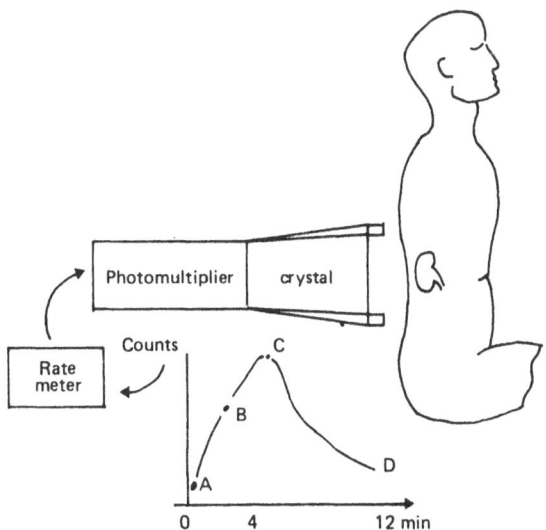

Figure 103. **Scheme of radio-isotope renography**

297

lesion such as obstruction or infection. *Retrograde pyelograms* can be used to define a site of obstruction more precisely. If the kidneys are of normal size, then *renal biopsy* may provide useful information as to the prognosis or mode of therapy.

The *isotope renogram* is of accessory value in selecting causes of unilateral renal hypertension and in the evaluation of urinary tract obstruction. For this reason a brief description of this technique will be given.

The radioisotope renogram

Certain substances such as phenol red, *p*-aminohippurate and sodium iodohippurate are excreted so well by the proximal tubules of the kidneys that their rate of excretion is a measure of renal plasma flow. Therefore the isotope derivative of the latter, namely sodium [^{125}I]iodohippurate, has become the standard agent for isotope renography (Figure 103). After an intravenous injection the uptake and excretion by each kidney is monitored by a separate collimated scintillation-counter linked to a ratemeter that makes a record on a chart.

In the case of urinary tract obstruction the excretory phase is prolonged and it is possible to tell whether it is unilateral or bilateral, (Figure 104).

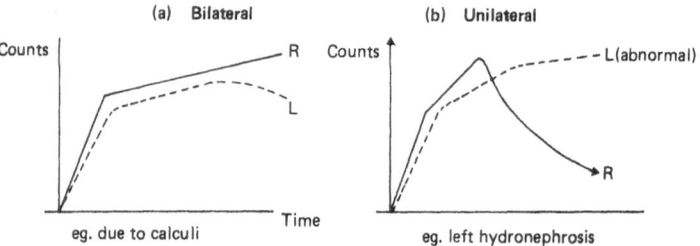

Figure 104.   Urinary tract obstruction revealed by the renogram

If there is a renal artery stenosis, then this will be detected by the delayed renal uptake phase (A-B-C) as in Figure 31. When there is poor function of one kidney only, say due to pyelonephritis, this should also be easily recognized (Figure 105).

CLINICAL PROBLEMS AND CRF PHYSIOLOGY

Each aspect of the chronic renal failure syndrome can be specified and treated accordingly. As nephrons become damaged, renal function declines so that there is an inability to excrete urea, uric acid, acid metabolites, sodium and potassium; each of these factors may influence the management. Clearly a

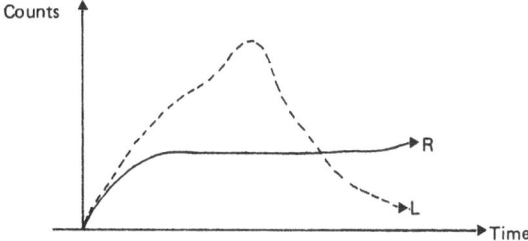

Figure 105. Abnormal function due to pyelonephritis: small non-functioning right kidney.

decrease in nephron mass reduces the capacity of the kidneys to excrete waste products and there is a failure to produce erythropoietin. It also shows up as an acidosis, which is consequent upon an inability of the tubules to excrete sufficient titratable acid and to produce ammonia. A reduced number of nephrons means that there is a tendency to salt retention, but at the same time there is an increased solute load to the remaining intact nephrons. There is thus a high flow down the remaining tubules and this will limit the reabsorption of water so that there is now an incapacity to concentrate the urine and an inability to conserve sodium. Glomerular damage, therefore, causes salt retention, while tubular damage causes salt loss. The idea that remaining nephrons can be regarded as behaving normally (Platt) became known as the 'intact nephron hypothesis', but they nevertheless suffer from 'work fatigue'.

The CRF syndrome can therefore be specified in the following terms:

(1) *Fluid and electrolyte problems*
  (a) glomerular insufficiency leading to retention of salt and water, acid and uraemic metabolites;
  (b) occasional water intoxication or hyperkalaemia;
  (c) tubular dysfunction leading to the production of urine of fixed osmolality close to that of plasma; therefore polyuria and a tendency to dehydration. Salt depletion can occur.

(2) *Cardiovascular problems*
  (a) hypertension;
  (b) congestive heart failure or pulmonary oedema;
  (c) arrhythmias;
  (d) pericarditis.

(3) *Immunosuppression and susceptibility to infection* on account of uraemic metabolites.

(4) *General uraemic features*
  (a) yellow-brown skin with pruritus, red eyes, brown nails and anaemia;

(b) anorexia, vomiting or hiccups, colitis;

(c) Kussmaul's acidotic respiration;

(d) muscle twitching, convulsions and/or coma, peripheral neuropathy.

(5) *Haemopoietic dysfunction*

Anaemia, purpura and bleeding problems.

(6) *Skeletal*

(a) dwarfism and renal osteodystrophy

(b) metastatic calcification when $Ca \times P > 75$ (mg%)

Fluid and electrolyte problems

Considering the energy expended it is clear that the most important function of the kidneys is the reabsorption of sodium. Control over this process is largely intrinsic to the kidney and is referred to as 'glomerulotubular balance'. This means that even in remaining nephrons there is a relationship between the filtered load of sodium and the fraction of filtered sodium that is reabsorbed in the proximal tubules. Since the remaining nephrons are inevitably subjected to solute load, an inflexible situation develops so that while the upper limit of sodium excretion is lower than normal, it also becomes easy for the diseased kidneys to run into negative sodium balance.

In general patients require salt restriction. However, they are in delicate balance—too high an intake readily causes oedema, and too low an intake results in salt depletion. The latter becomes evident as a loss of tissue turgor, a falling blood pressure and a rise of the blood urea. In this situation intravenous replacement with normal or hypertonic saline is required. Usually a patient can be placed on a 22 mmol sodium intake, and his input gradually adjusted to match his daily sodium excretion.

This applies also to the water intake. On the one hand the patient can become dehydrated and on the other he may become waterlogged. Thus, by trial and error, water input is increased above the basic '500 ml/day plus urine output' while a close eye is kept on body weight, appearance of oedema and the plasma electrolytes. When the weight rises and the plasma sodium falls, the patient's water intake has reached its optimum.

There is also a tendency to retain potassium, so the intake should be fixed on the low side, at 50 mmol/day, for instance. The serum potassium still has to be monitored frequently, especially so at times of infection or operative procedures that might increase tissue catabolism. If the level exceeds 6.0 mmol/l, then oral calcium–resonium 15g q.i.d. is required; this is preferable to simple resonium-A which, when absorbing potassium, can release so much sodium that the body cannot cope with the load. *Such mixtures as Mist, potassium citrate are absolutely contraindicated.* The emergency treatment of hyperkalaemia is to administer:

(1)   50 ml/50% dextrose and 20 U insulin i.v., or
(2)   50 ml/1 M lactate + 20 ml calcium gluconate i.v., or
(3)   intravenous 2.4% sodium bicarbonate,

and meanwhile arrangements should be made for dialysis.

The protein intake has to be severely curtailed. Although a normal person might eat 100 g/day protein, many patients usually consume some 60–70 g (1 g/kg); but when the GFR is reduced to 5 ml/min, the protein intake should be cut to 0.5 g/kg or 40 g/day. When the GFR is only 3.0 ml/min, the patient can only take 20 g/day protein and this is given as the G–G diet (page 304).

Cardiovascular problems

Hypertension should be treated vigorously but an initial lowering to a diastolic blood pressure of 100–110 mmHg is advisable. There is no worse situation than producing such severe hypotension that the patient keels over when he stands and when lying fails to pass sufficient urine!

There are now many hypotensive drugs from which to choose (page 84). Methyldopa or guanethidine are both familiar and reliable, and selective beta-blocking drugs are being used more. For refractory cases hydrallazine at a dosage of 25–50 mg three times a day or diazoxide 100–200 mg t.i.d. can be tried (cf. page 84).

Diuretics are always used. The very large-dose Lasix tablet (500 mg) has the advantage that it allows a little liberality with fluid intake in the patient with a very low GFR, but it is important to be vigilant for latent diabetes, iatrogenic gout and concurrent antibiotic nephrotoxicity.

Hypotensive agents

Guanethidine need only be given once a day as, in fact, its half-life is 5 days in the body. Loading can be made with a single large dose of 80 mg but soon maintenance can be as little as 10 mg/day. In view of its long life, dosage alterations should only take place fortnightly. Its action is to block the normal release of catecholamines that are caused by sympathetic nerve stimulation. This happens because it is taken up into nerve endings by the normal 'amine pump' and there it binds to the noradrenaline storage vesicles and causes their discharge. It is useful for severe hypertension and is effective in small dosage when given together with a diuretic. A variety of drugs such as the tricyclic antidepressants and chlorpromazine interact with guanethidine! It has little toxicity apart from the postural hypotension which comes on with exertion.

Diazoxide acts by causing direct relaxation of the smooth muscle of arteriole walls. In structure it is closely related to the thiazide diuretics, but it does cause sodium and water retention.

Diazoxide   *Chlorothiazide*

note the diuretic sulphamoyl group

On account of its liability to bind to albumin, when the 300 mg dose is given intravenously it must be injected rapidly so as to reach receptors in the arteriolar walls first. It is particularly effective for hypertensive encephalopathy, but the hypertensive crisis of a phaeochromocytoma or of monoamine oxidase inhibitor therapy should be treated with the alpha-blocking drug phentolamine or labetolol. Diazoxide can also be given orally (100–200 mg t.i.d.); side-effects are hyperglycaemia and also hirsutism, extrapyramidal symptoms, and occasional anorexia and vomiting.

Susceptibility to infection

In the early 1950s it was recognized that the survival of renal allografts is prolonged by the uraemic state *per se*. Immunoglobulin levels are normal and antibody responses are seldom impaired, but cellular immune reactions are depressed and likewise the capacity of the polymorphs to phagocytose bacteria. There is impaired *in vitro* reactivity of lymphocytes to antigens and likewise in the mixed lymphocyte culture (MLC). Indeed this is so apparent that the MLC may give false-negative results in the pretransplantation work-up of a potential live donor. MIF production and type IV delayed hypersensitivity skin reactions are also depressed, but PHA stimulation of lymphocytes seems to be normal. Urea is not the toxin and the nature of the suppression has yet to be established. There is no impairment of DNA and RNA synthesis.

Bone disease and calcium metabolism

Even modest reductions in glomerular filtration lead to phosphate retention, which in turn tends to depress the serum calcium, so there is an increased output of parathormone, and osteitis fibrosa develops insidiously. Additionally when PTH acts on the proximal tubules it leads to urinary bicarbonate loss and this exacerbates the metabolic acidosis.

In fact hypocalcaemia is the normal feature of chronic renal failure, although an occasional patient will be seen with hypercalcaemia due to established hyperparathyroidism. The hypocalcaemia does not cause tetany unless the acidosis is suddenly relieved.

Reversible causes of renal insufficiency

These may be part of, or be confused with, chronic renal failure.

Salt depletion
The patient complains of listlessness and fatigue and may have cramps. Later he becomes confused and stuporose, and tremors and twitches occur; hyponatraemia will be found. Therapy is to give saline so as to restore the deficit. Assuming that 60% of the body weight is extracellular fluid: m.mol sodium required = $(135–110 \text{ mmol/l}) \times 0.6 \times$ wt (kg).

Hypercalcaemia
Hypercalcaemia impairs renal function, even when not so severe as to cause 'nephrocalcinosis'. The patient may complain of conjunctivitis, and corneal calcification will be seen by means of a slit lamp. Treatment depends on the cause. In the case of vitamin D intoxication ingestion must be stopped and calcitonin might be given. Dialysis can always correct an acute hypercalcaemia, but in chronic hypercalcaemia parathyroid resection may become necessary (for other measures see page 231).

Chronic alkalosis
Patients with pyloric stenosis lose a great deal of stomach acid by vomiting, and at the same time they may be taking large amounts of milk and alkali. Chronic alkalosis *per se* results in a lowered glomerular filtration, and patients can in fact become very uraemic.

Added to this is the fact that in alkalosis there is loss of body potassium. The typical renal lesion of hypokalaemia is a tubular defect with inability to concentrate the urine and polyuria, and there is a vacuolar change in the tubules and tubular proteinuria.

It has to be emphasized, however, that chloride depletion is the key factor in this situation. So potassium chloride repletion will normalize the renal function.

Obstructive nephropathy
Back-pressure in an obstructed urinary tract leads to renal insufficiency, since ultimately a rise of pressure in the renal tubules will be transmitted to

Bowman's capsule (p. 6) so there is impaired urinary filtration. The situation is often complicated by infection in the urinary tract, by dehydration or by heart failure.

The principle of treatment is to establish urinary drainage and to treat infection. In order to gain time nephrostomy or ureterostomy tubes may have to be inserted. This can be done by a percutaneous procedure; a high-dose intravenous urogram is given, and a needle inserted into the renal pelvis under local anaesthesia. A flexible catheter is then inserted over the needle or through it according to the size; such a Longdwel catheter can be left in for weeks, but may need frequent washouts to remove blood clot and debris. During this time the patient could need peritoneal dialysis.

An important medical point is that after relief of obstruction there is a 'post-obstructive diuresis' with attendant losses of water and electrolytes so that sodium, chloride and potassium replacement must be monitored.

The patient can be investigated meanwhile in order to localize the site of obstruction in preparation for definitive surgery.

GENERAL ASPECTS OF MANAGEMENT OF CHRONIC RENAL FAILURE

Emphasis has been placed on the need to assess the CRF patient for those features which can be reversed, namely salt and water depletion; urinary tract infection; overdosage from sedatives, antibiotics or antiemetics; or chronic alkalosis.

Having done this, each aspect of treatment should be considered according to the features of the syndrome.

Retention of urea nitrogen and toxic metabolites

Protein restriction will be necessary to relieve gastrointestinal symptoms when the blood urea exceeds 25 mmol/l (creatinine 700–800 μmol/l). A protein intake of half normal, namely 0.5 g/kg per day or 40 g/day is then given. If nausea continues, Torecan 10 mg t.i.d. will help.

When the GFR is down to 3 ml/min the patient can only tolerate a 20 g protein diet of high biological value. The essential amino acids can be remembered by the mnemonic '*any help in learning these little molecules proves truly valuable*'—arginine, histidine, isoleucine, leucine, threonine, lysine, methionine, phenylalanine, tryptophan and valine. Except for methionine and tryptophan the minimum requirement of essential amino acids is provided for by consumption of two eggs, or of one egg and 200 ml (6 oz) of milk/day. Tryptophan itself occurs in vegetable protein and is therefore provided by rice, potatoes, fruit and vegetables. In this way the protein intake becomes 20 g/day. An additional half-egg should be allowed for every 3 g of protein that are being lost by a patient with advanced nephrotic syndrome. This is basically the Giordano–Giovannetti (G–G) diet.

Bread has to be made with wheatstarch, and cornstarch can be used in puddings. The diet is low in iron, which is usually given as a supplement, as also are tablets of methionine. At the same time the calorie intake must be boosted by taking the low protein (Rite diet) bread, Caloreen (a polymerized glucose that gives 4 kcal/g), low protein pasta and Hycal, a glucose rich drink. Fats are an excellent source of calories and thus a liberal allowance of butter is made and oil is used for frying. Cream is added to fruit and puddings. So by these means the calorie intake should be 3000 kcal/day. In a situation where there is no spare protein, urea and ammonia can be shown to be reincorporated into protein. Urea-nitrogen becomes available as it is hydrolyzed to ammonia in the gut and reabsorbed for use by the liver. The raised blood urea of uraemic persons is sufficient to supply an extra 4–7g of potentially utilizable nitrogen.

Variations on the low protein diet have been devised. In Birmingham frozen dried dialyzed egg powder, which is low in potassium, has been used. In Freiburg a 25g potato–egg diet is given, consisting of 50% potato and egg protein, 10% milk protein and then 40% vegetable and cereal protein. The minimum calorie content of 2100 calories can be boosted by means of medium-chain triglycerides, and by use of linoleic acid which is useful in combating the hyperlipidaemia with its adverse vascular effects.

Although a patient can live on a 20g protein diet supplemented with essential amino acids in tablet form, they develop malnutrition as shown by a lower serum albumin, low transferrin and haemoglobin values and also low ratios of essential to non-essential amino acids. In theory one can boost the diet by feeding ketoacid analogues since all but two of the essential amino acids (lysine and threonine) can be synthesized in this way.

In practice the patient should stay on 40 g/day protein as long as possible, and in reality this means early dialysis.

Salt and water balance

As indicated above this runs on a knife-edge, so that intake has to be adjusted starting from the basic 22 mmoles sodium, and fluid intake equal to 500 ml/day urine output. Some patients will need high-dose diuretics, while others require supplementation with slow sodium, or, as an aid to correction of acidosis, with sodium bicarbonate 1g t.i.d.

Potassium

A normal intake of 100 mmol/per day can be readily reduced to 50 mmol/day, but even on a low protein diet it becomes difficult to reduce potassium intakes below 30 mmol/day. Hyperkalaemic patients are really ready for dialysis but meanwhile should take calcium–resonium 15g b.d.

Haemopoietic system

Iron, folic acid and vitamins are given routinely. A decision to transfuse with blood is difficult since there is a risk of circulatory overload, transmission of hepatitis antigen and of sensitization to transplantation antigens (cf page 410).

Bone disease

The general approaches are as follows:

(1) *Lower the plasma phosphate*
When the plasma phosphate exceeds 7 mg% (2.3 mmol/l) then aluminium hydroxide should be given to bind phosphate in the gut. This will lower the plasma Ca x P product, which is known to cause metastatic calcification if it exceeds 75. A major problem is that aluminium can have long-term toxicity; also if the plasma phosphate is lowered too far, then hypophosphataemic osteomalacia will result.

(2) *Promote calcification*
The serum calcium can be raised by giving large doses of oral calcium as calcium carbonate 1g t.i.d.; additionally there are the following possibilities:
(a) vitamin D, calciferol tabs. forte 1.25 mg (50 000U) 1–4/day;
     calciferol injection in oleate 300 000U per ml/week;
     dihydrotachysterol (AT10) 0.25– 4.0 mg/day;
     1,25-dihydroxyD3: 0.5–1.0 μg/day;
     1-α-hydroxyvitamin D_3: 1–2 μg/day.

(3) *Subtotal parathyroidectomy* if the serum calcium persistently exceeds 12.0 mg% (3.0 mmol/l).

More detailed discussion of bone disease follows—pages 318–325.

METABOLIC CHANGES IN URAEMIA

Uraemic toxins

Various aspects of chronic uraemia suggest that the accumulation of toxins together with acidosis interfere with normal glucose metabolism, and the production and use of ATP by cells. There is insulin resistance and therefore impaired glucose tolerance which shows up as an elevated blood glucose, blood insulin and growth hormone levels (a 'pseudo-diabetes'). Actual penetration of glucose into cells is normal but there appears to be impairment of intracellular utilization. There can be impaired glycolysis, as shown for example by the red cell in a uraemic environment. The intracellular pH of the red cell is not well stabilized and the effect is likely to be due to inhibition by acidosis of hexokinase, inhibition of phosphofructokinase and inhibition of pyruvate kinase, as much as a direct effect of toxic metabolites (Figure 106). By way of compensation pentose phosphate shunt activity within the red cell is increased; this maintains levels of reduced glutathione. In other cells impaired pyruvate utilization can be demonstrated so there must be reduced activity of enzymes within the Kreb's cycle. Phenols and phenolic acids might do this, as they inhibit malate dehydrogenase.

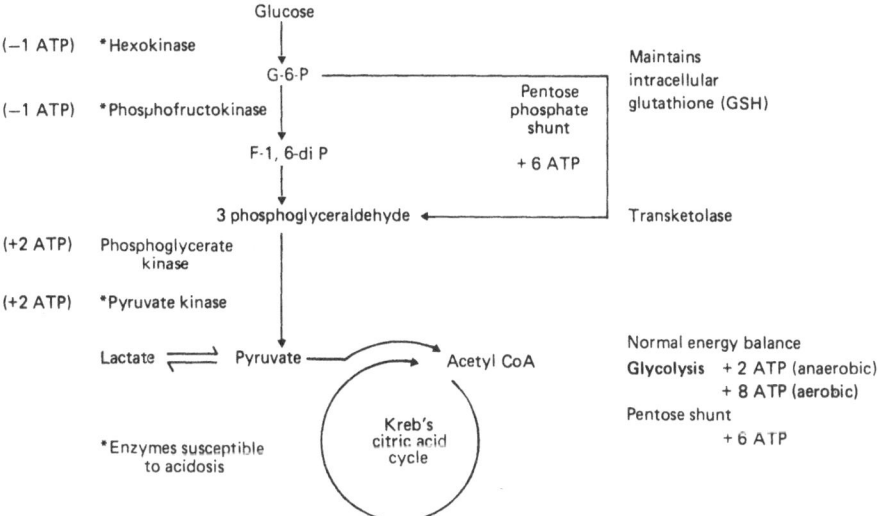

Figure 106.   Glucose metabolism and possible sites of inhibition in uraemia

The *acidosis* of uraemia is certainly one cause of impaired glucose metabolism. It is well known that glycolysis is impaired by acidosis but accelerated by alkalosis. Acidosis within the cell acts in particular to prevent the action of phosphofructokinase, and the consequent accumulation of the G6P will cut down the activity of hexokinase by feedback inhibition. ATP accumulation due to an ATPase defect will also inhibit phospho-F-kinase.

The effect that acidosis might have depends on the type of cell. In erythrocytes or macrophages there is marked permeability to carbon dioxide or to H^+/HCO_3^-. Commencing at an initial intracellular pH of 7.2 for a plasma pH of 7.4, the intracellular pH can be shown thereafter to be markedly dependent on extracellular pH. However, in the more organized cells, which are essential to body metabolic homeostasis, there is such good intracellular buffering that the intracellular pH is actively regulated. In these cells (for example muscle) the pH can remain normal even in advanced uraemia.

Urea and creatinine alone are not toxic even in high concentration. Creatinine, however, is converted by gut bacteria to methylguanidine:

creatinine → creatine → methylguanidine + acetic acid.

Methylguanidine has emerged as one of the most definite of the uraemic toxins. It is certainly an inhibitor of the Na–K ATPase of cells and it also appears to be capable of causing uncoupling of oxidative phosphorylation. Each of these facts may be relevant to the claim that methylguanidine acts as a natriuretic factor in advanced uraemia.

In addition to the guanidine derivatives, the many potential toxins which accumulate in uraemia include organic acids and a variety of *products of the intestinal flora*—dimethylamine and trimethylamine, aromatic amines, the phenols and the indoles. Inhibition of glycolysis and of oxidative phosphorylation have been shown repeatedly in animal experiments. The toxins uraemia are shown in Table 31.

Table 31   Potential toxins in uraemia

Bacterial products
    Amines—dimethylamine
    Indoles
    Phenols and phenolic acids (also from vegetable foods and tyrosine)

Food intake
    Hippuric acid and other aryl acids—fruits
    Phenols and phenolic acids—coffee and tea
    Myoinositol
    Vitamin A
    Toxic metals—aluminium, magnesium

Endogenous
    Methylguanidine
    Guanidino-succinic acid
    Some 'middle molecules' (molecular weight over 1200)
    Parathormone or its accompanying hypercalcaemia
    Acidosis and accumulation of potassium and magnesium

The *phenols* are lipid soluble and they can enter cells. Even at low concentrations they inhibit cerebral enzymes, they are absorbed by mitochondria and they uncouple oxidative phosphorylation; they also impair phosphate transfer across cell membranes. Compounds derived from the catechols (which are diphenols) and other simple phenols too can cause inhibition of the vital Na–K ATPase pump of cells. However most phenols are conjugated by gut, liver or brain to less toxic glucuronides.

Inhibition by phenols or like compounds would accord with the observation of diminished ATPase activity in uraemic red cells (Smith and Welt) and their elevated sodium and diminished potassium content as in the 'sick cell syndrome'. Uraemic red cells have a defective sodium efflux (Villamil *et al.*, 1968) and similar changes have been identified in neurones (Gaertner *et al.*, 1972). Uraemic red cells are also poor at incorporating phosphorus-32 with ADP to form ATP. This probably reflects inhibition of glycolysis.

Both phenols and guanidinosuccinic acid have been found to be effective *inhibitors of platelet aggregation* at concentrations found in uraemia. In general platelet inhibition is consequent upon a rise of intracellular cAMP content. The exact mode of action of these agents has yet to be explained; they could be inhibitors of ATP synthesis. The phenols can act by de-activation of prostaglandin synthetase.

The *derivatives of hippuric acid* (the arylacids) are also considered to be highly toxic. Indeed they are known to cause sodium loss by the proximal tubules of the kidney, so that they and methylguanidine (perhaps together) have claim to being the 'third factor' natriuretic substances of the uraemic state.

All these compounds including those of higher molecular weight, the 'middle molecules', are discussed below in relation to effectiveness of dialysis (Chapter 13, p. 379).

Bacterial metabolism of choline and lecithin is an important source of *trimethylamine*, and part is demethylated in the liver to dimethylamine; both should normally be excreted in the urine. Concentrations in the intestine are raised in uraemia but fall when broad-spectrum antibiotics are administered. Means of adsorbing such toxins in the bowel are discussed on page 378.

The effects of uraemia, being the summated effects of the toxins, are evident clinically as defective cerebration with impairment of cerebral oxygen consumption, and a paroxysmal slow-wave activity on the EEG. There is muscle weakness, in part due to vitamin D resistance and in part due to a metabolic toxin. There is also a peripheral neuropathy which appears to be related to an elevated serum parathormone level. It has been thought that inhibition of the enzyme transketolase of the pentose-phosphate shunt is relevant to uraemic neuropathy, since its activity provides NADPH and NADH for fatty acid, and hence myelin synthesis. In fact it has been claimed that guanidinosuccinic acid will inhibit transketolase both in red cells and the brain. The nerves in uraemia show segmental demyelination presumably due to Schwann cell dysfunction, but little axonal damage. Another candidate for defective myelination is the substance myoinositol; this accumulates in uraemia yet conversely its deficiency explains the neuropathy of diabetes. The striking tendency to cardiac arrhythmias can be explained by a combination of acidosis and potassium retention. Impairment of ATPase, which means the production of 'sick cells' by virtue of intracellular sodium accumulation and a reduced potassium, is clearly applicable to neurones and to muscle. This is evident from the decreased membrane potential of uraemic muscle (–90 mV inside normally) and of sick red cells (which normally have an inside potential of –10 mV).

It is relatively easy to suggest how the toxic metals can impair neuronal function. The binding of calcium ions to acidic phospholipids has been dealt with above. These acidic phospholipids, such as phosphatidylserine and also phosphatidylcholine, are important for the maximal activation of Na–K ATPase and thus for sodium and potassium ion fluxes as an action potential passes along a nerve fibre. Indeed the influx of sodium, which is part of the action potential, is followed by the influx of calcium ions. In the case of phosphatidylcholine (lecithin) it is known that metals displace calcium in the order:

$$Al^{3+} > Cu^{2+} > Mg^{2+} > Ca^{2+} > Na^+$$

This would indeed account for the cerebral toxicity of either aluminium or copper.

Glucose and lipid metabolism in chronic renal failure

Premature atherosclerosis has become a principal worry for those managing the chronic renal failure patient or the renal allograft recipient.

There are three aspects to the hypertriglyceridaemia and elevated levels of prebeta-lipoprotein (VLDL):

(1)   There is increased *mobilization of fatty acids* from the fat depots, and thus increased synthesis of triglycerides in the liver under the influence of raised serum insulin levels.

(2)   This is worsened by the *high carbohydrate intake* which is necessary in chronic renal failure, by the high dialysate glucose and acetate levels, and at the renal transplant stage by corticosteroid administration.

(3)   There is also uraemic *inhibition* of plasma and fat depot *lipoprotein lipase*, so that chylomicrons and VDL particles can accumulate in the plasma and cause lactescence.

Figure 107 indicates, but does not explain in detail, the various aspects of hypertriglyceridaemia, which is characteristically the cause of a type IV hyperlipidaemia profile although the patients are often thin. The raised levels of plasma insulin which occur, almost *pari passu,* with the reduction in insulin

310

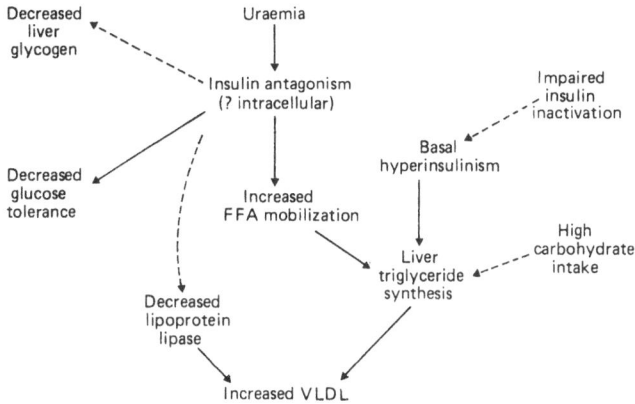

Figure 107. Summary of the lipid abnormalities of uraemia

sensitivity are in part due to a reduced catabolism in the renal tubules owing to the reduction in the glomerular filtration rate. They also arise as a result of 'insulin resistance'.

In untreated CRF impairment of glucose utilization can lead to a decrease hepatic glycogen, which actually renders the patient liable to hypoglycaemia.

Progression of nephritis or the nephrotic syndrome and the serum lipids

There is no doubt that a proportion of adults with symptomless haematuria or proteinuria and a high percentage of patients with the nephrotic syndrome are progressing towards chronic renal failure. The situation is worse if there is uncontrolled hypertension. In all these situations deterioration is easily measured by the rise of serum creatinine and by the fall of the endogenous creatinine clearance. A high plasma fibrinogen carries a bad prognosis, for not only does it indicate a worse state of the nephritic process, as indeed does the ESR, but a high fibrinogen also signifies a liability to vascular complications such as stroke, coronary thrombosis and deep vein thrombosis.

Additionally the level of the serum lipids portends the patient's fate in terms of vascular complications. High lipids, platelet aggregation, increased coagulation factors and accelerated atherosclerosis with thrombosis go together. The same patients have low anti-thrombin III and raised F.S.F.

As a generalization cholesterol is elevated up to ten times the normal in nephrotic patients and the higher it is, the lower is the serum albumin. Triglycerides are also elevated so that most patients are classified as type IIb, but very high triglycerides are only found in the worst cases. High density lipoprotein (HDL) (175 and 320 000) levels tend to be lowered in nephrosis, since like albumin these smaller particles are lost in the urine. Indeed, because there is some mechanism whereby albumin loss leads to increased lipoprotein synthesis by the liver, urinary loss of HDL might turn out to be the missing link (Figure 109).

The raised cholesterol correlates inversely with a lowered serum albumin, and in turn with the degree of proteinuria (Figure 108). The levels of plasma cholate are also raised.

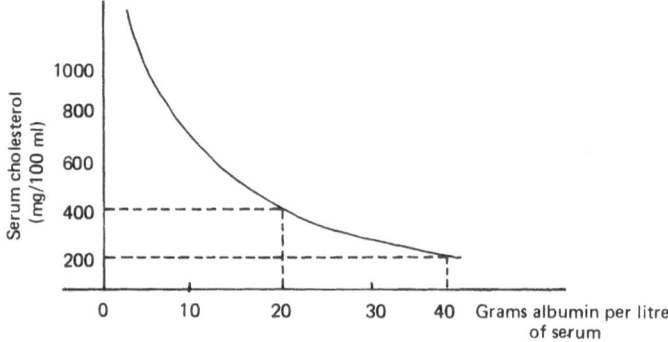

Figure 108.   Relation of serum cholesterol to the serum albumin

Fasting levels of fatty acids tend to be on the high side in nephrosis but the normal range is wide (300–1200 μmol/l). Since at the same time the serum albumin is low, the ratio of non-esterified fatty acids (NEFA)/albumin, which should be 0.77 in normal subjects, becomes 1.13 in the nephrotic patients; therefore there is more free fatty acid available to the tissues. The attachment of additional fatty acid to lipoproteins tends to accelerate their electrophoretic mobility.

The liver normally removes some 30% of the NEFA at a single passage. It uses them to form triglyceride, by attachment to that glycerol which is derived from a-glycerophosphate generated by glycolysis. That these fatty acids are being used to synthesise lipoproteins becomes obvious when carbohydrate is provided in abundance. So when a nephrotic patient is given a glucose infusion, it does not suppress the NEFA release as would occur in a normal patient, but demonstrates instead an increase of the hypertriglyceridaemia. There are other indications that a patient's carbohydrate intake influences the lipoprotein pattern in nephrosis, rather in the same way as it is now well established that a high carbohydrate intake leads on to a type IV hypertrigly-ceridaemia in quite normal people.

There has been some concern about the activity of lipoprotein lipase of the capillary endothelium in nephrotics. Its function is to hydrolyse VLDL, breaking it down to the cholesterol-rich LDL and liberating triglyceride. Defective function of this enzyme would exacerbate a hypertriglyceridaemia, but in effect it is normal in the majority of nephrotic patients; the enzyme is defective in uraemia.

On account of their hypertriglyceridaemia nephrotics are prone to premature atheroma, and for this reason attempts should be made to lower their lipids. As far as possible their carbohydrate and fat intake should be kept to defined limits and they will benefit from the administration of clofibrate. The dosage of this drug, however, has to be monitored in renal insufficiency, because if it accumulates a myopathy will occur (Figure 109).

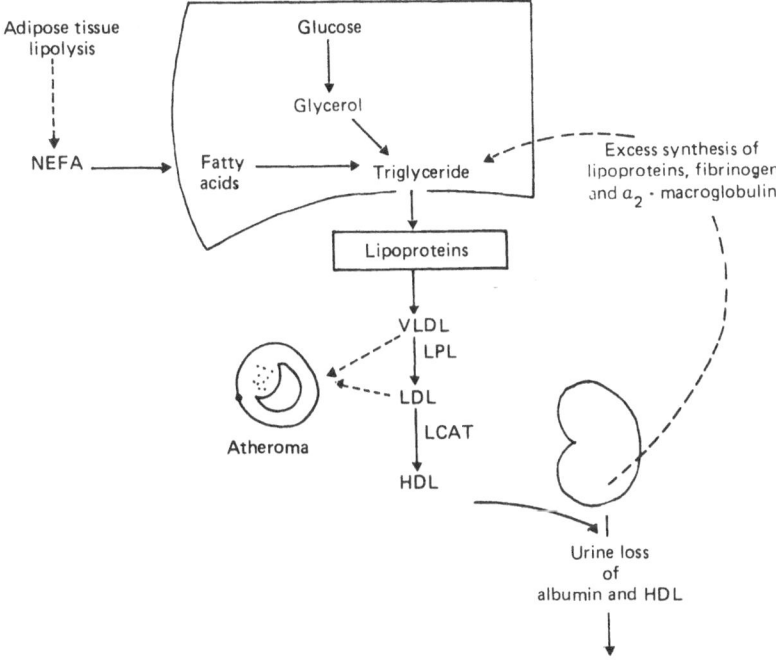

Figure 109. Lipid abnormalities in the nephrotic syndrome

The cycle is initiated by urinary loss of proteins including albumin and HDL, resulting in increased synthesis by the liver of new albumin, together with other proteins. Those of high molecular weight such as lipoproteins, fibrinogen and a_2-macroglobulin accumulate in the plasma; the excess lipoproteins are atherogenic.

Additionally there can be tissue hypothyroidism in nephrotics on account of a 25–30% urinary loss of thyroxine, either bound to albumin or as thyroxine-binding globulins. T3 levels are lowered in many chronic illnesses.

Anaemia in chronic renal failure

There is a refractory normocytic normochromic anaemia which is related to the degree of nitrogen retention. The haemoglobin falls by 2 g/100 ml for each 50 mg/100 ml increment of the blood urea. The possible mechanisms are as follows:

(1) *A refractory anaemia due to lack of erythropoietin,* which can also be exacerbated by protein deficiency, and by shortened red cell life span, and toxic marrow suppression in undialysed patients.

(2) *Superimposed blood losses* in the process of dialysis, due to physician investigations, and due to the uraemic bleeding defect of undialysed patients.

(3) *Other specific defects,* such as failure of iron absorption; folate deficiency; dialysis hypersplenism; infection or pyelonephritis; and microangiopathic haemolytic anaemia in accelerated hypertension.

The anaemia is caused principally by lack of erythropoietin, which is a glycoprotein hormone normally produced by the kidneys. It acts synergistically with testosterone to cause differentiation of erythroid stem cells in the bone marrow. Indeed it was noted originally by Jacobson that bilateral nephrectomy completely abolishes an animal's erythropoietic response to bleeding or to injections of cobalt; in the human situation bilateral nephrectomy should also be viewed with caution. There is no evidence at all that dialysis can restore the ability of damaged kidneys to produce ERP.

In addition many uraemic patients may have been through a period of conservative therapy requiring a very low protein diet. Even when allowed onto dialysis and an allowance of 60 g/day protein, the combined effects of nausea, infection, and previous adaptation to a low intake may mean that many patients only take some 45 g/day protein. Such patients can be identified by their low serum transferrin values.

In undialysed patients there is undoubtedly impaired red cell survival due to a metabolic defect. In turn this can be consequent on the metabolic acidosis and the accumulation of uraemic toxins. Inhibition of erythrocyte glycolysis is shown by impaired glucose and phosphate uptake. There can also be impaired activity of the hexose monophosphate shunt (cf page 307), and hence an increased liability to oxidation of the haemoglobin, as is evident from the low reduced glutathione concentrations and increased methaemoglobin and sulphaemoglobin concentrations that correlate with Heinz body formation. A reduction of transketolase activity can also be shown. Even in normal red cells 1% of the haemoglobin is converted to methaemoglobin and the uraemic cell has higher concentrations owing to its inability to cope with oxidative stresses. Accumulation of methaemoglobin in turn impairs the delivery of oxygen to the tissues; accumulation of sulphaemoglobin makes the cells more rigid so that they are removed from the circulation by the spleen.

Blood loss at dialysis is at least 20 ml. Dialyser residual volume blood losses have been known to account for as much as 500 ml/month and this is more than the inactive bone marrow of the uraemic patient can stand. A new dialyser is only acceptable if the residual blood volume is less than 10 ml—a burst coil during dialysis, for instance, can mean a blood loss of 350 ml. Physician investigations also have to be seen in perspective.

There have been claims in the past that the gut of the uraemic patient does not absorb iron. In fact the impression of poor isotopic uptake by the gut is really a reflection of the low rate of erythropoiesis, since it is this which regulates the amount of iron that crosses the mucosal barrier. It is also of note that the 20 g Giovannetti diet provides only 10 mg/day iron, so it is standard practice to give iron, folic acid and vitamin B supplements to chronic renal failure patients.

There is also an anaemia of infection which, of course, may be compounded with that of chronic renal failure. It can be seen in pyelonephritis, in which the degree of anaemia is more than would be anticipated from the degree of nitrogen retention. Sometimes the reticulocyte counts are raised before the stage of chronic renal failure, and this should indicate that the patient is taking oxidant drugs such as sulphonamides, phenacetin and other analgesics. Additionally some types of nepthritis may have their own more specific anaemia, as is the case when a positive Coomb's test due to C3 fixation on erythrocytes is found in hypocomplementaemic nephritis.

Microangiopathic haemolytic anaemia has been discussed on p. 275. It is particularly likely to occur in the context of accelerated hypertension or rapidly progressive nephritis with endocapillary proliferation. A trial of heparin should be considered, although experience seems to indicate that this may control the haemolytic process without arresting the decline in renal function.

The treatment of the anaemia of uraemia should therefore be basically as follows:

(1) Aim to keep the PCV at 22–30%, but because of the risk of hepatitis transmission (and of allograft recipient presensitization) keep transfusions to a minimum.
(2) Good regular dialysis is required (24–30 h/week).
(3) The patient should have a high protein intake (60 g) with supplementary iron and folic acid.
(4) Laboratory investigations and dialysis blood losses must be curtailed.
(5) Avoid oxidant drugs such as sulphonamides and antimalarials.

(6)   Give a weekly injection of testosterone, 250–500 mg.

(7)   Keep up the iron stores with intravenous Imferon—with due regard to haemosiderosis. Serum ferritin estimations help.

(8)   If bilateral nephrectomy is unavoidable, the patient should be transplanted early.

Two factors account for the bleeding defect of acute uraemia:

(1)   There is a reduced aggregation of the platelets, and hence a failure to release factors III and IV. Both phenols and guanidinosuccinic acid play a part in this, as does prostacyclin production.

(2)   There is an increased fragility of cutaneous blood vessels, so the bleeding time can be prolonged.

       On the other hand there are other features of 'hypercoagulability':

(1)   Raised levels of plasma fibrinogen and of factors V and VIII.

(2)   Increased resistance to heparin, and plasma antithrombin III is raised.

(3)   Fibrinolytic activity is decreased, owing to an increase of antiplasmins.

Vitamin D metabolism and chronic renal disease

Vitamin D, which is absorbed from the bowel or formed in the skin, is hydroxylated in two steps to its active form: (a) in the liver to become 25-hydroxycholecalciferol, and then (b) in the kidneys to 1,25-dihydroxy-cholecalciferol (Figure 110).

To date the physiological functions of the various forms of vitamin D appear to be as follows:

(1)   *Cholecalciferol (vitamin D₃).* This is the form that is absorbed from the gut or is made by ultra-violet light in the skin and is stored in fat and muscle.

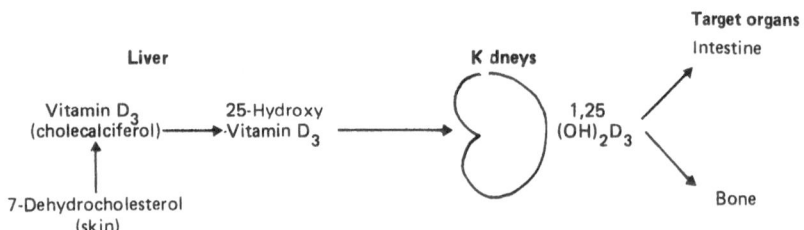

Figure 110. **Summary of the activation of vitamin D**

(2)   *25 HCC* (plasma level 5–50 μg/l). This is a major circulating form that plays a part in bone mineralization, and which also mediates renal tubular reabsorption of phosphate.

(3)   *1,25 HCC* (plasma level 0.02–0.04 μg/l). This is the active hormone that controls intestinal absorption of calcium and phosphate, and also remodelling of bone. It will therefore raise the serum calcium and depress the serum parathormone (PTH).

In addition it is now known that 1,25 HCC determines the appearance of a 24-hydroxylase enzyme which will convert 1,25 HCC to 1,24,25 HCC. This 24-hydroxylation heralds inactivation and excretion of the vitamin from the body.

This same enzyme is involved in other control mechanisms for while in hypocalcaemia 1,25 HCC is the major form in the blood, in hypercalcaemia 24,25 HCC appears instead. This is because PTH stimulates the 1-hydroxylase but represses the 24-hydroxylase. Thus vitamin D is present in an active form when parathormone production is high; this will explain why gut absorption of calcium is then increased.

In like manner hypophosphataemia stimulates 1-hydroxylation and represses 24-hydroxylation. Conversely high levels of intrarenal phosphate stimulate conversion to 24,25 HCC, which is now thought to play a part in increasing calcium absorption by the gut (Table 32).

Table 32 Summary of factors affecting Renal production of 1,25-dihydroxycholecalciferol (or 1-hydroxylase activity)

Stimulatory	*Inhibitory*
Low calcium diet ⎤	High calcium or strontium diet
⎬ low plasma Ca^{2+}	
Vitamin D deficiency ⎦	Vitamin D treatment
Low phosphate diet/ (low plasma phosphate)	High phosphate diet
Parathormone	Parathyroidectomy
Oestrogen, prolactin	

Finally, the problems in the interpretation of serum parathormone levels should be noted. An antibody which reacts with the carboxyl (C-terminal) end of the molecule will detect the large amounts of circulating inactive hormone fragments that are a particular feature of the uraemic patient. This will give quite different assay results from an antibody which detects the N-terminal end of the molecule. This is because the parathormone (PTH) secreted by the glands undergoes cleavage in the circulation into at least three distinct fragments; so the immunoreactive parathormone (iPTH) detected may vary.

BONE DISEASE

In dealing with bone disease it is important to have correct definitions. The bone is made of numerous 'osteones', each of which consists of an Haversian canal and its associated bone lamellae. These walls are remodelled by the combined activities of osteoblasts and osteoclasts, as in the structuring of the walls of a citadel (Mellanby).

Osteoporosis refers to a diminished amount of calcified tissue and can either be due to 'mineral osteoporosis' or reduced production of bone matrix ('matrix osteoporosis').

Osteomalacia appears when the normal reabsorption of calcified bone continues and yet the newly formed replacement matrix remains uncalcified, so that the bone becomes softened.

Often while they are still on conservative therapy, and certainly by the third year of haemodialysis, all patients have some bone disease. Progression of the mixed bone disease of chronic renal failure is often observed. It classically consists of (a) changes due to hyperparathyroidism, and (b) osteomalacia due to vitamin D resistance.

Secondary hyperparathyroidism due to phosphate retention

The phosphate retained as the number of nephrons diminishes causes a depression of the serum calcium. Therefore the parathyroid glands secrete increased amounts of parathormone, so that the calcium tends to return to normal or supra-normal. However the homeostasis is achieved at the expense of hyperparathyroid bone disease which is characterized by 'osteitis fibrosa'. The parathyroid glands themselves show secondary parathyroid hyperplasia and on occasions a gland will form an autonomous tumour, so-called 'tertiary hyperparathyroidism'. At this stage parathyroidectomy becomes necessary.

This sequence of events was neatly confirmed by Bricker and Slatapolsky by experiments in dogs which were subjected to partial nephrectomy of variable degree:

phosphate retention $\longrightarrow$ secondary parathyroid activity $\longrightarrow$ raised PTH $\longrightarrow$ osteitis fibrosa

In fact immunoreactive PTH values can be shown to be elevated in early chronic renal failure, when patients still have GFRs of 40–60 ml/min. The effects of parathormone are (a) to increase bone reabsorption by stimulation of osteoclastic activity, and (b) to decrease the renal tubular reabsorption of phosphate.

These factors are seen in Figure 111 which also emphasizes the other aspects of the bone disease problem. The multiple factors which influence the renal production of active vitamin D (as a hormone) have been discussed above.

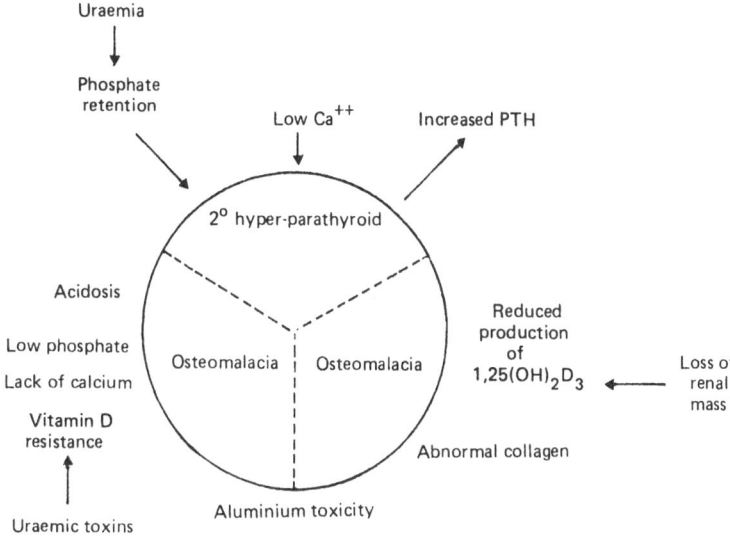

Figure 111. Factors contributing to renal bone disease

The histological features of the osteitis fibrosa which indicate increased parathyroid activity are increased osteoclastic resorption in the lacunae on the mineralized bone, replacement of the old bone by fibrous tissue so that the medullary trabeculae are eroded, and formation in that fibrous tissue of new woven bone (Figure 112).

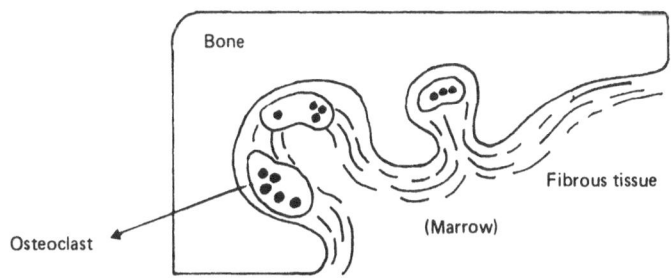

Figure 112. Representation of the histology of osteitis fibrosa

The radiological appearances include subperiosteal bone resorption, cyst formation, and sometimes alternating sclerosis and porosis of the vertebrae— so-called 'rugger-jersey' spine. Erosions occur typically on the periosteal surfaces of the distal and middle phalanges on their radial side, and also at many subperiosteal, subchondral and subtendinal sites. Common places

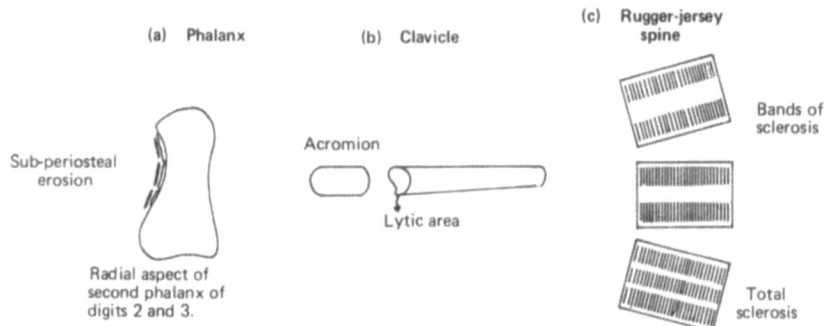

Figure 113. Radiological features of secondary hyperparathyroidism in uraemia

include the symphysis pubis, the sacroiliac joints, the lesser trochanters of the femora, the medial upper third of the tibiae, the proximal humeral metaphyses and the lateral ends of the clavicles (Figure 113).

Trabeculae of relatively small diameter increase in number, such that the components can hardly be distinguished, and it is this overall process which corresponds to the bony sclerosis. In the skull, areas of sclerosis alternate with areas of bone resorption, so that the vault may appear dense and featureless, although in some areas there may be cysts. Destruction of the middle third of the distal phalanges results in a telescoping of the soft tissues and the clinical picture of pseudo-clubbing. In those patients in whom the 'calcium x phosphorus product' is elevated, there is metastatic calcification in the media of arteries and calcinosis in the soft tissues. Moreover in patients with an elevated phosphate there can be calcium deposition in the skin, cornea and conjunctivae.

Vitamin D resistance and osteomalacia

Both hypocalcaemia *per se* and lack of 1,25 dihydroxcholecalciferol cause osteomalacia, or an inability to calcify newly formed osteoid (Figure 114). It has been known for a long time that patients with chronic renal failure have 'vitamin D resistance'. (cf vitamin D, page 316) The biochemical sequence is now more fully appreciated. It is that cholecalciferol, which is formed in the skin by ultraviolet light or which is absorbed from dairy produce in the food, is hydroxylated first in the liver to 25-hydroxycholecalciferol (see Figure 110). Thereafter it should be further hydroxylated in the kidneys to 1,25 dihydroxycalciferol; this is the active 'hormone' which stimulates absorption of calcium from the gut and which is also the direct cause of bone calcification. There is thus accumulation of osteoid when there is hormone deficiency in uraemia. Uraemic toxins may play some part in vitamin D resistance.

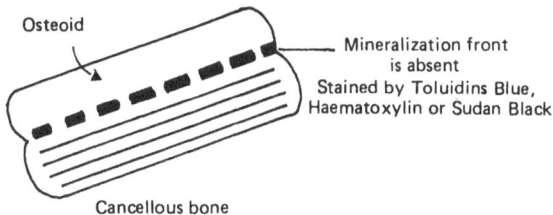

Osteoid

Mineralization front
is absent
Stained by Toluidins Blue,
Haematoxylin or Sudan Black

Cancellous bone

Figure 114. The osteomalacia of chronic renal bone disease

Such patients suffer from bone pains, as in true non-renal osteomalacia, which are readily passed off as 'rheumatism' or 'fibrositis'. There is often an accompanying proximal myopathy, which is responsible for a waddling gait and difficulty in mounting stairs. When osteoid predominates there is an elevation of the serum alkaline phosphatase, and the urine calcium is conspicuously low. Conversely when there is osteitis fibrosa, the plasma hydroxyproline correlates with the number of bone resorption areas.

In the adult the combined picture of osteitis fibrosa with osteomalacia leads to the radiological mixed picture as described above; but children with renal failure quite characteristically fail to grow and show the features of 'renal rickets' (Figure 115). This means that there is a failure to calcify the epiphyseal cartilage with a consequent proliferation and disorganization of the chondrocytes.

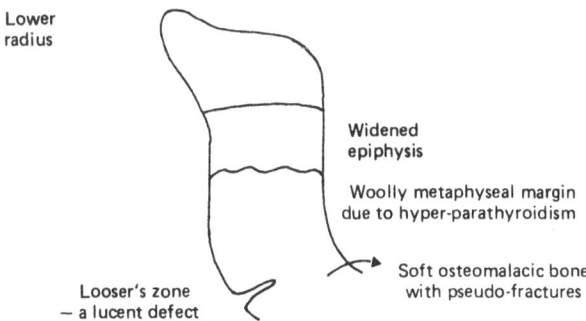

Lower
radius

Widened
epiphysis

Woolly metaphyseal margin
due to hyper-parathyroidism

Soft osteomalacic bone
with pseudo-fractures

Looser's zone
– a lucent defect

Figure 115. Renal rickets

The problems resulting from bone disease are summarized in Table 33.

In such patients it is clear that orthopaedic intervention is often required. Thus rupture of the quadriceps tendon retards the ability to extend the knee, and demands surgical repair. When calcific deposits are large and painful,

321

Table 33

Children	Adults	Post-transplant
Small stature Rickets—bowing of bones, knock knees and slipped upper femoral epiphyses	Osteomalacia and secondary hyper-parathyroidism Fractures Soft tissue calci-fication and ruptured tendons	Bone disease heals, but there can often be aseptic necrosis of the femoral head, which is the result of steroid therapy
	Acute arthritis—either due to uric acid, calcium deposition, or sepsis	

they will have to be excised. Open reduction of fractures and internal fixation with pins, plates and screws is often necessary, even though the softened bones lead to many technical problems.

The investigation of bone disease

X-ray features
X-rays are not sensitive enough for the detection of bone decalcification, which often means a loss of 40% of the skeletal calcium before demineraliza-tion is detected. One helpful early sign of osteodystrophy is the ring calcification between the toes in the dorsalis pedis artery.

Bone density
Photon absorption is a more sensitive technique for assessment of bone density. For this the distal end of a long bone is scanned with a collimated beam of photons from a 200 mCi iodine-131 source. Clearly there is dense bone over each cortex with a lesser density over the medulla.

Neutron activation analysis depends on the fact that there is in bone a small amount of calcium-48 which is activated by neutrons to calcium-49, a gamma-emitting isotope with a half-life of 8.8 min. The technique is used on the hand, which grasps for 10 000 seconds a container rod holding a neutron source of americium-241 and beryllium-9. The emitted spectrum is then quantitated.

Calcium kinetic techniques
Whole body calcium kinetic isotope techniques measure only exchangeable pools of calcium and are difficult to interpret. They can be dismissed as being of no practical use.

Biochemical measures used for assessment

(1) The serum alkaline phosphatase that correlates with the amount of osteoid but can also be indicative of osteitis fibrosa.

(2) The plasma hydroxyproline that correlates with resorption areas of osteitis fibrosa.

(3) A Ca × P product which is of note when in excess of 70 (mg%), for such values lead to ectopic calcification.

(4) Serum aluminium level. (see below) and tap water Al content.

Serial bone biopsies

Lastly one has to consider the use of serial bone biopsies, although these are unpleasant. Techniques of micromorphometric measurement of the decalcified samples have been evolved so that quantitation is made of the following indices:

(1) total volume of bone and mineralized bone
   (% measured area) of an iliac section

(2) volume fraction of osteoid (% of measured area)

(3) osteoclastic surface resorption ⎤
(4) surface endosteal fibrosis   ⎦ indicating hyperparathyroidism.

In fact, osteoclastic surface resorption and endosteal fibrosis both correlate with serum PTH values. Osteoid volume is found to be greater in those hyperparathyroid patients with a greater degree of acidosis. This is taken to mean that the hyperparathyroid state itself worsens acidosis (cf page 302).

Chronic acidosis

One point, which has not so far been emphasized, is that in chronic renal failure there is a steady positive balance of hydrogen ions, namely a chronic acidosis, which some authors still think will contribute significantly to the dissolution of bone. This is the case in renal tubular acidosis.

Parathyroid autonomy

Various forms of calcium infusion test have been devised in an attempt to measure the suppressibility of the parathyroids. Thus calcium at 15 mg/kg can be infused over a 4 h period, during which measurements of the plasma hydroxyproline are made. It is suggested that those patients who show a fall of plasma hydroxyproline during calcium infusion have retained parathyroid control, and that their osteitis fibrosa should therefore respond to dialysis against a higher calcium dialysate concentrate of 1.8 mmol/l (1.5 mmol/l is used).

Treatment of bone disease in chronic renal failure

The treatment is summarised on page 306.

Clearly the objectives in treatment must be to:

(1)   lower the serum phosphate and to increase calcium absorption from the gut; but avoid toxic accumulation of aluminium;

(2)   deal with the abnormality in vitamin D metabolism;

(3)   lower the PTH and suppress the parathyroid glands.

In practice oral aluminium hydroxide or carbonate is given to *bind phosphate* in the gut, so that it is not absorbed. Additionally the plasma phosphate can be lowered by increasing the frequency of dialysis, and the calcium can be elevated by dialysing with a bath calcium of at least 1.5 mmol/l (6.0 mg%). Indeed it has been shown that when the bath calcium is 1.8 mmol/l there is a net accumulation of calcium by the body, but when the bath calcium is 1.5 mmol/l there is a loss.

Both the plasma calcium and phosphate have to be closely monitored. Hypophosphataemia is a real risk which *per se* can cause hypophosphataemic osteomalacia. This could be one answer to the 'dialytic bone disease'. More commonly it is due to aluminium toxicity (Figure 111).

The plasma PTH falls automatically as the serum calcium rises. Other approaches have been tried. One way is to increase the magnesium of the dialysate to 1.5 mmol/l. Magnesium is thought to inhibit the secretion of PTH in much the same way as calcium does. If parathormone is lowered, then it is assumed that bone erosion is lessened.

Vigorous *calcium replacement* either by oral supplements or by high bath concentrations can, of course, lead to hypercalcaemia, with symptoms of nausea and vomiting. The dangers inherent in vitamin D administration are also great, for the plasma calcium can rise rapidly with little warning and then remain high for some 2–3 weeks after the vitamin D has been discontinued. If the hypercalcaemia is persistent, then the development of a parathyroid tumour can be suspected and exploration of the neck may be necessary.

Renal *dialysis per se* certainly does not cure renal osteodystrophy, but it does lead to some amelioration of the 'vitamin D resistance'. At the same time one has also to be aware that a low protein diet is another factor which worsens bone disease by causing matrix osteopenia.

Vitamin D 50 000–200 000 units /day used to be given for osteomalacia. Now that it is known that the patient's own diseased kidneys cannot produce 1,25 dihydroxy-vitamin D_3, the logical therapy is to give this at a dosage of 1–5 μg/day. This is still on trial and current therapy is still with dihydro-tachysterol or the new synthetic analogue 1-alpha-hydroxychole-calciferol at a dosage of 1–2 μg/day. This has to be hydroxylated to 1,25 $(OH)_2$-D_3 before it is effective.

Other causes of bone thinning such as *immobilization osteoporosis*, and that osteomalacia which occurs when patients are given microsomal enzyme-inducing *drugs* such as the anticonvulsants and phenobarbitone, must also be borne in mind. Likewise the possibility of *aluminium*-induced bone disease in those areas where tap water aluminium is high is very real.

Sensitivity to calcitonin is, in fact, retained in uraemic patients, so that there will be a degree of protection against osteoclasis. Measured calcitonin levels are lower in those uraemic patients who have a raised alkaline phosphatase and raised PTH levels indicative of osteitis fibrosa, so *calcitonin* might have therapeutic potential. In fact when there is elevated plasma calcitonin after nephrectomy, bone disease tends to heal.

Ultimately it is hoped that all patients will receive a *renal transplant*, since this is the best guarantee of healing of bone disease. After a transplant the osteomalacia heals quite rapidly but the osteitis fibrosa persists for much longer, possibly because of the hyperplasia of the parathyroid glands. If the serum alkaline phosphatase is followed serially, it will be seen to fall in the post-transplant period but will then rise again for about a year while there is remodelling of the bones. In this early phase there is also hypophosphataemia due to phosphate loss as part of the post-transplant polyuria.

Although the serum calcium and phosphorus do return to normal, except in the occasional patient who persists with hypercalcaemia and needs a subtotal parathyroidectomy, PTH values tend to remain elevated in most patients. In fact this seems to relate to the time that they spend on dialysis prior to transplantation and is thus directly related to established bone disease. Continued administration of steroids, which will hinder gut calcium absorption, plays some part in this process.

REFERENCES

Physiology of renal failure

Cockroft, D.W. and Gault, M.H. (1975). Prediction of creatinine clearance from the serum creatinine. *Nephron*, **16**, 31

Cutler, S. and Ederer, F. (1958). Survival figures by the life table method. *J. Chron. Dis.*, **8**, 699

Dunstan, H.P. (1955). Functional interpretation of renal tests. *Med. Clin. N. Am.*, **39**, 947

Effersøe, P. (1957). Endogenous creatinine clearances and serum creatinine. *Acta Med. Scand.*, **156**, 429

Griffiths, H.J. (W.B. Saunders and Co.) (1976). *Radiology of Renal Failure*.

Jelliffe, R.W. (1971). G.F.R. with corrections for age and sex. *Lancet*, **ii**, 710

Kelsey Fry, I. (1971). Radiology in the diagnosis of renal failure. *Br. Med. Bull.*, **27** (2), 148

Lemann, J. (1965). Fixed acid excretion in renal acidosis. *J. Clin. Invest.*, **44**, 507

Muldowney, E.P. (1972). Parathyroid hormone and urinary acidification. *Q. J. Med.*, **61**, 321

Platt, R. (1952). Structural and functional adaptation in renal failure. *Br. Med. J.*, **1**, 1313

Siddiqui, J. (1971). Complications of renal failure. *Br. Med. Bull.*, **27** (2), 153

Hypertension in renal failure

Advances in renin–angiotensin. (1977). *Fed. Proc.*, **36**, 1753

Brown, J.J. (1969). Renin and control of blood pressure. *Nephron.*, **6**, 329

Fraley, E.E. (1972). Renal hypertension. *N. Engl. J. Med.*, **287**, 550

Page, I.H. and McCubbin, J.W. *Renal Hypertension.* (Year Book Medical Publishers), (Chicago: 1968)

Vertes, V. (1969). Hypertension in end-stage renal disease. *N. Engl. J. Med.*, **280**, 978

Pathogenesis of uraemia

Cohen, B.D. (1970). Guanidino-succinic acid in uraemia. *Arch. Intern. Med.*, **126**, 846

Giovanetti, S. and Barsotti, G. (1975). Uraemic intoxication. *Nephron*, **14**, 123

Grantham, J. (1976). Fluid secretion in kidney tubules (hippurates). *Physiol. Rev.*, **56**, 250

Sullivan, P.A. (1978). Cerebral transmitter precursors in renal disease. *J. Neurol., Neurosurg., Psychiat.*, **41**, 581

Teschan, P. (1970). Neurological aspects of uraemia. *Am. J. Med.*, **48**, 671

Tyler, H.R. (1975). Neurological aspects of uraemia. *Kidney Int.*, **7**, S 188

Wills, M.R. (1971). *Biochemical Consequences of Chronic Renal Failure.* (Aylesbury: Harvey, Millar and Metcalf)

Trace elements

Alfrey, A.C. (1975). *Kidney Int.*, **7**, S 85

Deleves, H.T. (1976). *Proc. Roy. Soc. Med.*, **69**, 11

Middle Molecules

Bergström, J. (1975). *6th Int. Congr. Nephrol.*, p. 600

Chronic renal failure (CRF)

Fürst, P. (1975). Separation techniques. *Kidney Int.*, **7**, S 45
Man, N.K. (1973). *Trans. Soc. Artif. Int. Org.*, **19**, 320
Migone, L. (1975). *Clin. Nephrol.*, **3**, 82
Nolpe, K.D. (1977). *Ann. Int. Med.*, **86**, 93

Phenols

Hicks, J.M. (1964). *Clin. Chim. Acta.*, **9**, 228
Jützler, G.A. (1968). *Arch. Klin. Med.*, **214**, 214
Kramer, B.H. (1965). *Clin. Chim. Acta.*, **11**, 363
Wardle, E.N. and Wilkinson, K. (1976). *Clinical Nephrol.*, **6**, 361

Uraemic toxins and platelet function

Horowitz, H.I. (1970). *Arch. Intern. Med.*, **126**, 823

ATPase

Minkoff, L. (1972). Brain sodium–potassium ATPase in uraemic rats. *J. Lab. Clin. Med.*, **80**, 71
Villamil, M.F. (1968). Sodium transport by red cells in uraemia. *J. Lab. Clin. Med.*, **72**, 308
Smith, E.K.M. (1970). The red cell as a model for uraemic toxins. *Arch. Intern. Med.*, **126**, 827

Methyl-guanidine

Giovanetti, S. (1968). *Experientia*, **24**, 341. *Experientia*, 1971, **27**, 1157
Gonella, M. (1975). *Clin. Sci.*, **48**, 341

Neurological complications

Asbury, A.K. (1963). Neuropathy. *Arch. Neurol.*, **8**, 413
Platts, M.M. (1977). Aluminium encephalopathy. *Br. Med. J.*, **4**, 657
Thomas, P.K. (1976). Neuropathy. *Eur. Dialysis and Transplant. Assoc.*, **13**, 109

Susceptibility to infection

Abrutyn, E. (1977). Granulocyte function in patients with chronic renal failure. *J. Infect. Dis.*, **135**, 1
Baum, J. (1975). *Kidney Int.*, **7**, S 147
Byron, P.R., Mallick, N.P. and Taylor, G. (1976). *J. Clin. Pathol.*, **29**, 765
McIntosh, J. (1976). Defective immune and phagocytic functions in uraemia and renal transplantation. *Int. Arch. Allergy*, **51**, 544

Carbohydrate metabolism

de Fronzo, R.A. (1973). *Medicine,* **52,** 469

Dzurik, R. (1975). Inhibitor of glucose utilization. *6th Int. Congress Nephrology,* 590

Hormones and metabolism

Feldman, H.A. and Singer, I. (1975). *Medicine,* **54,** 345

Anaemia of uraemia

Erslev, A.J. (1974). Management of the anaemia of chronic renal failure. *Clin. Nephrol.,* **2,** 174

Fried, W. (1973). Erythropoietin. *Arch. Intern. Med.,* **131,** 929

Klein, H.O. (1971). Kinetics of erythroblasts in patients with chronic renal failure. *Proc. Eur. Dialysis and Transplant Assoc.,* **viii,** 93

Loge, J.P. (1958). Anaemia with chronic renal insufficiency. *Am. J. Med.,* **24,** 4

Naets, J.P. (1975). Haematological disorders in renal failure. *Nephron,* **14,** 181

Torrance, J.D. (1975). Changes in oxygen delivery during haemodialysis. *Clin. Nephrol.,* **3,** 54

Yawata, Y. (1973). Tap water haemolysis. *Ann. Intern Med.,* **79,** 362

Bleeding defect

Castaldi, P.A. (1966). *Lancet.* **ii** 66

Eknoyan, G. (1969). *N. Engl. J. Med.,* **280,** 677

Horowitz, H.I. (1967). *Blood,* **30,** 331

Effects of bilateral nephrectomy

Stenzel, K.H. (1975). *Am. J. Med.,* **58,** 69

Bone disease

Aluminium and bone. Berlyne, G. (1972). Lancet **i** 564.

Bloom, W.L. and Flinchum, D. (1960). Osteomalacia caused by aluminium hydroxide. *J. Am. Med. Assoc.,* **174,** 1327

Doyle, F.H. (1972). Types of renal osteodystrophy. *Br. Med. Bull.,* **28,** 220

Ellis, H.A. (1976). Renal osteodystrophy histology. *J. Clin. Path.,* **29,** 502

Hosking, D.J. (1977). Renal osteodystrophy. *Br. Med. J.,* **2,** 110

Kerr, D.N.S. (1979). *Lancet,* **i,** 406

Lotz, M. (1968). Phosphate depletion syndrome in man. *N. Engl. J. Med.,* **278,** 409

Chronic renal failure (CRF)

de Luca, H.F. (1975). The vitamin D endocrine system. *Am. J. Med.*, **58,** 39
de Luca, H.F. (1976). The vitamin D endocrine system. *J. Lab. Clin. Med.*, **87,** 3
Slatapolsky, E. (1968). Control of phosphate excretion in uraemic man. *J. Clin. Invest.*, **47,** 1865
Tougard, L. (1976). Treatment with 1-a-Vit. D. *Lancet*, **i,** 1044

Lipids in chronic renal failure

Bagdade, J.D. (1968). *N. Engl. Med.*, **279,** 181
Bagdade, J.D. (1970). *Arch. Intern. Med.*, **126,** 875
Cramp, D.G. (1975). *Lancet*, **i,** 672
Hampers, C.L. (1970). *Arch. Intern. Med.*, **126,** 870
Lindner, A. (1974). Accelerated atherosclerosis on dialysis. *N. Engl. J. Med.*, **270,** 697
Losowsky, M.S. (1968). *J. Lab. Clin. Med.*, **71,** 736

Increased malignancy during chronic renal failure

Matas, A.J. (1975). *J. Clin. Pathol.*, **1,** 883

Acquired cystic disease in chronic renal failure

Dunnill, M.S. (1977). *J. Clin. Pathol.*, **30,** 868

12
Drug therapy in chronic renal failure and dialysis patients

In chronic renal failure those drugs which are normally excreted into the urine will accumulate within the body. Drugs which are liable to precipitate convulsions (lignocaine or largactil) are particularly likely to do so in the uraemic patient, and yet at the same time it is so easy to overdose the patient so that he becomes drowsy and even demented (as with phenobarbitone or Valium).

The basic principles of drug kinetics apply. Each drug has its own volume of distribution (Vd) and is eliminated at a rate, K, which can be a combination of a renal clearance constant K_r and an extrarenal or metabolic clearance K_m. Hence

$$\text{total body clearance} = \text{renal clearance} + \text{metabolic clearance}$$

$$\text{Vd} \times K \qquad \text{Vd} \times K_r \qquad \text{Vd} \times K_m$$

For example digoxin clearance = 21% per day renal + 14% per day by the liver.

It ought to be possible to draw up simple dosage tables (that can be carried around) for all those drugs commonly used in renal failure according to the type of scheme in Table 34. This is the basis of 'constant interval : reduced dosage therapy' (see below).

331

Table 34   Sample dosage table for drugs used in renal failure

Drug	*Per cent reduction of normal dose according to the GFR*							
GFR	80	60	40	20	10	5	0	ml/min
Digoxin	89	79	68	58	52	50	47	
Penicillin G	80	61	41	21	12	7	2	
Ampicillin	84	67	51	34	26	22	18	

Certain drugs, of course, have to be avoided completely in renal failure. These include the tetracyclines which cause acidosis and also increase protein catabolism, raising the blood urea. There is also furadantin which readily causes neuropathy, and digoxin which can be very dangerous in a patient with changing intracellular potassium balance. Lithium easily accumulates to toxic levels. The hypoglycaemic drugs should be used with caution.

Naturally drugs whose dosage need *not* be changed are those which undergo metabolic inactivation in the liver. They include *antidepressants:* codeine, morphine, propoxyphene, diazepam, quinine, warfarin, indomethacin, epanutin, and also the *antibiotics:* rifampicin, doxycycline, cloxacillin, ampicillin and chloramphenicol.

All those drugs normally excreted by the kidneys have to be reduced. Thus in the case of gentamicin (cf page 272) we can say broadly that adjustment will be on a 'fixed dosage : reduced time interval' approach, as shown in Table 35.

Table 35

Renal function	GFR	*Dosage adjustment Normal*
Normal	70 ml/min	80 mg/ 8 h
Moderate impairment	20–50 ml/min	80 mg/16 h
Severe impairment	10 ml/min	80 mg/48 h
		or after each dialysis

Similar adjustment applies to the paediatric dose which starts at 0.8 mg/kg three times a day. Indeed the basic principle is that 'a drug *level* in a patient with renal disease should be the same and should be reached after a similar time interval as in a patient with normal renal function'. The schedule in Table 35 follows from the fact that the serum half-life of gentamicin is directly related to the serum creatinine concentration (Figure 116) so that whereas the normal half-life is 2–3 h, it will be prolonged to over 60 h when

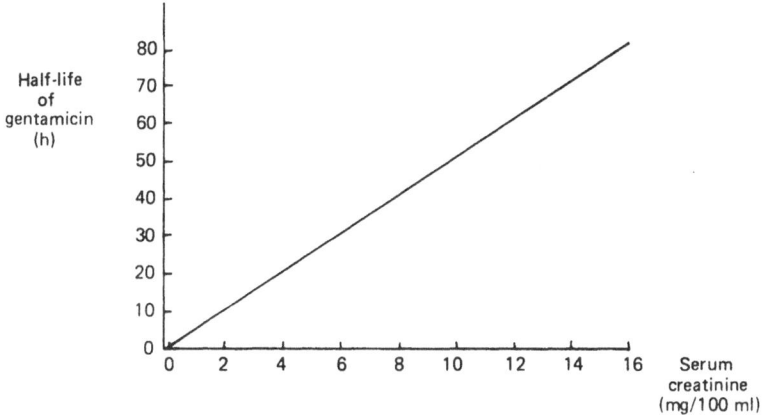

Figure 116. Gentamicin half-life and the serum creatinine

there is virtual anuria. As a generalization the half-life for gentamicin is given by the serum creatinine × 4; or one can use the 'rule of eight' referred to in acute renal failure therapy (page 272).

Many clinicians find it easier to think in terms of a half-life of a drug or protein. This is the time taken for the plasma level of the drug to fall to half of its original concentration (Figure 117). In fact, the 'elimination constant', K, is simply derived from the half-life:

$$K = \frac{\ln 2}{T\frac{1}{2}} = \frac{2.303 \log 2}{T\frac{1}{2}} = \frac{0.693}{T\frac{1}{2}}$$

The advantage of an elimination constant is that it can be summated $(K_r + \dot{K}_m)$ as in the equation above.

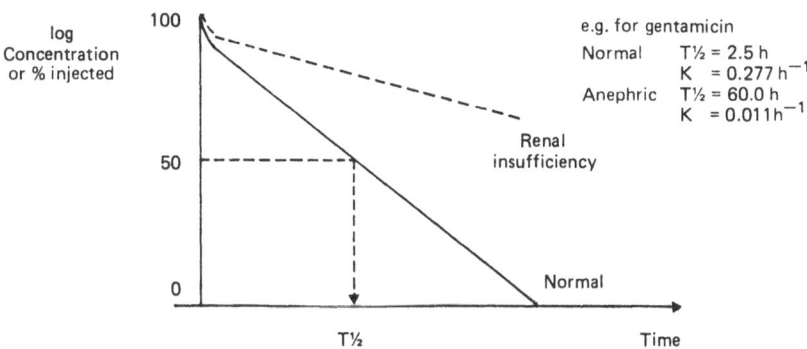

Figure 117. Decay of a drug or isotope is exponential

Kanamycin is another example, as a rough guide its half-life is thrice the serum creatinine in mg%. It has a normal half-life of 4.0 hours and thus is also normally given on an 8 h regime. When the creatinine clearance is reduced to 10 ml/min, its biological half-life becomes prolonged to 40 h. Therefore the dosage interval used with normal renal function now has to be multiplied by the ratio of the observed biological half-life to the original half-life:

$$\text{dose interval} \times \frac{\text{observed half-life}}{\text{normal half-life}} \text{ becomes } 8\,h \times \frac{40}{4} = \text{normal dose every 80 h}$$

Each antibiotic will have to be dose-adjusted in this manner; often it is quite simple. Thus amikacin sulphate, which acts against Gram-negative organisms, including *Pseudomonas,* has also a normal half-life of 2–3 h. On a rule-of-thumb basis it is suggested that the serum creatinine (mg%) should be multiplied by 9 to give the interval between dosages of amikacin at 15 mg/kg. So with a serum creatinine of 2.0 mg% the dosage interval is 18 h, and at a creatinine of 4.0 mg%, it is 36 h.

Table 36   Half-life and elimination constants of common drugs

	Normal half-life (h)	*Renal failure* (h)	*K:normal* (h^{-1})	*K:anephric* (h^{-1})
Ampicillin	0.5	13.0	1.15	0.05
Benzylpenicillin	0.15	7.2–10.5	4.6	0.46
Carbenicillin	1.0	14.0	0.69	0.04
Cephalexin	2.0	20.0	0.35	0.035
Cephaloridine	1.7	17.3	0.4	0.04
Cephalothin	0.5	2.0	1.38	0.35
Chloramphenicol	1.6–3.3	3.2–4.3	0.23	0.069
Chlortetracycline	5.6	7.0–11.0	0.12	0.063
Clindamycin	2.4	10	0.28	0.069
Colistin	4.5	10.3	0.15	0.067
Digoxin	40	86	0.017	0.008
Doxycycline	15	20	0.046	0.034

Table 36 Continued

	Normal half-life (h)	*Renal failure* (h)	*K : normal* (h^{-1})	*K : anephric* (h^{-1})
Erythromycin	1.4	5.0	0.71	0.14
Fluorocytosine	4.0–8.0	30.0–250.0	0.086	0.003
Gentamicin	2.0–3.0	60	0.27	0.011
Isoniazid	2.6	4.3	0.266	0.16
Kanamycin	4.0	48.0–96.0	0.173	0.007
Lincomycin	4.0	11.0	0.17	0.06
Methicillin	0.7	4.0	0.99	0.173
Oxacillin	0.4	2.0	1.73	0.35
Polymyxin B	7.0	72.0	0.1	0.01
Rifampicin	3.3	4.0	0.21	0.17
Streptomycin	2.0–3.0	52.0–110.0	0.23	0.006
Sulphamethoxazole	12	24	0.06	0.03
Trimethoprim	12	24	0.06	0.03
Tetracycline	8.5	60.0–100.0	0.08	0.008
Vancomycin	6.0	218	0.12	0.003

COMPENSATORY DOSAGE REGIMES

The fixed dosage, varying time interval approach to therapy

It will be apparent from the above discussion that this method is adopted for the various *antibiotics* having considerable nephrotoxic potential. The general method is to inject, and then to wait until blood levels have fallen before the next dose is given. In practice there are those drugs whose decay is dependent on the GFR since they are normally eliminated completely in the urine; there are those partially dependent on the GFR (vancomycin, for example); and finally there are those drugs eliminated in some other way, such as in the bile, so clearance is independent of the GFR (doxycycline or rifampicin).

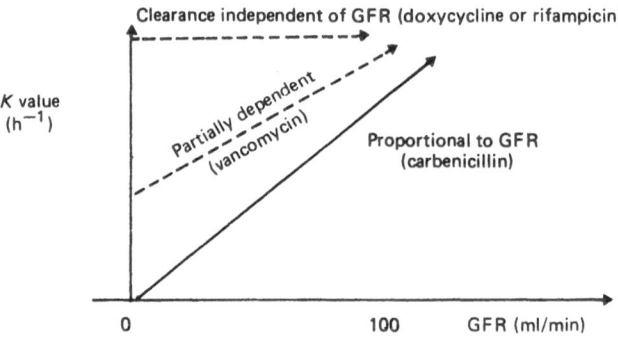

Figure 118. Relation of drug elimination to the GFR

If the original dose interval is T, then the new dosage interval T' can be calculated as a proportional change in the elimination constant:

$$T' = T \times \frac{K\,(\text{normal})}{K\,(\text{renal impairment})} \equiv T \times \frac{\text{observed half-life}}{\text{normal half-life}} \quad (\text{as above})$$

The whole process is facilitated by means of the table of elimination constants (Table 36), and graphical determination of the K value which should be used at a particular level of creatinine clearance (Figure 119).

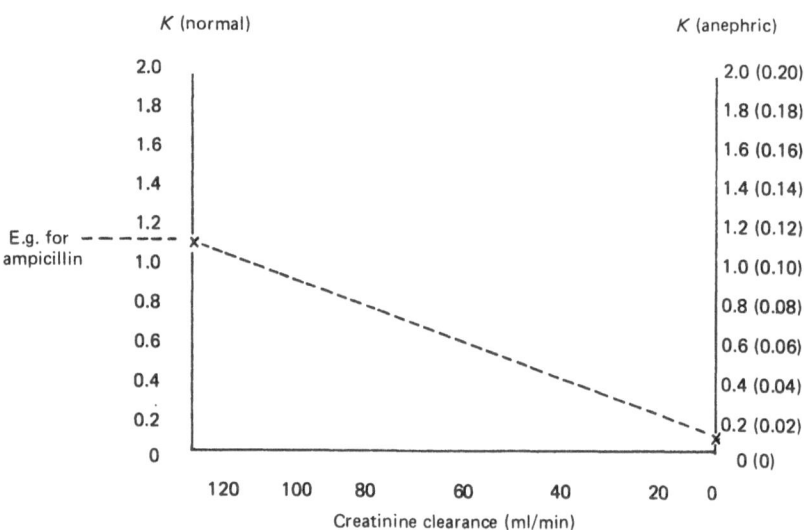

Figure 119. Graphical determination of elimination constants

Reduced dosage, constant interval technique

This has the advantage that there is much less oscillation in the drug levels. It is best applied to non-toxic drugs such as the penicillins and cephalosporins and also to digoxin.

In the case of *digoxin* 35% of the body content is normally lost each day by wastage of 21% via the kidneys and 14% by hepatic elimination, so the daily percentage loss is 14 + 0.21 x creatinine clearance. Hence the normal loading and maintenance doses should be calculated using this correction factor.

As for *carbenicillin*, it is usual to give 4 g i/v to achieve effective plasma concentrations of 100 mg/l. In the anephric patient the new dose D' will have to be adjusted according to the change in the elimination constants.

Thus

$$\text{new } D' = \text{old } D \, \frac{K \, (\text{renal})}{K \, (\text{normal})} = 4000 \times \frac{0.04}{0.7} = 250 \, \text{mg}$$

Constant infusion technique

When a drug is given by constant i/v infusion and its elimination follows first order kinetics, the time course t of the concentrations in serum (C) is given by:

$$C = \frac{K_o}{K_e V_d} \left[1 - e^{-K_e t)} \right]$$

where K_o is zero order rate of infusion,

K_e is first order elimination constant,

V_d is the apparent volume of distribution.

In the steady state the time becomes infinity so that the equation simplifies to:

$$C = \frac{K_o}{V_d K_e} = \frac{K_o}{V_d} \times \frac{T_{1/2} (r)}{0.693}$$

It is even easier to consider that the *steady state plasma level* is proportional to the dose D given during time T, and inversely proportional to the elimination rate K_{el}.

$$\text{plasma level} = \frac{D/T}{K_{el}} \equiv \frac{\text{steady state plasma infusion rate}}{\text{elimination constant of the drug}}$$

So in fact the dosage readjustment will be according to the ratio of the elimination constants

$$\text{dose readjustment} = \text{original dose} \times \frac{K \text{ in renal disease}}{K \text{ normal}}$$

(which is the same formula as used above).

Adjustments for dialysis

The customary technique is to measure arteriovenous drug concentrations across the artificial kidney under standard conditions of blood and dialysate flow. The whole process is facilitated by recirculating the dialysate. In that way it is only necessary to measure the rate of disappearance from the patient, and the rate of accumulation in the dialysate pool.

So when using gentamycin in an anephric patient:

plasma clearance = renal clearance (O) + non-renal (120 ml/hr) + dialyser
(1560 ml/h)   clearance   clearance
                                                                          (1440 ml/h)

Thus the plasma clearance while on dialysis is 1560 ml/h and in the interdialysis period is 120 ml/h. So it is usual to administer gentamycin post-dialysis.

Dosage in uraemia will thus be affected by dialysis which removes the aminoglycosides and penicillins and cephalosporins such as ampicillin, carbenicillin, cephalothin and cephalexin. Upon completion of dialysis, the proportion of drug that is estimated to have been removed should be replaced; for example, 70% of the standard dose of kanamycin should be read-ministered.

DRUG METABOLISM IN URAEMIA

The metabolic inactivation of many drugs takes place by hydroxylation, oxidation, reduction or hydrolysis by means of the cytochrome P450 system of the liver. The first stage makes the drug more polar (or water soluble) than the original drug. Then the drug is coupled to a much more polar compound such as glucuronide, sulphate or glycine so that it is readily excretable in the urine.

One can take, as a specific example, the conversion of phenol to its glucuronide. Phenols have a high lipid/water partition coefficient in their unionized form. Also at pH 7.4 only 0.5% is ionized since the pK is 10. On conversion to phenylglucuronide (pK 3–4) the product is polar and 99% ionized at pH 7.4, and so is unreabsorbable in the renal tubules. (Figure 120).

This is not the place for a detailed pharmacological discussion, but it is pertinent to enquire whether all the normal drug inactivation mechanisms are

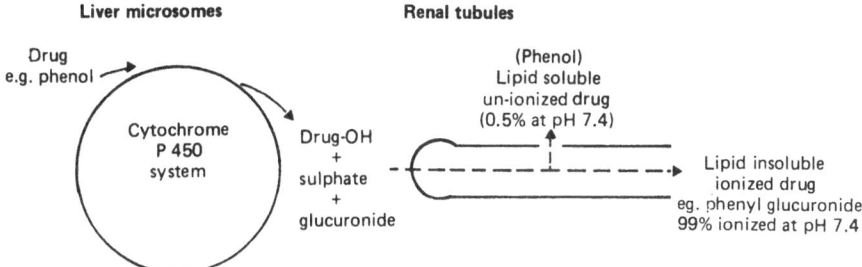

Figure 120. Conversion of phenol to its glucuronide

functioning in the uraemic patient. Otherwise one has to take account not only of poor urinary excretion (the K_r) but also of impaired metabolic inactivation (the K_m). Table 37 is a brief synopsis of the drug inactivation pathways and what is known of their function in uraemia.

Table 37 Drug inactivation pathways

Mechanism	Example of drug metabolized	Uraemia
Glucuronide formation	Chloramphenicol, indomethacin, salicylates, paracetamol,	Probably normal but not at high dose loads
	various hormones	
Hydrolysis	Insulin protease, procaine esterase,	Slower in uraemia
	plasma cholinesterase	Low in uraemia
Acetylation	Sulphonamides, isoniazid, PAS, hydrallazine	Definitely slow
Sulphate conjugation	Methyldopa,	Normal
O-methylation	Amines	Normal
Glycine conjugation	Benzoic acid	Slower

Although animal experiments point to a depression of microsomal oxidative functions, there are several papers which indicate that uraemic patients have an increase of drug oxidations so that antipyrine, the anticonvulsant Epanutin and vitamin D are inactivated more rapidly! The induction may be due to previous drug therapy.

DEALING WITH DRUG OVERDOSAGE

When faced with a comatose patient due to drug overdosage, it is important to identify the specific intoxicant rapidly either from witnesses or from analysis of the blood or the results of gastric lavage. Only then can specific antidotes or a logical treatment regime be instigated. Meanwhile oxygen and mechanical ventilation are required for respiratory failure and intravenous saline and plasma infusions for hypotension.

Coma is graded according to the following simple scheme:

Grade 1   Drowsy but responsive
Grade 2   Unconscious but responds to minimal stimulus
Grade 3   Unconscious but responds to pain
Grade 4   Unresponsive.

Clinical evaluation can give a clue as to the type of drug that has been taken (Table 38).

Table 38   Clinical evaluation of drugs

Drug	*Symptoms and signs*
Central nervous system (CNS) depressants	
Alcohol	Smell, drunken behaviour
Barbiturates, glutethimide, Librium, Valium, anti-histamines	Drowsiness, nystagmus and ataxia, and dysarthria passing to depressed respiration
Mandrax	Agitation, motor activity and tonic spasms
Salicylates	Sweating and tinnitus, vomiting, urine ferric chloride reaction purple
Antidepressants	
Tricyclic antidepressants	Dry mouth, mydriasis, hypotension, convulsions
Monoamine oxidase inhibitors	Headache, hypertensive crisis, arrhythmias
Phenothiazines	Drowsy, dystonic reactions, hypotension
Cholinesterase inhibitors phosphorus insecticides	Tight chest, mydriasis, respiratory distress, sweating and salivation Give atropine plus pralidoxime

Table 38 Continued

Drug	Symptoms and signs
Oxalic acid, antifreeze, etc., iron and copper salts	Pain in mouth and abdomen, sweating, vomiting and collapse
Hydrocyanic acid	Smell of bitter almonds. Give immediate cobalt edetate 600 mg i/v
Carbon monoxide	Smell of coal gas, pink mucosae
Heroin, morphia, methadone	Nodding drowsiness, shallow breathing, small pupils
Amphetamines and ritalin	Aggressive, dilated pupils
Atropine	Agitated, flushed dry skin, dilated pupils
LSD	Restless, dilated pupils, perceptual distortions

Choice of treatment

Peritoneal dialysis

Only useful for lithium salts.

Forced diuresis

Drug elimination by 'forced diuresis' of urine flow is indicated for acidic drugs that are non-ionized at pH 7 but ionized at pH 8.0 (such as phenobarbitone, barbitone, salicylates), or for basic drugs that are non-ionized at pH 7 but become ionized at pH 6.0 (such as amphetamine, amitriptyline, mepacrine, quinine and fenfluramine). The approach is, therefore, as follows:

First hour for alkaline diuresis	First hour for acid diuresis
500 ml/5% dextrose	1 l/5% dextrose
500 ml/2.4% sodium bicarbonate	500 ml normal saline
500 ml/5% dextrose	10 g arginine hydrochloride i/v over 30 min

Haemodialysis

This is applicable to the long-acting barbiturates phenobarbitone and barbitone as well as to salicylates. However, the short-acting barbiturates and other hypnotics need not be dealt with in this way. Haemodialysis is particularly recommended in the following situations:

Barbital > 30 mg%

Phenobarbitone > 20 mg%

Glutethimide or methaqualone > 3 mg%

Aspirin > 90 mg%

Ethyl alcohol > 300 mg%   methyl alcohol > 50 mg%

Carbon tetrachloride or ethylene glycol within first 48 h

Excess of bromide/thiocyanate/calcium or magnesium ions.

The many drugs not dialysed effectively are lipid soluble and attempts have been made to use vegetable oil as the dialysate in order to enhance their removal, e.g. Lipaphysan and 10% emulsion of evening primrose oil.

Table 39   Dialysable water soluble drugs

Sedatives

    Barbiturates—barbital and phenobarbitone
    Alcohols—methyl and ethyl alcohol, and ethylene glycol
    Glutethimide, methaqualone
    Phenelzine, tranylcypromine, pargyline (monoamine oxidase inhibitors)
    Anticonvulsants
    Heroin, amphetamines

Analgesics

    Aspirin and salicylates, propoxyphene

Metals

    xs. potassium, calcium, magnesium, sodium, mercury and arsenic

Halides

    Bromide and iodide

Antibiotics

    Nephrotoxic—kanamycin, gentamicin, neomycin, cephaloridine
    Streptomycin, tetracycline, sulphonamides, chloramphenicol, erythromycin
    Isoniazid

Coated charcoal haemoperfusion

Commercial charcoal columns (Haemocol) are now available. They consist of biocompatible polymer-coated activated carbon granules (about 300 g) in sodium chloride solution. They will absorb a wide range of organic molecules. Barbiturates, glutethimide, methaqualone, salicylates, ethchlorvynol and meprobamate can all be removed in this way, as also can the phenols and bile acids that might contribute to the adverse effects of hepatic coma (page 381).

This type of approach should be reserved for patients in grade 4 coma, those with high plasma levels, or those who are showing clinical deterioration in spite of adequate support procedures.

RENAL DISEASE CAUSED BY DRUGS

Drug-induced renal disease covers the whole spectrum of renal damage.

Drugs may cause acute nephritis, interstitial nephritis or nephrotic syndrome, acute or chronic renal failure and renal tubular dysfunction. Examples are readily obtained by reference to the antibiotics as shown in Table 40.

Table 40

Drug	Site of injury	Signs
Penicillin, methicillin	Acute interstitial nephritis	Azotaemia and proteinuria 15% eosinophilia
Neomycin, gentamicin and kanamycin	Tubular degeneration and necrosis	Azotaemia with albuminuria and casts
Cephaloridine Neomycin polymyxins Stale tetracycline	Proximal tubular damage	Fanconi syndrome
Demethylchlor-tetracycline	Inhibition of ADH	Nephrogenic diabetes insipidus
Amphotericin B	Distal tubular damage	Hypokalaemia, tubular acidosis and nephro-calcinosis

The polymyxins and polyenes are known to cause cell membrane damage. Amphotericin reduces renal blood flow and therefore creatinine clearance, and at the same time it allows the distal tubules to leak potassium and the back-passage of hydrogen ions. When given for aspergillosis it is given on a carefully controlled schedule (1.0 mg/kg by infusion on alternate days) and it has to be remembered that a total dose of 5.0 g will cause nephrocalcinosis. Potassium supplementation will be needed with only modest doses of amphotericin.

Some 20% of patients receiving colistin (polymyxin E) suffer renal damage; all patients receiving polymyxin B should be monitored for falling urine output and azotaemia as its potential for damage is even greater.

Table 41 classifies other drugs which damage the kidneys.

Table 41

Drugs causing vasculitis

Thiazides, sulphonamides

Nephritic syndromes with acute or interstitial nephritis
Sulphonamides, phenylbutazone, phenindione
Iodides
Thiazides

Nephrotic syndrome

Gold, bismuth, mercury, heavy metals and penicillamine
Tridione, phenindione, probenicid, tolbutamide, K perchlorate

Acute renal failure

Antibiotics and heavy metals
Dextran osmotic nephrosis
X-ray contrast media
Carbon tetrachloride or trilene

Chronic renal impairment

Phenacetin, aspirin and phenylbutazone
Heavy metals, such as lead

Uric acid nephropathy

Cyclophosphamide, 6 MP, nitrogen mustard

Diabetes insipidus

Demethylchlortetracycline (Ledermycin)
Lithium
Methoxyflurane
Glyburide

Note: It will be clear that some of these are direct toxicity effects and others represent hypersensitivity reactions.

High serum levels of IgE have been found in patients with drug-induced interstitial nephritis. When renal biopsies are examined there may be a linear deposition of IgG and C3 along the tubular membranes (for example, in methicillin nephritis). It appears that a dimethoxyphenylpenicilloyl hapten is bound to a structural protein of the kidneys. Additionally serum antibodies of IgG and IgM class can be demonstrated.

Iatrogenic renal dysfunction is only too common, as with retro-peritoneal fibrosis due to methysergide, but often the damage has also been caused by the patient administering his own medicaments. This applies to the nephrocalcinosis caused by alkaline stomach powders, to hypokalaemia caused by purgatives, and to analgesic nephropathy.

OTOTOXIC DRUGS

Hearing losses which hinder doctor–patient communication can occur in 10–15% dialysis patients. Drugs which damage the ears should be used with respect. They include:

Streptomyces-derived antibiotics—streptomycin, kanamycin, gentamicin and neomycin
Polymyxin and colistin, vancomycin
Salicylates
Quinine, chloroquine
Nitrogen mustard
Ethacrynic acid and frusemide.

REFERENCES

Anderson, R.J., Gambertolglio, J.G. and Schrier, R. *Clinical Use of Drugs in Renal Failure.* (Springfield, Ill.: C.C. Thomas) 1976
Appel, G.B. (1977). Nephrotoxic antimicrobials. *N. Engl. J. Med.,* **296,** 663
Bennett, W.M. (1974). A guide to drug therapy in renal failure. *J. Am. Med. Assoc.,* **230,** 1544
Cuttler, R.E. and Christopher, T.G. (1975). Drug therapy on dialysis. *Kidney Int.,* **5,** 516
Dettli, L. (1976). Elimination kinetics and dosage of drugs in renal disease. *Proc. Euro Dialysis and Transplant,* **13,** 603
Dettli, L., Spring, R., Habersang, R. (1970). Drug dosage in patients with impaired renal function. *Postgrad. Med. J.,* **October,** suppl. 32
Dettli, L., Spring, R. and Ryter, S. (1971). *Acta Pharmacol. Toxicol.,* 3S, 211

Kaye, D. (1974). Unpredictability of serum gentamycin levels. *J. Infect. Dis.*, **130,** 150

Kunin, C.M. (1967). A guide to the use of antibiotics in renal disease. *Ann. Intern. Med.*, **67,** 151

Linton, A.L. and Lawson, D.H. (1970). Antibiotic therapy in renal failure. *Proc. Euro Dialysis and Transplant Assoc.*, **7,** 371

Mathod, R.H. and Klein, W.H. (1969). Ototoxicity of ethacrynic acid. *N. Engl. J. Med.*, **280,** 1223

Matz, G.J. (1968). Ototoxic drugs and poor renal function. *J. Am. Med. Assoc.*, **206,** 2119

Rawlins, M.D. (1976). Drug distribution in renal disease. *Euro Dialysis and Transplant Assoc.*, **13,** 611

Reidenberg, M.M. (1977). Renal function and drug action. *Am. J. Med.*, **62,** 466

Welling, P.G. (1975). Prediction of drug dosage in renal failure. *Clin. Pharmacol. Ther.*, **18,** 45

Drug-induced renal disease

Curtis, J.R. (1977). *Br. Med. J.*, **2,** 375

Mukherjee, A.P. (1974). *Int. Urol. Nephrol.*, **6,** 225

Drug-induced encephalopathy

Taclob, L. (1976). *Lancet,* **ii,** 704

Dialysis for poisoning

Bloomer, H.A. (1966). Diuresis for barbiturate poisoning. *J. Lab. Clin. Med.*, **67,** 898

Lassen, N.A. (1960). Forced diuresis for barbiturate poisoning. *Lancet,* **ii,** 338

Rice, A.J. and Wilson, W.R. (1972). Rapid identification of drugs in body fluids of comatose patients. *Clin. Toxicol.*, **6,** 59

Schreiner, G.E. (1958). Haemodialysis in acute poisoning. *Arch. Intern. Med.*, **102,** 896

Shinaberger, J.H. (1965). Use of lipid dialysate for lipid soluble drugs. *Trans. Am. Soc. Artif. Int. Org.*, **11,** 173

Yatzidis, H. (1965). Charcoal perfusion. *Lancet,* **ii,** 216

13
Haemodialysis

This is (a) to remove toxic waste products from the body, and (b) to achieve the ultrafiltration of excess salt and water. The arrangement therefore is that blood circulates from the patient through a semi-permeable membrane so that small molecules can pass through into the dialysate solution, whose electrolyte composition is close to that of normal plasma. Urea and low molecular weight toxic products (of less than 1200 daltons) diffuse from the blood into the dialysate, whilst glucose and bicarbonate or acetate move in the opposite direction.

The patient's blood flows from a Teflon–silastic shunt, inserted as an arteriovenous connection at the wrist or ankle, or from needles inserted into a subcutaneous arteriovenous fistula which has been constructed in the forearm. After passing through the blood compartment of the dialyser the blood is returned via the venous connection back into the patient. The blood circuit has to be leakproof, not only to prevent loss of blood, but also to prevent the passage into the patient of bacteria and their endotoxins which may be present in the dialysate fluid. Coagulation is prevented by heparinization.

The basic features of any haemodialysis machine are shown in Figure 121, depicted so as to emphasize the various safety monitors.

347

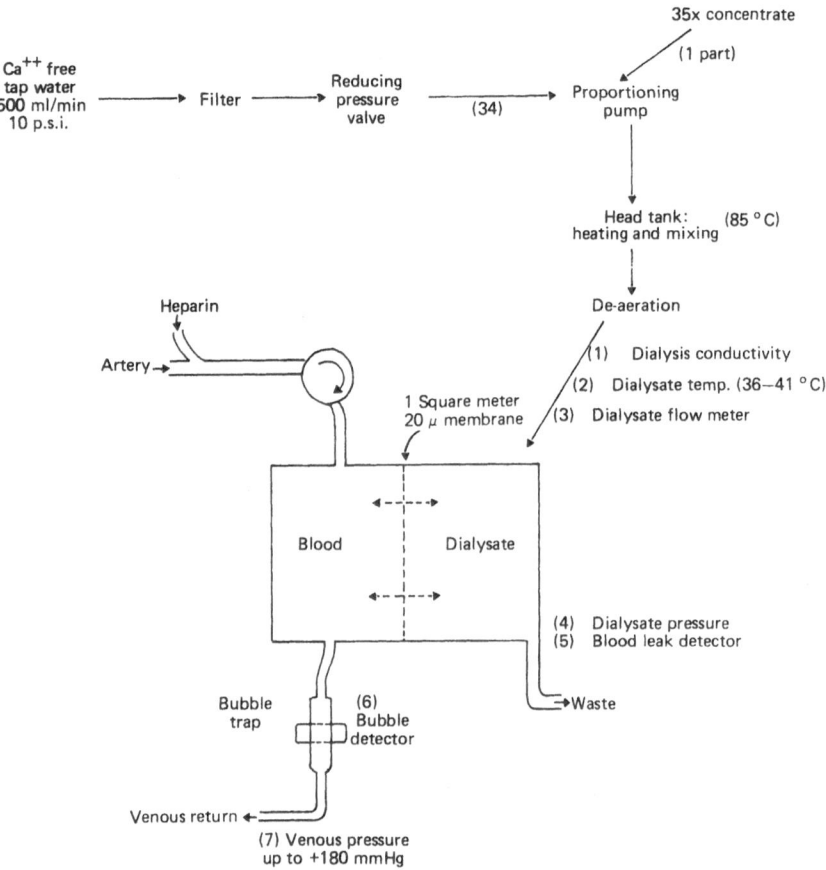

Figure 121. **Basic features of a haemodialysis machine and proportionating system.**

Dialysis procedure

Dialysis is used either for acute renal failure or for long-term maintenance of chronic renal failure patients. The initial problem of 'dialysis dis-equilibrium' has been explained above (p. 271).

Prior to use, the machine with its coil or Kiil is 'primed' by running through 2 litres of saline containing 2000 units of heparin. Then at the onset of dialysis 5000 units of heparin are injected smartly into the arterial line and thereafter a maintenance dose of 1000 U/h or 2000 U/2 h so that the patient's whole blood clotting time is maintained at 15–20 min.

According to the flow from the shunt the pump speed will be increased so as to deliver 200 ml/min of blood. Higher rates of ultrafiltration can be obtained by increasing the venous pressure to +50 to +150 mmHg (see Figure 123), but then, of course, the risk of a burst is increased.

If the venous pressure is actually higher than expected, then one should suspect (a) that there is clotting in the venous line, (b) spasm of the patient's vein, or (c) kinking of the venous line. If a coil bursts, as shown by the appearance of a tinge of pink in the dialysis fluid, then the immediate drill is to clamp off both bloodlines close to the patient and at the same time to stop the blood pump.

The dialysate

Filtered and softened ion-free water is mixed in a proportion of 34 parts to one part of dialysate concentrate (35x) in a proportioning pump. As the fluid is mixing its temperature is raised to 85–90 °C in order to sterilize it, and thereafter it is deaerated. Although sterilization is usually by heating, alternative chemical processes can be employed. The blended dialysate is then pumped through a conductivity cell which is sensitive to 1% changes in the sodium concentration. It passes to a constant head vessel of 750 cc capacity, where excess fluid overflows into a sump. By this time it has cooled to the temperature at which it will flow through the dialyser; this temperature is then monitored. The prepared dialysate is then drawn by a constant volume effluent pump through a negative pressure control valve and on to the actual dialyser at a rate of 450–500 ml/min, as indicated on the flow meter. After leaving the dialyser the fluid passes through a blood-leak detector, which monitors any haemoglobin in the fluid, and then it passes to waste.

The dialysate pressure is controlled by means of a pressure control valve within the range 0 to −150 mmHg. Its monitor is capable of detecting a 2% change in the pressure of the dialysate and will ring an alarm if there is deviation outside the set limits.

A thorough waterboard analysis should have been made on the source of tap water to any dialysis patient since he will be exposed to some 1000 litres week, compared with the mere 10–20 litres week consumed by a normal person. Iron which is derived either from the water or the pipes can precipitate in the filters as ferric hydroxide and cause great trouble. Moreover in hard water areas the calcium and magnesium has to be removed by 'softening' either by cation-exchange or by deionization. Certain metals which have a special affinity for cellophane and which may accumulate include lead, zinc and copper. A high aluminium content of the water is credited with the occurrence of bone disease in certain areas.

Dialysate concentrate which has been correctly diluted has the following composition:

349

sodium	133 mmol/l
potassium	1.5 mmol/l
chloride	103 mmol/l
acetate	35–40 mmol/l

The acetate is an appropriate substitute for bicarbonate. It is metabolized in peripheral tissues, such as fat depots and muscle, to acetyl-CoA in a proton-consuming reaction which therefore accounts for the buffering power. In patients with poor liver function bicarbonate is preferred.

$$\text{acetate}^- + CoA + ATP + H^+ \xrightarrow[\text{kinase}]{\text{thio}} \text{acetyl-CoA} + AMP + \text{pyrophosphate} + H_2O$$
$$\longrightarrow \text{bicarbonate}$$

Additionally there has to be calcium 1.5 mmol/l, magnesium at 0.4 mmol/l and there may be an occasional reason for adding phosphate (p. 324). The dextrose concentration is normally 11.0 mmol/l (200 mg%).

The blood circuit

Blood which leaves the patient's artery is heparinized and is driven by its own pressure as far as the blood pump. Pumps are of the occlusive rotatory type and can deliver 100–900 ml/min. After passing through the blood compartment the 'washed' blood finally emerges at the bubble trap, whose function is to prevent return of air into the patient's circulation. A bubble detector is placed so as to signal such an eventuality. Then there is a venous pressure monitor which is set at +50 to +180 mmHg. The higher the venous pressure the greater will be the amount of ultrafiltration in the dialyser. Indeed excess water is removed from the patient by clamping the efferent venous line so as to raise the pressure in the blood compartment and thereby to produce filtration under pressure.

Monitoring

The blood flow rate should be at least 200 ml/min. It is measured by injecting a bubble of 1 ml air into the arterial line and then timing its progress along a set distance to the T-junction on that line. So a transit time of 12 sec over a distance of 2 m might indicate a blood flow of 200 ml/min.

As in Figure 121, monitors and alarms, as listed below, are a vital part of the dialysis machinery:

(1)   Monitor of the sodium concentration, as dialysate conductivity ($\pm 1\%$).

(2)   Dialysate temperature in the range 36–42 °C.
(3)   The dialysate flow meter (up to 500 ml/min).
(4)   The dialysate pressure (0 to −150 mmHg).
(5)   The blood leak detector.
(6)   The venous line bubble detector.
(7)   The venous line pressure monitor.

When a monitor is activated an alarm sounds and the machine is automatically switched off until checked by an attendant.

Types of dialyser

There are three main types of artificial kidney (Figure 122):

(1)   *Kiil-flat board dialysers* in which the membranes separate blood and dialysate compartments, arranged as in a sandwich.
(2)   *Coil dialysers* in which blood flows through membranes wrapped around a drum which sits in a bath of dialysate (the original scheme of Kolff and van Noordwijk, 1946).
(3)   *The capillary (hollow-fibre) dialyser,* which is a coil packed with hollow capillary fibres made of regenerated cellulose or of cuprophan. Cuprophan is cupra-ammonium processed cellulose, and is highly permeable to small molecules. The blood passes through the capillaries around which is the dialysate fluid. It is possible to apply a high intracapillary pressure to achieve ultrafiltration.

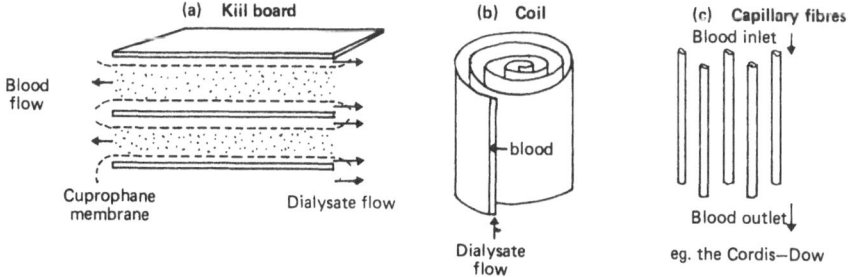

Figure 122. Types of dialyser

For special ultrafiltration a capillary fibre unit (eg XM-50 membrane) can be used in its own circuit or in series with the artificial kidney. Otherwise, as explained above, a high venous pressure is applied to the blood compartment by clamping. Anticipated results are shown in Figure 123. Thus an increase in blood flow causes an increase in ultrafiltration, especially when the venous pressure is also elevated so as to increase the transmembrane pressure.

351

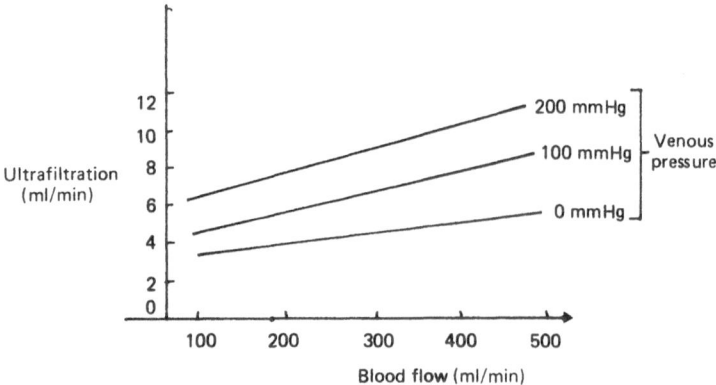

Figure 123. Ultra-filtration during dialysis

The Kiil board dialyser

The Watson–Marlow dialyser (see Figure 122a) has three boards so that when membranes are inserted between each pair, there is a blood flow channel on each side of the centre board.

The blood flows through the two membrane compartments in a direction opposite to the dialysate fluid, which is actually in the grooves on the boards. The volume of each blood compartment is 60–85 ml. The actual dialysis is determined by (a) the rate of blood flow, and (b) the pressure within the dialysate compartment. These important factors are illustrated in Figure 124.

After each dialysis the membranes are discarded. The dialyser is then rebuilt with fresh membranes which are sterilized in 2% formalin, and the

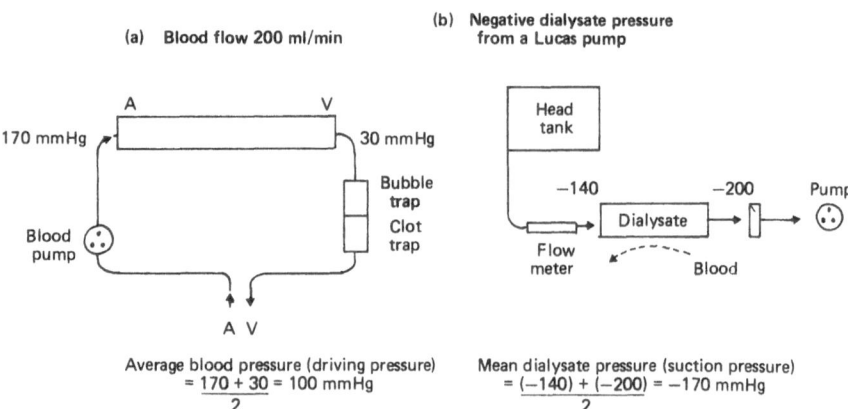

Figure 124. Role of blood and dialysate pressures

whole dialyser is washed through with heparinized saline prior to use. Formalin contamination of blood causes severe rigors, so it is essential to do routine tests for formalin contamination by using Clinitest tablets which give a violet colour.

Since it is important to avoid membrane leaks, which mean loss of blood, immediately after assembly and before the dialyser is filled with fluid, the membranes are tested by applying an air pressure of 300 mmHg with a sphygmomanometer bulb. The fall in pressure should not exceed 20 mmHg over a test period of 3 min.

The Gambro-Lundia—This is a flat bed dialyser which forms a disposable rectangular box. For the 1 m² variety the priming volume is low at only 90 ml. Dialysance is good.

The Rhone-Poulenc (RP)—This is another flat plate disposable dialyser. Dialysance for smaller molecules is not so good but paradoxically it is better for middle molecules. These observations are better appreciated when viewed in the standard manner as shown in Figures 127 and 129.

The coil dialyser
The twin-coil Kolff dialyser (see Figures 122b and 125) consists of two tubular membranes wound around a central core. Blood is pumped in at the centre of the coil and flows around centrifugally before exiting at the outer side. The coils of the cellophane tubing are separated by plastic mesh and the dialysis fluid is pumped up through these interstices from below upwards.

When dialysing with a coil a typical blood flow rate may be 200 ml/min and the dialysate flow rate 500 ml/min. The mid-coil transmembrane pressure is about 200 mmHg, and is calculated as the mean of the difference of pressure

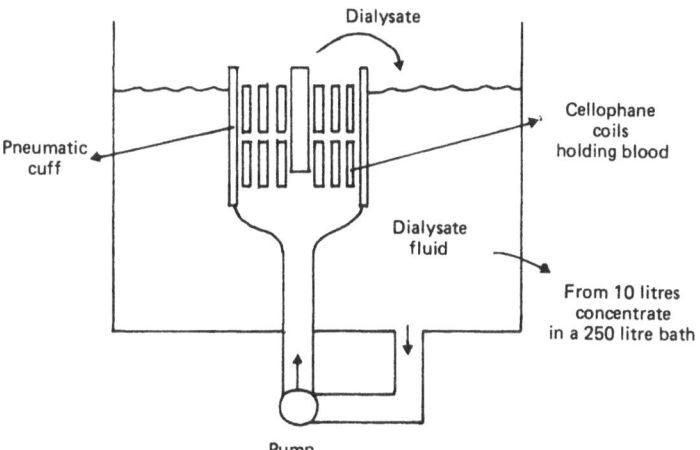

Figure 125. A coil dialyser

between the arterial line (150 mmHg) and the venous return line (set at +50 mmHg) minus the pressure midway between the top and bottom of the dialyser coil.

These figures are derived using a closed container and a negative dialysate pressure system as illustrated in Figure 126. With an open container the mid-container dialysate pressure is zero. The transmembrane pressure, which is important as it determines the rate of ultrafiltration, then depends solely on the mean blood pressure.

Since the membrane at the arterial end of the coil is subject to the greatest hydrostatic stress, it is here that the coil tends to rupture; the mean rupture rate for coils during dialysis is as high as 6%. In part the susceptibility to rupture is because the tubular membrane is not supported, although some support is provided by the inflatable cuff that surrounds the Ultra Flo 100 coil or by a rigid jacket as in the case of the EX03 coil.

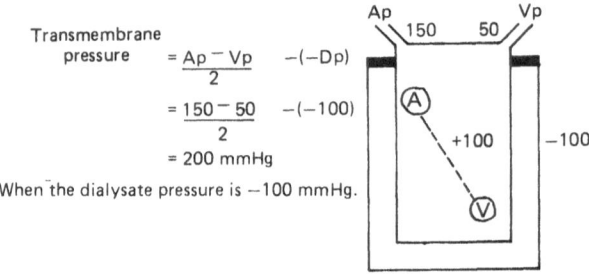

Figure 126.   **Illustration of trans-membrane pressure (EX 03 coil)**

Capillary dialyser (Figure 122c)
The Cordis-Dow—This is a capillary hollow fibre dialyser (Figure 122c), to which a high pressure can be applied in order to achieve ultrafiltration. Clotting within the fibres can be a problem, but dialysance of molecules is good, especially in the Cordis 5 for 'middle range molecules' (Figure 129).

Vascular access

The Quinton–Scribner shunt
This is merely a silastic U-shaped loop, whose join can be parted to form arterial and venous connections to the dialysis machine, and whose far ends fit into the artery and vein respectively by means of Teflon cannulae. Its simplicity is deceptive if the cannulae are at all angulated in relation to the vessels. Indeed it is essential that this shunt should be embedded in correct alignment in a subcutaneous position.

When handling a shunt, *strict asepsis* must be maintained as infection is hazardous and endocarditis may follow. Thrombosis is a result of poor flow; in turn this may be because of poor positioning, hypotension or hyper-coagulability. The latter can be controlled to a degree by heparin, by warfarin anticoagulation, or by a platelet inhibitory drug such as sulphinpyrazone.

The shunt is placed in the radial artery at the wrist and in the adjacent cephalic vein, or more commonly in the posterior tibial vessels at the ankle. In this way the arm is reserved for a fistula.

The Brescia–Cimino arteriovenous fistula

This is formed by anastomosing the side of the radial artery at the wrist directly to the cephalic vein. The high flow in the forearm veins will then cause distension and thickening over the course of 4–6 weeks, so that they become pulsatile and are amenable to venipuncture by needles or by cannulae and can be connected to the dialysis machine.

For children or patients who have lost their distal sites an antecubital fistula can be created. Alternatively a loop of saphenous vein can be transplanted to the forearm to form a connection from the radial, ulna or brachial artery into an adjacent vein. Again time is required for full matura-tion of the circuit. Thereafter repeated venipuncture must be performed with care because of the risks of aneurysm formation, perivascular haematoma and stricture formation.

Yet another possibility is a bovine carotid artery heterograft (BHG), which is immunologically inert and conveniently stored until required.

Single needle dialysis

In acute renal failure it is sometimes the policy to insert a Seldinger catheter into a femoral artery as the arterial line and to use a venous return into a vein on the patient's arm. This system can only be tolerated for a short time.

In routine dialysis the insertion of two needles into a fistula can be a painful and sometimes difficult process, requiring considerable skill on the part of the nurse or doctor. The Gambro single needle utilizes time or pressure cycling, so as to alternate the blood flow between withdrawal and return of blood.

Dialyser performance and comparisons

Ultrafiltration (cf. haemofiltration page 382)

It has been emphasized above that this depends on the transmembrane pressure. Filtration is very important for the removal of the excess fluid from a patient whose fluid intake has to be restricted owing to a poor urine output. Indeed patients on regular haemodialysis are usually allowed 1 litre of water intake as food or drink. Since water loss by evaporation or in the stools is about 500 ml/day, such patients will accumulate fluid at the rate of 500 ml/day. So when there is a 3-day gap between dialyses, patients will be expected to gain the equivalent of 1.5 litres in weight. In fact many will gain 2 kg or more. This fluid has to be removed at the next dialysis or else the blood pressure will rise.

A reasonable rate of ultrafiltration is in the range 200–500 ml/h fluid at a transmembrane gradient of 200 mmHg. Ultrafiltration rate can be measured during dialysis by consideration of the patients weight loss. A Datex bed-weighing system is used in conjunction with a calibrated chart recorder. Measurements are carried out during the second hour of dialysis at a constant blood flow rate of 200 ml/min. The ultrafiltration rate is measured over 20 min periods at varying transmembrane pressures (Figure 123).

Similar measurements can be made for the purpose of dialyser evaluation in a closed circuit system. A blood flow of 200 ml/min is used. Dialysate flows at 500 ml/min from a graduated cylinder through the dialyser. Depending on the type of dialyser, either the dialysate negative pressure control is altered or the blood outlet pressure, so that transmembrane pressure is adjusted according to the formula:

$$\text{transmembrane pressure} = \frac{(P_b \text{ in} + P_b \text{ out})}{2} - \frac{(P_d \text{ in} + P_d \text{ out})}{2}$$

Volume reduction in the graduated cylinder is plotted against time, so that the ultrafiltration rate can be determined.

Clearance and 'dialysance'

The 'clearance', namely the amount of plasma/min that is cleared of a particular substance, is a familiar concept. For urea, uric acid, creatinine, potassium and phosphate it is simply determined by taking arterial and venous blood samples 1 and 6 h after the onset of dialysis.

Thus

$$\text{Clearance} = \frac{\text{blood flow (ml/min)} \times (\text{arterial concentration} - \text{venous concentration})}{\text{arterial concentration}}$$

'Dialysance' incorporates additional consideration of the amount of the substance under study that is already in the dialysis fluid.

$$\text{Dialysance} = \frac{\text{blood flow (Q) ml/min} \times (C_A - C_V)}{C_A - C_{\text{dialysate}}}$$

In fact the dialysance is flow dependent within the normal blood range of 200–300 ml/min, as Figure 127 shows.

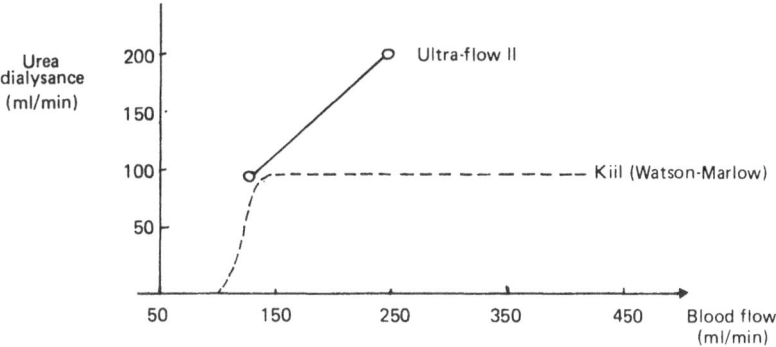

Figure 127. Dialyser performance at different flow rates

The clearance of a molecule will depend on its molecular weight. Urea (molecular weight 60) has a high clearance of at least 80 ml/min on a Kiil board and 150 ml/min in a Kolff-type coil dialyser. On the other hand vitamin B_{12} (molecular weight 1355) has a dialysance of only 20 ml/min in a coil. Those molecules with a molecular weight in excess of 1000 are known as 'middle molecules' and their dialysance is poor, although it is increased both by high surface area and by high permeability membranes (Figure 128).

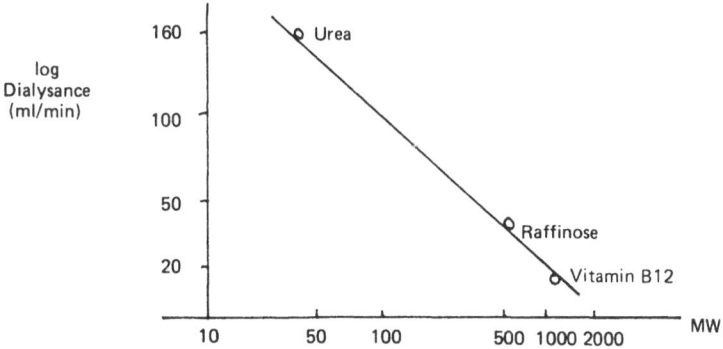

Figure 128. Dialysance and molecular weight

In general dialysance is closely related to molecular size, as shown above, but for phosphate it is less than expected. Phosphate has an actual molecular weight of 95, but its dialysance corresponds to that of a molecule of 210 daltons, for presumably its charge hinders diffusion through the membranes. The dialysance of phenols is one-half that of creatinine. This is probably due both to their lipophilicity and to their protein binding.

When measuring dialysance (or clearance) in a dialyser evaluation

357

circuit, dialysance is calculated at varying blood flow rates (in the range 100–300 ml/min) at a constant dialysate flow rate of 500 ml/min. In the case of a coil a high dialysate recirculation rate is required, and this can be obtained by using a Lucas recirculating mingle pass unit (RMPU).

In vivo clearances are made in the second hour of dialysis in view of the fall-off in performance that can occur during the first hour. Blood flow is varied by means of the blood pump and is measured thrice by bubble transit time over a 200 cm segment of the arterial line. Arterial and venous line urea and creatinine values are easily measured by an autoanalyser. The clearance results conform to a curve of the form:

$$\text{Clearance} = \frac{Q}{a+b.Q} \quad \text{where } a \text{ and } b \text{ are constants.}$$

A line can be fitted by the method of 'least squares' approximation.

The clearances of higher molecular weight ('middle molecule' substances) can be measured by isotopes such as ^{14}C sucrose (340 daltons, ^{51}Cr EDTA (380), ^{3}H vitamin B^{12} 1355 daltons) or by a dye that is easily quantitated colorimetrically such as bromsulphthalein (molecular weight 835).

The performance of the newer dialysers (Figure 129) has been evaluated by such techniques, particularly with respect to the clearance of middle molecules (up to 1500 daltons). In view of the supposed toxicity of 'middle molecules' (see below) the trend has been toward dialysers with a larger surface area. Yet in the hope that they will one day be portable there has also been research on smaller editions. Thus the *Haemomicro-Nephros* is a parallel flow dialyser which is less than 0.3 m in length and only 50 mm in width or depth! Its 62 dialysate channels and 61 blood compartments are formed from a single folded sheet of cuprophan 11.5 μm thick.

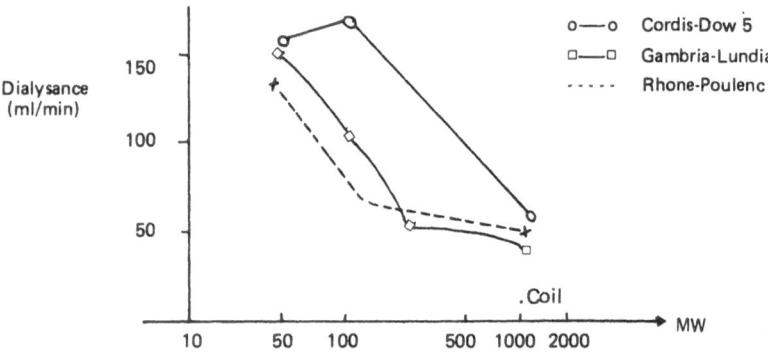

Figure 129. Dialysance of newer dialysers

358

Priming volume
This is the volume of blood that is needed to fill up the machine at the onset of dialysis, and which, if saline were not substituted, would result in a blood volume deficit for the patient. Adult priming volumes can be in the range 250–400 ml. Adjustment is clearly needed for children (of less than 30 kg weight), for whom one has the choice of a single layer standard Kiil (priming volume 175 ml) or of a Meltec Kiil of surface area 0.6 m^2 with a priming volume of 80 ml. Less than 10% of the blood volume must be in the dialyser. The one-layer Mini-D takes 10 ml and Gambro mini-minor 25 ml blood.

Residual blood loss
At the end of a dialysis blood is washed back into the patient using 5% dextrose. During this time the Kiil board is placed vertically and a coil in a horizontal position; even so the blood left within the dialyser can amount to 10–15 ml. This is small but cumulative losses become significant—at least 1.5 litres/year.

Blood losses can be quantitated either by using chromium labelled red cells, or, by washing the used machine with distilled water in order to find the original amount of blood as calculated from the haemoglobin concentration of the recirculating water. In this latter case the saline remaining in the used dialyser is recirculated through a 1 l bottle of 0.04% ammonia. The residual blood volume is then given by the formula:

$$RBV = \frac{h\,(1000 + \text{circuit volume (ml)})}{200\,H}$$

where h is the haemoglobin concentration of recirculated residual fluid, and H is the haemoglobin concentration of the patient's arterial blood at the end of dialysis. This is diluted 1/200 in 0.04% ammonia solution.

If the patient has actually been injected with chromium-labelled red cells, at the end of dialysis the washed dialyser is simply taken and is counted in a specially constructed shield counter in relation to a reference sample.

Clotting of blood components
In part residual blood loss is determined by the amount of thrombus deposition within the dialyser. Thrombus is quite apparent on the cuprophan membranes of flat plate dialysers. Closer examination shows adherent platelets, fibrin strands and trapped red cells in spite of adequate heparinization (Figure 130). In fact an appreciable fall in platelet counts and hence a concomitant serotonin release occurs in the course of each dialysis. Studies of the venous effluent of dialysers in action show that there is increased release of platelet factor IV, a reduction of Hageman factor XII, and that there is foreign surface activation of kallikrein esterase.

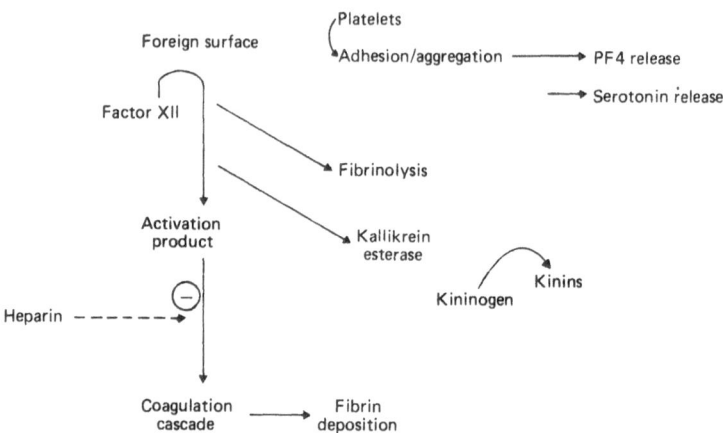

Figure 130.   Activation of coagulation on a foreign surface

Apart from their thrombogenicity, dialysis membranes have a tendency to so alter polymorphs that on their return to the body they adhere to the endothelium in the lungs and activate the complement cascade. The result is a leucopenia shortly after the onset of dialysis, accompanied by a fall of C3 and C4 complement components.

Additionally mechanical pumps cause damage to red cells, in the same way as turbulence in coil dialysers causes damage.

Coil bursts
These form another major problem which contributes to blood loss. The risk is, however, negligible with the flat plate dialysers which utilize cuprophan membranes in sheet form.

Management of the dialysis patient

In the chronic renal failure patient the indication for dialysis is disabling irreversible uraemia. In effect this will mean a creatinine clearance of less than 3 ml/min (but less than 6 ml/min if the patient is hypertensive), a urine output of less than 500 ml/day, or a urinary urea output of less than 6 g/day. The urinary urea should be multiplied by 3 to give the amount of protein that is being catabolized.

Patients do better if they start on a dialysis programme early without having to wait for a long period on a low protein diet. Clearly local strategic considerations will play a role in decision-making and it is often usual to start patients initially on weekly peritoneal dialysis. In this time an arm fistula can be constructed, and the patient's social background and psychological outlook can be assessed.

In the case of chronic renal failure patients the normal twin-coil dialyser, which holds 250 litres of dialysate, will be used for a 6 h run. With the flat Kiil board dialyser a patient will be dialysed for three sessions per week, each of at least 10 h, although these times are now being shortened. So in some centres a long dialysis is now 6–9 hours three times weekly, as excess fluid and salt and most of the toxic metabolites can be removed by three times weekly haemodialysis of 6 h per session.

Conservative management is usually possible for a time, but one has to realize that the patient on a very low protein intake is developing malnutrition, and that the chronic retention of uraemic metabolites will predispose to neuropathy and bone disease. The typical uraemic symptoms of anorexia, nausea and vomiting, and hiccup occur with a blood urea level of 200 mg% (33 mmol/l), and some symptoms and the anaemia will often appear when the blood urea is above 100 mg%.

It is reasonable to conclude that dialysis should be instituted, even without a phase of protein restriction, when creatinine clearances are falling from 10–5 ml/min. Indeed normally if the creatinine clearance is reduced to 5 ml/min the protein intake has to be reduced to 40 g/day, and when only 2.5 ml/min this can only be 20 g/day in the form of the Giordano–Giovanetti (G – G) diet. Principles of dietary management have been discussed above as part of the management of the chronic renal failure patient (p. 304).

When dialysis starts, fluids may have to be restricted to as little as 500 ml/day but the patient who is still passing poor quality urine may be allowed 1 litre. In the interests of strict control over hypertension and avoidance of pulmonary oedema, sodium restriction will also be mandatory, except in a few patients who have a sodium-losing state. Potassium intake has to be monitored, as fatal hyperkalaemia might easily develop. This means that the patient has to avoid all soft drinks, fruits, chocolate and instant coffee, as well as all salt substitutes. Once on the dialysis regime protein intake can be liberalized at 1 g/kg. Those patients who have been on protein restriction for too long can be identified by their low serum transferrins and their low serum albumin; they are also anaemic. Supplementation of the water soluble vitamins B and C is necessary in order to correct losses through the dialyser.

Complications in the course of dialysis

Headache

At the onset of dialysis too vigorous or prolonged treatment will cause 'dialysis dis-equilibrium'. Urea is being removed rapidly from the extracellular fluid, and yet less readily from the brain substance, so the result is an osmotic swelling of the brain, which results in headache and vomiting (Figure 131). Cardiac arrhythmias may also be precipitated. It has to be

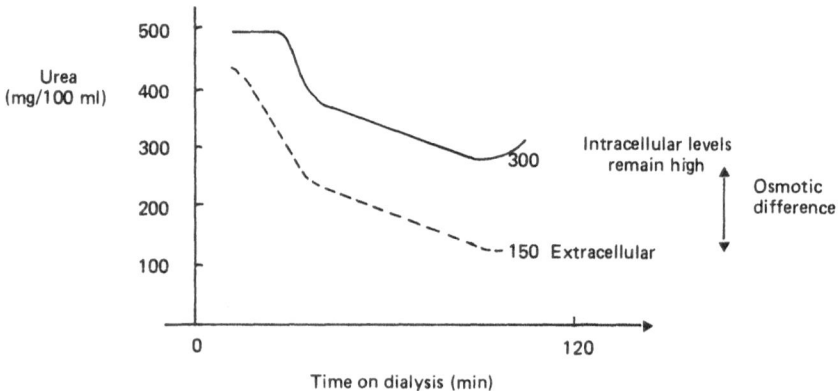

Figure 131. Comparison of intracellular and extracellular urea levels

remembered that hypertension is another frequent cause of headache. On occasion it may also be the first sign of an intracranial haemorrhage such as subdural haematoma. Persistent headache must therefore be taken seriously.

Pyrogen reaction
Bacterial contamination of the dialysis fluid and absorption of endotoxin will cause malaise, rigors, pyrexia or hypertension. The immediate treatment is to take a blood culture and Limulus lysate assay sample, and to administer hydrocortisone. Formalin contamination can produce similar symptoms. Other causes of pyrexia include an elevated dialysate temperature, and blood or plasma protein reactions.

It is also of note that when protamine sulphate is given at the end of dialysis to neutralize heparin, an anaphylactoid reaction often ensues, since the protamine–heparin interaction activates the complement system.

Hypotension
This may occur at the onset of dialysis if the patient is 'bled into the machine', or towards the end of dialysis when the ultrafiltration rate has been too great. In this latter case fluid replacement with saline is required.

A hypoalbuminaemic and thus plasma volume-depleted patient is a particular risk. It is important always to be on the lookout for a burst coil or a gastrointestinal bleed.

Cramp in the leg muscles
This is caused by poor circulation due to removal of too much fluid. The treatment is therefore to infuse saline or 50 g mannitol.

362

Chest pain
Haemodialysis patients have premature coronary artery disease. They should not be allowed to smoke. Angina is common but dialysis bone disease, gout or pericarditis all contribute to chest pains.

Abdominal pain
Gastrointestinal upsets are common in uraemia and these patients often have a duodenal ulcer. Pain can result from the constipation induced by taking aluminium hydroxide. Occasionally it might be due to pancreatitis or a bleed into the retroperitoneal tissues.

Hard water syndrome
This occurs when there is failure of the deionizer or water softener. Hypercalcaemia then causes nausea and vomiting, pruritus and metastatic calcification.

Electrolyte disturbance or metal intoxication
Hypernatraemia can be seen on the rare occasion when there is a failure of the proportioning pump, so that the dialysate fluid is overconcentrated. Conversely, *hyponatraemia* will result from too much dilution with water. Both *copper and zinc intoxication* have been known to arise due to contamination of plumbing systems. Aluminium absorption can account for osteomalacic bone disease and dialysis dementia.

Air embolism
This is due to the sucking in of air at some weak point in the dialysis circuit. It is an emergency situation, for which the following drill should be adopted:

(1)   discontinue dialysis;
(2)   place the patient head down with his right side uppermost, so that air tends to stay in the right ventricle;
(3)   infuse volume expanders to maintain the blood pressure;
(4)   give 100% oxygen for several hours;
(5)   administer dexamethasone to prevent cerebral oedema.

THE LOGISTICS OF DIALYSIS
Survival

Survival on chronic renal dialysis is related to age, and the degree of vascular disease that a patient has. Representative figures are:

3 year survival: age 15–35 70%; age 35–55 65%; age 55+ 45%;
10 year survival: average 15–25%

Therefore selection for dialysis is determined by stringent criteria, which are only likely to be relaxed when economic pressures diminish. Currently it costs £10 000 per annum for each patient on dialysis.

The type of chronic renal failure patient

This can be judged from the following represesentative figures:

Chronic glomerulonephritis	40%
Polycystic kidneys	10%
Malformations	10%
Pyelonephritis	15%
Alport's syndrome	5%
Nephrosclerosis/gout	5%
Rapidly progressive nephritis	5%
Diabetes	3%
Others	about 10%

Contraindications for dialysis

Even within these categories, the following are usually regarded as reasons for rejection:

(1) Cardiovascular disease that has resulted in a stoke or myocardial infarction, even though hypertension, left ventricular failure, or congestive heart failure are not barriers to acceptance. Peripheral arterial disease also makes dialysis impossible.
(2) Disablement by advanced peripheral neuropathy or renal bone disease.
(3) A coexisting lethal disease such as diabetes or gout which is accompanied by vascular disease or blindness.

Personality and suitability for dialysis

A high level of education and psychological and family stability are all favourable factors for the individual on dialysis, as each aids rehabilitation;

much also depends on how well adjusted the patients are. Almost all patients with chronic renal failure complain of lack of energy, and loss of interest and ambition. However, while well-adjusted persons minimize their losses, those less well adjusted become irritable, anxious and aggressive. Inevitably there is apprehension about income and support, and the feeling that accepting charity is socially or personally degrading. A good helper with the dialysis procedure, preferably a spouse or relation, is of inestimable value, but even this person will have to cope with loss of sleep and physical and mental tension. Life for patient and helper can become simply a question of concentrating on the patient staying alive. Dialysis patients need to follow active and productive lives, but whether they have friends, social contacts or interests will depend very much on their personality. It is all too easy for them to become tied to their machines.

Home dialysis

Most patients use a Kiil board or a disposable dialyser in the home. Clearly the house will have to be suitable or be reconstructed in the following way:

(1)   A telephone is essential.
(2)   Room space and waterproof floor covering of 7.4 to $9.2 \, m^2$ is required.
(3)   The electrical supply must give a 13 amp and a 30 amp socket for heat-sterilizing machines.
(4)   A water pressure of around 137 kN/m^2 will be needed for the proportionating unit. (i.e. 20 lbs per square inch)
(5)   On the water line there has to be a course filter and a pressure-reducing valve.
(6)   After the pressure-reducing valve there must be a domestic water softener.
(7)   The drains must be able to accommodate some 30 litres/h effluent fluid.

Dialysis or transplantation?

In Europe some 40 patients per million develop chronic renal failure each year and 16 patients per million are accepted for dialysis and transplantation. Some 120 patients per million are already surviving by means of either dialysis or transplantation. In fact, only 30–50% of chronic renal failure patients get onto a dialysis programme and of these less than one-quarter receive a transplant.

Clearly all chronic renal failure patients might hope for a return to normal health; but the chance of this is very small. It is important that both doctor and patient appreciate what is in store for the patient, whether he elects for a period of dialysis followed by transplantation, or whether he stays on home dialysis. If the transplant outcome is poor, the patient will die or revert to dialysis in any case. If the transplant is successful, the patient can look forward to a better quality of life, although maintenance immunosuppressive drugs with the attendant risk of bacterial and viral infections are always present. On dialysis some patients can survive for 10 years, but the 5 year survival is only 50–70%. Death is usually due to vascular problems or to infection. It is, however, reassuring to know that dialysis survival is far superior to that on dietary and medical support alone (Figure 132). The type of renal disease makes little difference, although those with polycystic kidneys have less anaemia, and perhaps less bone disease. Some 40% of both children and adults have glomerulonephritis. Hereditary and congenital conditions are now replacing pyelonephritis as the next major affliction of children.

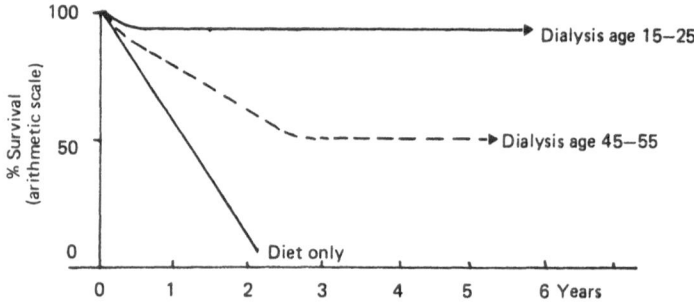

Figure 132. Dialysis survival compared with conservative therapy

Dialysis takes a considerable amount of time and effort. Coagulation problems mean that there is a gradual loss of shunt sites, and there is development of cardiovascular disease due to accelerated atherosclerosis. Continuing anaemia means restriction of exercise and working capacity, so most patients spend two-thirds of their non-dialysis time at passive activities, whilst only one-third of their time is put to use as active work. Patients are often infertile, and bone disease tends to progress. These disadvantages must be set against the potential complications of transplantation, where there is commonly a slow decline in function of the transplant kidney; in the long term patients can develop hypertension, either due to the chronic rejection process, or sometimes on account of stenosis of the artery.

Living donor survival after transplantation is 80% at 2 years and 65% at 5 years. Cadaver kidney figures are much poorer, with a 60% survival at 2 years, and only 45% at 5 years. Thus on a short-term basis of 2–3 years the chances on dialysis are better than with a transplant. In effect, since the waiting time for a kidney is 2 years in many centres, the patients do, in fact, come to know exactly what life on dialysis means, and the more stoical adjust to it so that some may return to work, meanwhile learning from their colleagues what are the risks of transplantation. Ultimately loss of shunt sites, fistula problems and worsening bone disease may mean that the patient is obliged to take his chance with a cadaver transplant. Transplant survival figures are shown in Figure 133 below. Although actual cadaver kidney survival has been poor, with respectable immunosuppressive regimes the patients should survive.

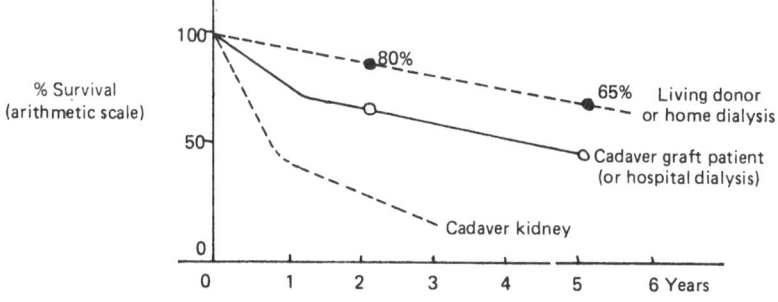

Figure 133. Patient survival with a renal transplant

The chance of being alive after 5 years of therapy is as good with home dialysis as it is with a living related donor graft. Dialysis patients who have problems remain on hospital programmes and as a group fare worse. Thus full rehabilitation is only achieved in 50% of hospital dialysis patients, as compared with 70% of home dialysis patients and 85% of patients with a successful allograft.

Several factors contribute to the poor survival of cadaver grafts:

(1)   First year losses are in the range 26–62%, with a mean of 40%. Although the occurrence of post-transplant acute tubular necrosis is said not to be an adverse factor, a prolonged warm or cold ischaemia time and the occurrence of 'perfusion nephropathy' (page 392) are bound to be harmful.

(2)   The age of the recipient is also relevant, since at 2 years the survival of grafts given to patients under 40 is about 40%, whilst for patients who are older the graft survival is only 25%.

(3)   Clearly the art of transplant matching is important (see p. 406); the 3 year survival of cytotoxic negative patients is over 40%, but the figures are much poorer when the cytotoxic cross-match is positive.

MEDICAL PROBLEMS ASSOCIATED WITH LIFE ON DIALYSIS

Hypertension

The initial dialyses have to be of short duration so as to avoid dialysis dis-equilibrium. The aim, nevertheless, is to remove salt and water so that the patient comes down towards his 'dry weight'. With the reduction of the extracellular fluid and sodium, hypertension will become more easy to control. Meantime severe salt restriction and hypotensive agents will be required. In the final event it is often found that there is a narrow margin between the reduction of weight that produces normotension, and that needed to achieve a 'dry weight'. At this stage the patient manifests symptoms of postural hypotension.

Most patients have volume-expansion hypertension due to salt and water overload. This is particularly obvious in anephric patients, whose blood pressure is very sensitive to the degree of hydration. Overhydration will cause a rise of blood pressure, due in part to an increase of the cardiac output and in part to an elevation of the peripheral vascular resistance. As salt and water is removed, so control of blood pressure becomes easier because of the removal of salt from the smooth muscle of the arterial walls.

There are a few patients whose renin secretion is inappropriately high. This does not rule out a response of their blood pressure to haemodialysis alone, but since they are mainly patients with vascular damage causing juxtaglomerular ischaemia, they often need bilateral nephrectomy. This is a serious step as the mortality is 20%. Added to this, such patients invariably have refractory anaemia and polyneuropathy is more common. It should also be remembered that even with a GFR of 1 ml/min the kidneys are still making some contribution to solute excretion.

When nephrectomy is contemplated, patients must be taken off beta-blocking drugs at least 1 week beforehand. After the operation there is a risk of bleeding at the operative site so 'regional heparinization' will be required for a time. This means that a dialysis is performed by infusion of heparin into the arterial line, and conversely protamine is infused into the venous line, so that there is neutralization of heparin as blood returns to the body. Unfortunately it is fraught with snags and is seldom satisfactory, particularly as it is inevitable that some heparin will be returned to the patient. Also the neutralization of heparin by protamine creates a complement-activating reaction with liberation of kinins in the blood.

Anaemia

Uraemic anaemia has been discussed on page 315. The dialysis patient normally receives supplements of oral iron and folic acid. Additionally an anabolic steroid, such as Decadurabolin 50 mg i.m. every third week, is an important supplement, since it works in synergism with the patient's declining levels of erythropoietin. Only those patients with polycystic disease are free of anaemia symptoms, as they usually have increased ERP production. It helps if patients can be placed on a normal protein intake, for then they will synthesize their own transferrin in adequate amounts.

Heart size and function

The cardiac output in CRF is increased from 6 to 15 litres/min.

Cardiac size

This quite clearly correlates with the degree of hypertension, together with the extra 20% increase in cardiac output that accompanies the establishment of an arteriovenous fistula, and also with the extra output necessary on account of anaemia.

Cardiomyopathy

This is described in a minority of dialysis patients. The possibility of alcoholism should not be overlooked. Thus an occasional uraemic patient will be found to have chronic heart failure and cardiomegaly and an increased ventricular volume, yet no evidence of hypertensive hypertrophy. The velocity of myocardial shortening during contraction can be shown to be decreased and the ventricular end-diastolic pressure is increased. Such patients do badly and so far no improvement with dialysis has been claimed.

Pericarditis

This occurs in some 50% of undialysed patients. Even among stable chronic renal patients some 10% may develop symptoms in the form of chest pain with fever; the chest X-ray shows a globular or pear-shaped heart. These patients are usually not as well dialysed as it might seem. Cytomegalovirus disease should also be considered.

Fibrinous pericarditis may give rise to haemorrhage or cardiac tamponade. Ultrasound helps with the diagnosis of an effusion. In fact the classical Kussmaul's sign, with elevation of the jugular venous pressure on inspiration, and the paradoxical pulse with a pressure drop of over 10 mmHg on inspiration are signs found only in those patients who are developing tamponade. The alternative hazard is that a fibrinous pericarditis may progress to a chronic constrictive pericarditis.

There is still discussion about the cause of uraemic pericarditis. Although uric acid elevation is a feature of some cases, this is not always so. Some cases may be caused by a bleed during dialysis heparinization, and others might be due to intercurrent bacterial or viral infection. In any event it usually reflects poor control of the uraemia.

The basic treatment is to give the patient intensive dialysis under regional heparinization, to try the effect of indomethacin 50 mg q.i.d., or perhaps an intrapericardial injection of triamcinalone, and lastly to resort to partial pericardiectomy.

Vascular disease

Premature atherosclerosis is a particular feature of chronic dialysis patients and those who are newly transplanted. The incidence, however, is said to be less in those who have maintained a renal transplant for up to 10 years and who are using only small doses of corticosteroids. Certainly steroids do worsen the hyperlipidaemia that these patients have.

The accelerated atherosclerosis may be attributed to a combination of hyperlipidaemia and hypertension. There is increased triglyceride synthesis in chronic renal failure patients who are on a high carbohydrate intake, and additional lipaemia due to uraemic inhibition of lipoprotein lipase. Such patients also have calcification of the media of the large arteries, which is seen in 40% of patients at the onset of dialysis and in 100% by 5–7 years. Calcification of the dorsalis pedis artery along the great toe is seen on early radiographs.

Abnormal lipid levels almost always increase with the duration of life on dialysis. There are some claims that this situation can be combated by lowering the dialysate glucose.

Neurological complications

Uraemic encephalopathy
This is a feature of the undialysed patient. There is cerebral oedema with neuronal degeneration and proliferation of astrocytes. The EEG changes are non-specific, but there is diffuse and focal slowing (cf PDE).

Progressive dialysis encephalopathy (PDE)
This condition has only come to light in recent years. Its appearance seems to parallel the use of aluminium hydroxide for lowering the blood phosphate; an increased brain and bone content of aluminium has been demonstrated.

The four features of PDE are (a) dementia with memory impairment and disorientation, (b) speech disorder in the form of global dysphasia or mutism, (c) myoclonic jerks, and (d) behavioural disturbance manifest as agitation or paranoia. PDE evolves slowly, whereas uraemic encephalopathy is an acute condition. The EEG is different, since in PDE there are distinctive rhythmic

370

delta and frontocentral spike and slow waves. At autopsy lacunae can be found in the basal ganglia and thalamus.

When a patient with dialysis dementia is first seen, the possibility of chronic drug intoxication must always be considered. Diazepam or phenobarbitone with Epanutin overdosage are strong possibilities.

Peripheral neuropathy

There is segmental demyelination and axonal degeneration. The symptoms are more commonly those of a distal sensory neuropathy than a motor defect. Thus often the patient has restless legs with paraethesiae and burning of the skin, and only a little muscle weakness. In fact, less than one-fifth of patients have symptomatic neuropathy, but many are discovered by the routine use of nerve conduction studies, vibration sensitivity, EMG, and nerve morphometry. The changes tend to correlate inversely with the time on dialysis. Neuropathy is certainly worse in those with elevated PTH levels.

Infections

Impaired leucocyte function in uraemia leads to infections; humoral antibody responses are seldom abnormal.

An even more serious hazard is serum hepatitis B virus infection, normally spread by blood products. Staff and patients must have routine screening tests for hepatitis B antigen, gloves and protective clothing must be worn at all times, all blood must be screened, and transfusion requirements should be kept to a minimum. Patients cannot be accepted in transit from other units.

Chronic renal failure patients often have anicteric hepatitis which means that they carry the virus antigen in their blood, but they may or may not show elevated serum transaminases and alkaline phosphatase. Hyperimmune gammaglobulin is now available for administration to contacts, but unlike the situation with hepatitis A virus, ordinary gammaglobulin fraction is not effective.

Bone disease

This has been discussed on page 318, so only a brief summary of therapy will be given here.

(1) Reduce the serum phosphate so as to raise calcium and depress the PTH:
    (a) by a low milk diet;
    (b) with Aludrox 2 tabs. q.i.d. (*NB* this may have long-term toxicity).
(2) Elevate serum calcium by increasing the gut calcium load by administration of:

371

(a) Calcium carbonate powder 1 g t.i.d. (400 mg calcium t.i.d.);
(b) Calcium gluconate tabs. 4 q.i.d. (400 mg calcium q.i.d.); and by raising the dialysate calcium above 6.0 mg%, (2.5 mmol/l) or magnesium to 1.5 mmol/l.

(3) Give vitamin D or analogues:
   (a) vitamin D 50 000–200 000 units/day;
   (b) 1,25-dihydroxy. D_3 0.5–1.0 μg/day;
   (c) dihydrotachysterol (DHT) 0.25–4.0 mg/day.
   (d) 1-a-hydroxyvitamin D_3 1–2 ug/day.

(4) Avoid anticonvulsants if possible.
(5) Transplant as soon as possible.

Gouty arthritis

Chronic renal failure patients often develop secondary gout, although some do have primary gout. Today the problem is easily dealt with by use of the xanthine oxidase inhibitor allopurinol, which is given at a dose of 2 × 300 mg/day, but even so an occasional case of podogra will occur. The synovial fluid must be examined for crystals of diagnostic significance. Monosodium urate crystals are linear and needle-shaped. Under polarizing light they show birefringence, so that they are yellow when lying parallel to the slow vibration component and blue when at right angles to it. When there is 'pseudogout' there are rhomboid-shaped calcium pyrophosphate crystals.

Hard water syndrome

Headache and vomiting during the last hours of dialysis suggest a 'dis-equilibrium syndrome'. However, when dealing with home dialysis patients one must be aware that failure of the water softener also causes headache and vomiting, which on this occasion is probably due to hypercalcaemia. It can also lead to pancreatitis.

Ascites

There are a few haemodialysis patients who show ascites when they are fluid-loaded. The cause is not actually known; in some the peritoneal membrane may have become altered during previous peritoneal dialysis, but it is also possible that there is some natriuretic factor in the blood which causes the membrane to leak sodium. It is, of course, assumed that coincidental cirrhosis has been excluded.

Gonadal dysfunction

Patients on chronic haemodialysis are infertile and can be shown to have oligospermia due to low basal testosterone levels, which do not respond to chorionic gonadotrophin. Additionally many are impotent.

Hypersplenism syndrome

Some patients on dialysis develop the hypersplenism triad of anaemia, leucopenia and thrombocytopenia. The spleen is enlarged and they have a high transfusion requirement. Naturally the depressed bone marrow of the uraemic patient cannot compensate for this degree of red cell sequestration; the only cure is splenectomy. Note, however, that many of these patients have been Australia-antigen positive and that the problem is not seen in many centres.

Shunt clotting

Shunt life is influenced by infection and by clotting. Occasionally a problem shunt may be the cause of infected pulmonary emboli or of endocarditis. Not only do dialysis patients have high blood lipids, high blood clotting factors and a marked tendency to platelet aggregation, which all combine to produce 'hypercoagulability', but, of course, any additional local factor in the shunt will cause local thrombosis. Malalignment of the shunt cannulae, or stenosis near a cannula tip, is commonly found when an arteriogram or venogram is performed on the problem shunt. The result is a poor blood flow that makes dialysis difficult.

This type of patient therefore should be well heparinized during dialysis, assuming that there is no contraindication, and is normally given oral warfarin anticoagulant. Consideration might also be given to use of a platelet inhibitor—aspirin being the most effective, since it also stimulates fibrinolysis. However it provokes gut irritation and allergy. Sulphinpyrazone is now recognized to reduce shunt clotting and thrombus formation on dialysis membranes.

Bleeding problems

The occasional nose bleed in the hypertensive patient is to be expected. In chronic renal failure patients there is an everpresent risk of subdural haematoma; it has been said that it can happen in 5–10% of dialysis patients. Occasionally it may be bilateral. The predisposing factors include hypertension, convulsions, head trauma, aneurysms associated with polycystic disease, and, of course, uraemic bleeding or anticoagulation.

Headache is the most prominent complaint but vomiting, convulsions, or progressive confusion or coma are all likely. In order to establish the diagnosis an encephalogram, bilateral carotid angiography and thereafter burr holes will be required. Those patients whose condition allows a postponement of surgery for 5–7 days have a better survival prognosis. A high index of suspicion is required for the diagnosis of this condition.

Ectopic calcification

As already described this occurs when the Ca x P product (mg%) exceeds 75. In the past phosphate was lowered by means of aluminium hydroxide (2–6 g/day with meals). Now alternative therapy is available in the form of the diphosphonates, such as EHDP. This is given orally as 500–600 mg/day, as two equal doses taken 2 h before meals. Therapy is continued for 6–9 months.

Renal cyst formation

This phenomenon is now recognized as a sequel to long-term dialysis. It has no relationship to polycystic disease. The cysts probably result from small haematomata, which occur as a result of the anticoagulation during dialysis.

SPECIAL FACETS OF CHRONIC RENAL FAILURE SUPPORT

Dialysis in children

As already mentioned, dialysers should take no more than 10% of the patient's blood volume. One-layer small priming volume paediatric dialysers are now available. As in adult dialysis a good blood flow is essential, and this necessitates good vascular access. A modified Scribner shunt can be placed halfway up the arm or leg, but the groin is best avoided because of the risk of causing infection or limb ischaemia. The Buselmeier shunt, a U-tube with access points, allows higher flow rates.

Dialysis dis-equilibrium is more easily induced in children. Early symptoms include headache, nausea or vomiting, chest or abdominal pain and muscle cramps. A high bath glucose content helps to prevent this, as also does the infusion of 1 g/kg of mannitol.

Weight monitoring of the amount of fluid removed by ultrafiltration is of great importance. If the patient has salt and water overload, some 10% of the body weight can be removed, but in nephrotic children the infusion of albumin is necessary in order to allow this.

Conversely at the end of dialysis the volume of fluid infused back into the patient must not exceed 10% of the blood volume for fear of inducing severe hypertension and pulmonary oedema. Ultrafiltration may have to be continued until this is possible.

Psychosocial problems are likely to be greater with children. The child may show withdrawal and lack of communication, or the parents are likely to become overprotective.

Another problem is growth impairment—a reduction of growth will always occur when the GFR is less than 25 ml/min or when the calorie intake is below 80% normal. Even after transplantation children may not catch up because their growth potential diminishes with age.

When the weight of a child is corrected for the expanded extracellular fluid, height for weight is unusually low in dialysed children, although it can be improved by calorie supplementation. The 'height for weight index' using the 50th percentile should, of course, be 1.0 in normally nourished children but is quite often lower. There is no real evidence for a defect in growth hormone secretion but that hormone acts via somatomedin (the 'sulphation factor'); values of this can be low. The roles of both renal osteodystrophy and renal acidosis have been mentioned. Children with renal tubular acidosis often have to be treated with alkali as early as 1 month of age, if they are to attain normal growth.

Peritoneal dialysis

This simple but perverse technique requires the insertion of a flexible catheter into the peritoneal cavity, so that dialysate fluid can be run in and out. Waste products diffuse across the peritoneal membrane and are readily eliminated. It is normal to run in 2 l at a time over a 15 min period, then to allow 30 min dwelling time, and thereafter 15 min for evacuation into a closed drainage system as shown in Figure 134.

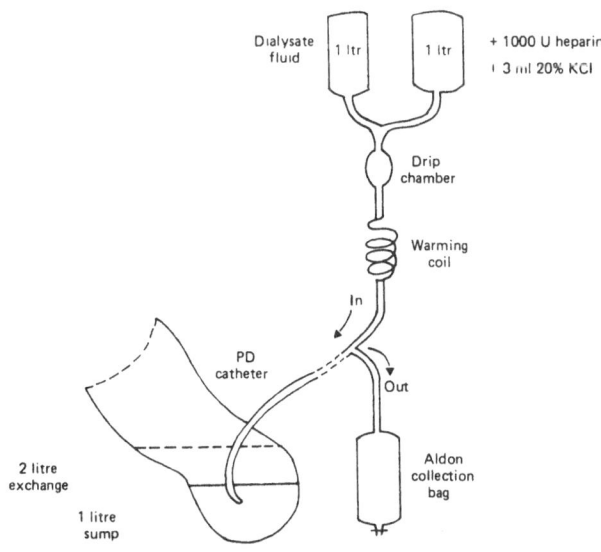

Figure 134. Peritoneal dialysis system

The dialysate fluid contains sodium 140 mmol/l; chloride 100 mmol/l; calcium 5 mmol/l and magnesium 1.5 mmol/l, and to it is added potassium according to requirements. If 3.0 ml of 20% KCl are added to each 2 l of fluid, this will give a final concentration of 4.0 mmol/l. The standard dialysate fluid used by most units contains acetate anions at 40 mmol/l, since this is inimical to the growth of bacteria and is readily converted by the body to bicarbonate. Normally a low glucose concentration of 1.36% is used, but if the patient is to be dehydrated then each cycle is made up of one bottle of 1.36% and one bottle of 6.36% glucose. Heparin 500 units is usually added to one bottle in each cycle to prevent fibrin formation in the catheter.

Insertion of the catheter is only difficult if the patient has adhesions from previous peritonitis or has had numerous dialyses. Phenoperidine 2 mg with Droperidol 10 mg i/m can be used as premedication and is given 1 h beforehand. It is vital to ensure that the patient's bladder has been emptied. There is always a slight risk of perforation of the patient's bowel, but this is normally avoided by filling the abdomen with fluid before inserting the catheter into the patient's pelvis.

Dialysis is usually continued for 48–72 h, although it may be more comfortable for the patient at night to drain the abdomen and spigot the catheter. During an average dialysis a patient may in fact lose 40 g protein, and some 10 g of amino acids, for the peritoneum is much more permeable than a dialysis membrane. For this reason peritoneal dialysis has the theoretical advantage that it removes 'middle molecules' more efficiently. In return even a low glucose solution may contribute 100–200 g to the patient's intake. When using high glucose fluids, it is wise to monitor the blood glucose and to give insulin as required. The volume of fluid delivered, the volume drained and the cumulative fluid balance are always carefully recorded.

Infection is a grave hazard and for this reason cultures of the effluent fluid should be sent to the laboratory each morning. The incidence of positive cultures increases with the length of dialysis. One way of anticipating infection is to monitor the lysozyme content of the fluid; a rise of 7.5 μg/ml and over indicates that polymorphs are being mobilized to deal with bacteria, that often are of the *Pseudomonas* type. Abdominal pain is common due to disturbance of the bowel, cold fluid or hypertonic solutions but peritonitis should always be kept in mind. Gentamycin 20 mg or tetracycline 50 mg can be added to each cycle.

There is always a slight amount of blood in the first effluents, but if the haematocrit is over 1% a serious bleed from a vessel must be suspect. It does not usually result from the bleeding diathesis of uraemia.

Another major problem is wetness of the lung bases, and thus potential bronchopneumonia, because uraemic patients have impaired polymorph function.

The Tenckhoff indwelling catheter is used for long-term chronic peritoneal dialysis, particularly for those who lack vascular access or for those who cannot be trained for haemodialysis. The procedure is less expensive, and the patient may sleep better than with haemodialysis, if an automatic dialysate fluid recycling machine is used. Such catheters clearly are subject to obstruction. The usual heparin 500 units/l dialysate fluid is added but, in addition, 3000 units of heparin are left in the peritoneal cavity at the end of a dialysis.

Dialysis of low molecular weight uraemic toxins

Urea and creatinine have a high clearance through dialysers. They are really indicators of protein and muscle catabolism, and have little toxicity. However, patients may be said to be poorly dialysed when the post-dialysis creatinine values exceed 7 mg% (600 μmol/l). Indeed it is found that above these values patients have appreciable retention of phenols and other potential toxins that can be protein bound. Although the mean molecular weight of phenols is about 150, their clearance is only half that of creatinine owing to their lipid solubility; 4-hydroxy-phenylacetic acid is the most abundant phenolic acid. In fact, free phenol levels are of the order of 1×10^{-4} M and bound phenols have a level of 4×10^{-4} M. These are levels which are sufficient to cause inhibition of cerebral enzymes, if those phenols cannot be conjugated by the liver to sulphates and glucuronides. Usually this is the case. However there is now some evidence that phenol glucuronide has toxicity. Organic acids such as hippurates alter transport systems.

Table 42 gives estimates of levels of hippurates in post-dialysis serum, and in the bath water of a 100 litre bath (Kramer *et al.*, 1965; Jutzler *et al.*, 1968).

Table 42

	Final serum level	*Bath level at end of dialysis*
Hippuric acid	1750 μg%	700 μg/100 ml
o-OH-Hippuric acid	20	8
m-OH-Hippuric acid	160	64
p-OH-Benzoic acid	70	28

Note: It would appear that the hyperlipidaemia of uraemic patients has considerable relevance to the dialysance of toxins, for the above ratios show that even at the end of dialysis the serum:dialysate levels are roughly 3:1. Lipophilic compounds do not dialyse well.

'Middle molecules'

The dialysance of molecules with a molecular weight over 1000 is poor, as Figure 128 shows. The toxicity of these compounds was postulated by the Seattle group in 1971.

There are indeed many claims that peptides in the range 1300–1700 daltons are responsible for uraemic neuropathy. It is also claimed that patients with neuropathy can benefit from peritoneal dialysis, since this does not impose a molecular size limit. Dialysis machines have, therefore, been made with a high surface area and a high permeability. The removal of 'middle molecules' depends on an increase in the area of the dialysing surface, rather than blood flow or dialysate flow rate. Thus dialysers have been developed with a surface area of 3.9 m² in the 'Triple HFAK IV' and at the minimum 1.4 m² in the 'Double EX-21'. These dialysers have such a high rate of ultrafiltration (400–600 ml/h) that saline replacement at 30 min intervals is necessary, and even so there is a risk of severe hypotension.

Positive evidence for 'middle molecules' is still scanty but the suggestion has certainly stimulated much effort for separation of the various uraemic toxins. Foremost in this field is Furst who has developed a technique for high speed gel filtration of plasma. The type of pattern obtained is illustrated in Figure 135. Peak 5 represents phenols, guanidines and organic acids, peaks 7 and 8 represent 'middle molecules' and peak 9 includes compounds of high molecular weight 40 000–50 000. The toxicity of phenols and guanidines has been discussed already. The middle molecules are peptides which are said to be capable of causing inhibition of haemopoiesis and of lymphocyte transformation and cytotoxicity in cultures of fibroblasts. Chemical details are not yet available.

The French school (Funck–Brentano) use a different technique of Sephadex G-15 chromatography and therefore their peaks differ. Those designated b2, b4, b5 and b6 correlate with neuropathy.

Gastrointestinal sorbents

Creatinine, uric acid and urea all leak readily into the gastrointestinal tract and the urea is broken down to ammonia. Unlike starch itself oxystarch is not catabolized in the gut. Oxidation of the starch is achieved by periodate, resulting in a polymeric dialdehyde with the following type of structure.

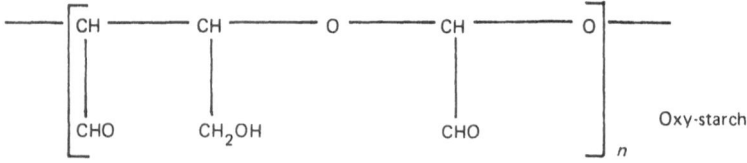

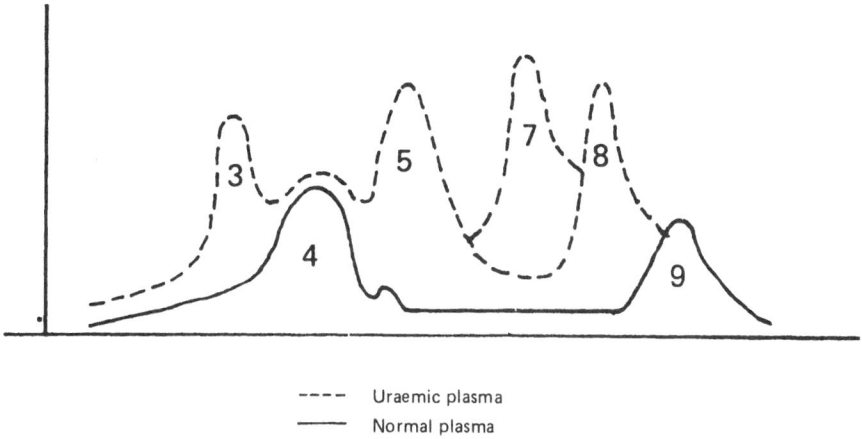

---- Uraemic plasma
—— Normal plasma

Figure 135.   Gel filtration of uraemic molecules

At ammonia concentrations of 10 mmol/l, the oxystarch will absorbe 9%/wt of ammonia. Therefore, when 20 g/day are given orally in four divided doses, patients can either be maintained on a low protein diet prior to dialysis or peritoneal dialysis frequency can be reduced.

Charcoal has been given by mouth for many years for various types of poisoning, and also aluminium hydroxide to remove phosphate, and sodium polystyrene sulphonate to remove potassium. Many other ideas are in a developmental stage. Urease can thus be microencapsulated to protect it from proteolytic enzymes and if there is zirconium phosphate within the same membrane, the ammonium is absorbed releasing bicarbonate which is then lost as carbon dioxide and water. It is possible also to incorporate an enzyme system so that the ammonia is converted to glutamine.

Oral capsules which contain bacterial enzymes derived from *Serratia* or *Pseudomonas* have been given to institute biodegradation within the gut; in this way blood levels of urea, creatinine and guanidine derivatives can be lowered.

The alternative procedure which deserves consideration in some patients is the *provocation of diarrhoea*. A warmed solution containing mannitol 180 mmol/l is ingested at the rate of 200 ml every 5 min for a period of 3 h. This causes a profuse diarrhoea which lowers the blood urea nitrogen by some 35 mg%. When used three times weekly in combination with a 30 g protein diet, patients can be kept tolerably well under primitive conditions.

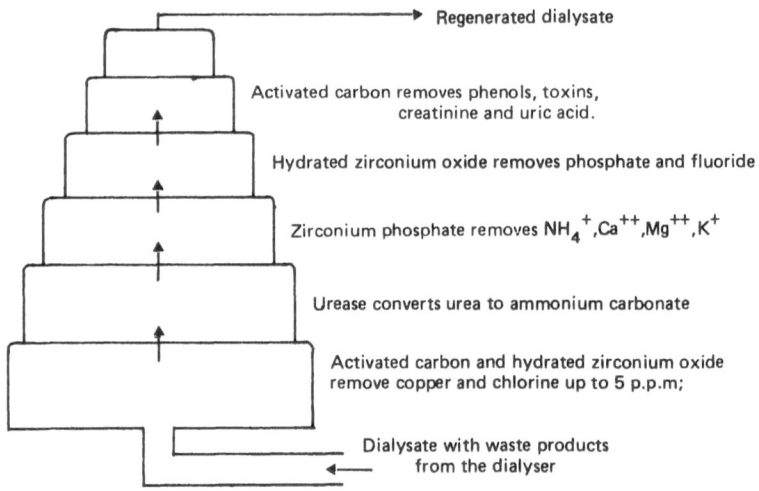

Figure 136. **A Redy dialysate sorbent regenerator**

The sorbent regeneration of dialysate (Redy system)

Problems with housing, architecture, plumbing and government departments often make the installation of permanent dialysis facilities in the patient's home very difficult. In the last 5 years a welcome advance has been the development of a system for dialysate regeneration, consisting of a multilayer cartridge which combines enzymatic hydrolysis of urea with ion-exchangers and sorbents (Figure 136). Uraemic metabolites are removed as the dialysate circulates through the sorbent cartridge. In fact, the 5 litres of dialysate fluid recirculate through a disposable cartridge which contains activated carbon, zirconium phosphate and oxide, and also urease. The carbon removes creatinine, uric acid, guanidines, phenols and any drugs; ammonium, calcium, magnesium and potassium are exchanged for sodium and hydrogen ions on the zirconium phosphate, and the zirconium oxide removes phosphate and anions. It is also possible to use a similar system for peritoneal dialysis, but a continuous flow peritoneal dialysis will only be possible when a double lumen peritoneal catheter is available so as to allow concurrent infusion and drainage.

Haemoperfusion—the ACAC kidney

Activated charcoal was used by Yatzidis to remove uraemic products as early as 1964. It is now apparent that its use is even greater in hepatic and hepatorenal failure, since charcoal will absorb not only urea, uric acid and creatinine but also indoles, phenols, guanidines and organic acids; Thus it absorbs all possible toxic products, with the exception of ammonium. The current problem, however, is that charcoal tends to cause platelet aggregation and thus hypotensive reactions and coagulation. Indeed as a general rule the adherence of plasma proteins to a foreign material will produce a 'thrombogenic membrane'. Much depends on the nature of the coagulum, since the higher the albumin content of the absorbed layer, the less is its thrombogenicity. Clearly one approach would be to separate the plasma from the cellular elements of the blood, before perfusion over charcoal. Also a haemodialyser has been constructed with high porosity membranes that allow passage of the serum proteins but not the cells.

Meantime Chang has pioneered the ACAC (albumin-coated activated charcoal) microcapsule artificial kidney. This contains 300 g of coconut or peat-activated charcoal granules encapsulated in cellulose nitrate and coated with albumin so as to reduce platelet damage. The membrane coating does not close off the pores so the absorbent quality of the charcoal is fully retained. In fact microencapsulation with polyhydroxyethyl methacrylate (polyhema) reduces platelet losses further, as does encapsulated petroleum pitch charcoal. Moreover, biocompatible Amberlite resins (XAD-2,4 and 7) can also be used to absorb protein-bound toxins such as bilirubin and bile salts, and also endotoxins.

Since many drugs such as barbiturates, benzodiazepine, digitalis, salicylates, glutethimide and methaqualone are readily absorbed by charcoal, renal units and poisons centres should have facilities for haemoperfusion. The principle of the perfusion circuit is shown in Figure 137.

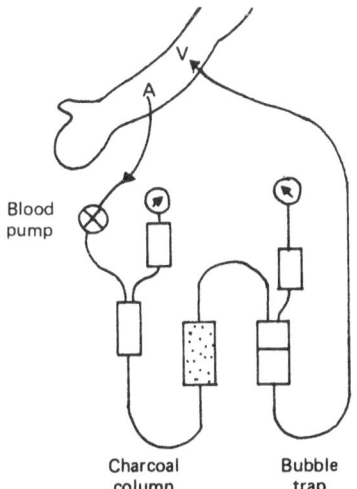

Figure 137. Haemoperfusion system

Since the resistance to flow is only 10 mmHg, a blood flow rate of 200 ml/min is easily obtained without a pump. Middle range molecules (600–1300) are readily removed. In fact even for these molecules there is a linear relationship with clearances of 100–200 ml/min over a blood flow range of 100–300 ml/min.

In theory the combination of haemoperfusion with ultrafiltration should be ideal for either uraemia or hepatic coma. In fact 2 h of haemoperfusion alone is as effective as 6 h of dialysis (assuming that there are no setbacks). Comparisons have also now been made of ACAC perfusion with ACAC/ultrafiltration (haemofiltration) using the new polyacrylonitrile (PAN) membrane, which has a permeability up to 15 000 (molecular weight of lysozyme). It is formed of copolymer of acrylonitrile with sodium methollyl-sulphonate and the pores are ten times the size of those in the cuprophan membrane (Table 43).

Table 43

	ACAC perfusion	*ACAC/ultrafiltration*
Creatinine clearance	230 ml/min	220
300–1500 molecular weight	20	110
Phosphate	0	20 ml/min

Whereas conventional haemodialysis with a cuprophan membrane has no effect on the state of hepatic coma, dialysis using the more permeable PAN membrane leads to an improvement both of consciousness and of the EEG.

Haemofiltration

Figure 138 shows a Gambro dialyser in a circuit which is designed to filter plasma from the blood simply according to the driving pressure; this process mimics the process of glomerular filtration and is called 'haemo-ultrafiltration'. More commonly an RP6 dialyser with an acrylonitrile membrane is used and this filters all molecules, small or large up to 40 000 daltons, with the same velocity depending on the applied filtration pressure. With a transmembrane pressure of 500 mmHg and a blood flow rate of 300 ml/min from a fistula the rate of filtration of plasma is about 66 ml/min, which is about half that achieved by the glomeruli. At each session 18–20 litres of fluid are filtered, so it is imperative to replace fluid by means of modified Ringer-lactate. More of this fluid is used if it is infused before the filter (which actually seems to be to the patient's advantage), than if it is infused after the filter.

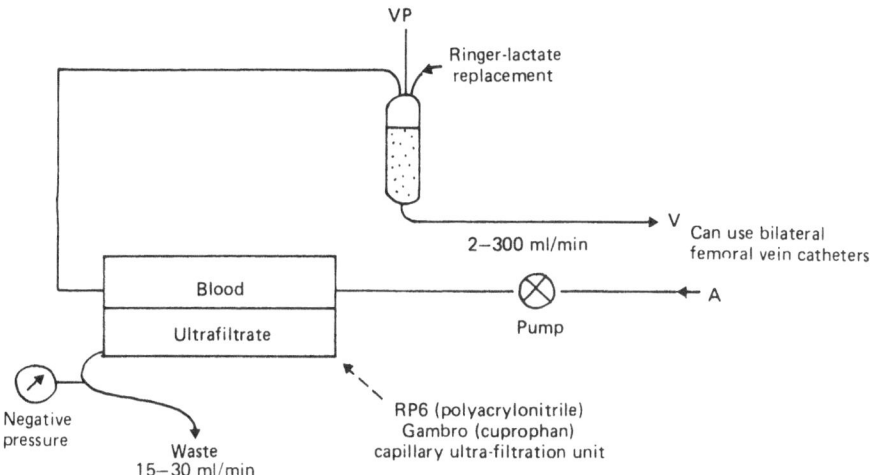

Figure 138. Haemofiltration circuit

Unlike haemodialysis (see Figures 128 and 129) the clearance of molecules of all sizes (60–5000 daltons) is the same at 60 ml/min. The patient is subjected to an iso-osmolar dehydration, so there are no water shifts and it is well tolerated; 1–2 litres of fluid can be removed each hour.

As in the case of glomerular filtration, the actual filtration can be expressed as:

$$Q = A \times K_p \quad \text{(hydraulic pressure – osmotic pressure)}$$

where Q is the flux rate (ml/min), A the area of the membrane and K_p its porosity.

Although the process has to be instituted three times a week, there are distinct advantages:

(1) All equipment is disposable and costs are lower.

(2) There is no dialysate and no risk of bacterial infection.

(3) There are no osmolarity problems.

(4) All molecules, including middle molecules, are removed physiologically.

(5) Patients feel better, anaemia and neuropathy improve, and hyper-triglyceridaemia remits, although in fact each session produces much platelet damage.

(6) Hypertension is easily controlled, without provoking hyperreninaemia.

(7) Serum phosphate is readily normalized and aluminium hydroxide therapy is thus not required.

The same technique is applicable to the removal of diuretic-resistant oedema fluid, as for example in hepatic disease.

ASSESSMENT OF THE DIALYSIS PATIENT: IS DIALYSIS ADEQUATE?

In Europe there are over 1000 dialysis centres, over 300 centres which cater for transplantation, 300 for home dialysis, and some 150 which run long-term peritoneal dialysis. In Britain almost ten people per million are on dialysis and the same number are alive with renal transplants.

As discussed above it is important to know how to assess dialysers, for example according to pore size, membrane surface area, blood flow rate, dialysance and how they are to be used for most effective dialysis according to the frequency and duration of that procedure.

It is equally important to know how to look at the patients, appraising them in terms of:

(1) *Patient survival.* A good survival will be 80% at 5 years of dialysis.
(2) *Rehabilitation.* It is expected that 60% patients will be working.
(3) *Fitness.* This is detailed below. Patients should not be suffering from obvious malnutrition (protein–calorie deprivation); most patients of 40–55 kg weight are grossly debilitated.
(4) *Objective clinical measures.*
     (a) What is their degree of anaemia? The PCV should be at least 25%.
     (b) How much bone disease do they have?
     (c) What are the motor nerve conduction velocities?

In practice patients on home dialysis are seen in the clinic at least every 4 months, so that they can be examined in detail and technical problems discussed. A record is kept of potential fistula and shunt sites. The work-up extends to pretransplant investigations, which will include a serum pseudo-cholinesterase, which can be low in CRF, so that quite often patients can remain paralysed after reversal of anaesthetic muscle relaxants.

Other features are considered in detail in the sections below.

Adequacy of dialysis

A patient should come off dialysis with a blood urea of less than 13 mmol/l (80 mg%) or a serum creatinine of less than 5 mg% (440 μmol/l). Representative figures in good units are shown in Table 44.

Nutrition

The patient's intake of calories, protein, vitamins and minerals should be checked. Brief note is made of:

Table 44

	Pre-dialysis		Post-dialysis	
Urea	150±25 mg%	(25 mmol/l)	45±15 mg%	(7 mmol/l)
Creatinine	14± 2	(1240μmol/l)	4±1.5	(350 μmol/l)
Uric acid	9± 2	(0.54 mmol/l)	2.5±1.0	(0.15 mmol/l)

(1)   the dry weight, height, skinfold thickness and muscle bulk;
(2)   growth and maturation of children;
(3)   biochemical indices such as the serum albumin and transferrin, the blood haemoglobin, and the red cell and serum folate;
(4)   any sepsis of the skin, shunt site or mouth? Is dental attention needed?

Vascular status

(1)   Hypertension. Is the patient down to his dry weight? If he is still hypertensive, is he getting adequate hypotensive therapy? In refractory hypertension check the sodium balance and renin levels.
(2)   Has there been trouble with angina, congestive heart failure or pericarditis? An ECG is essential.
(3)   What are the fasting lipids? Is the patient smoking?
(4)   Have there been frequent episodes of shunt clotting?

Is there renal bone disease?

(1)   Pains in the feet are an early indication.
(2)   A skeletal radiographic survey and bone biopsy should be performed yearly.
(3)   Check the serum calcium, phosphate and alkaline phosphatase monthly and PTH quarterly.
(4)   Bone density should be measured when possible.

The nervous system

(1)   Weakness indicates myopathy, and numbness and tingling indicate peripheral neuropathy.
(2)   Check short-term memory and neurological reflexes. Is there impotence?
(3)   **Arrange:**

385

(a) motor nerve conduction velocity 3-monthly on ulna and peroneal nerves;

(b) EEG for slow waves of 3–7 Hz as compared with the total waves of 3–13 Hz, for this index correlates inversely with adequacy of dialysis;

(c) the visceral evoked response (VER) of the electrical activity in brain measured by scalp electrodes to show that delay which correlates with the serum creatinine;

(d) tests of mental agility such as basic arithmetic problems or a 'trail-making' test.

Social status, working capacity and home dialysis problems

(1) How does the family cope? Have there been machine or water softener problems?

(2) Has there been dis-equilibrium, underdialysis, infection or hepatitis?

(3) Is there any TB risk?

(4) Is work rehabilitation in progress?

REFERENCES

Requirement and provisions

Brand, R.A. (1971). Incidence of uraemia and requirements for maintenance haemodialysis. *Br. Med. J.*, **1**, 249

Gurland, H.J. *et al.* (1976). Combined report on regular dialysis and transplantation. *Proc. Eur. Dialysis and Transplant Assoc.*, **13**, 3

Pincherele, G. (1977). Services for patients with chronic renal failure in England and Wales. *Health Trends*, **vol. 8**, 41

Wing, A.J. (1977). Treatment prospects in renal disease. *Br. Med. J.*, **2**, 881

Distribution of nephrological services for adults in Britain. *Br. Med. J.*, (1976). **4**, 903

Dialysis technique

Baillod, R. (1965). Overnight dialysis in the home. *Proc. Eur. Dialysis and Transplant Assoc.*, **2**, 99

Clark, P.B. (1966). The Scribner shunt for haemodialysis. *Br. Med. J.*, **2**, 1200

Farrell, P.C. (1974). Haemodialyser reuse. *Kidney Int.*, **5**, 446

Farrell, P.C. and Stewart, J.H. (1976). Treatment with the artificial kidney. *Med. J. Aust.*, **1**, 160

Kerr, D.N.S. (1974). Which dialyser? *Nephron*, **12**, 368

Kjellstrand, C.M. (1972). Anticoagulation during dialysis. *Surgery,* **72,** 630

Levy, N.B. (1974). The quality of life on dialysis. *Lancet,* **i,** 1328

Muir, W.M. and Martin, A.M. (1971). Which kidney machine? *Br. J. Hosp. Med.,* **November.** (Equip. suppl.).

Silverstein, M.E. (1974). Treatment of severe fluid overload by ultra-filtration. *N. Engl. J. Med.,* **291,** 747

Whelpton, D. (1974). *Renal Dialysis.* (Sector Publishing Ltd.)

Wing, A.J. and Magowan, Mary. *The Renal Unit.* (London: MacMillan Press) 1975

Haemodialysis in children

Anderson, J., Lee, H.A. and Stroud, C.E. (1965). Technical aspects of regular dialysis in children. *Br. Med. J.,* **2,** 446

Broyer, M. (1972). Technical aspects of regular dialysis in children. *Acta Paediatr. Scand.,* **61,** 677

Peritoneal dialysis

Chan, J.C. and Campbell, R.A. (1973). For children. *Clin. Paediatr.,* **12,** 131

Craddock, P.R. (1977). Granulocyte adherence changes during haemodialysis. *N. Eng. J. Med.,* **296,** 769

Drüeke, T., Le Pailleur, C. (1977). Uraemic cardiomyopathy. *Br. Med. J.,* **1,** 350

Gordon, E.M. (1972). Gastric assessment, *Lancet,* **i,** 226

Jones, J.H. (1971). *Br. Med. Bull.,* **27,** 165

MacGregor, R.R. (1977). Granulocyte adherence changes during haemodialysis. *Ann. Intern Med.,* **86,** 35

Marmion, B.P. (1972). Hepatitis control. *Br. Med. Bull.,* **28,** 169

Mitchell, T.R. (1971). Oxygen affinity in chronic renal failure. *Br. J. Haematol.,* **21,** 463

Peachy, J. (1969). Automatic peritoneal dialysis. *Biomed. Eng.,* **4,** 460

Richet, G. (1970). Drug intoxication in renal failure. *Br. Med. J.,* **2,** 394

Scheuer, J. and Stezoski, S. (1973). Uraemic cardiomyopathy. *J. Mol. Cell. Cardiol.,* **5,** 287

Siriwatratanananta, P. (1978). Defective chemotaxis in uraemia. *J. Lab. Clin. Med.,* **92,** 402

Snydman, D.R. and Bregman, D. (1977). Hepatitis B (occurrence). *J. Infect. Dis.,* **135,** 687

Torrance, J.D. (1975). Oxygen affinity in chronic renal failure. *Clin. Nephrol.,* **3,** 54

Dialysis technique

Babb, A.L. (1971). Genesis of the square-meter hour hypothesis. *Trans. Am. Soc. Artif. Int. Org.,* **17,** 81

Blagg, C.R. (1974). In Edwards *Drugs and the Kidney.* Prog. Biochem. Pharmacol., **9,** 239

Editorial (1976). Hepatic haemoperfusion. *J. Am. Med. Assoc.,* **235,** 12

Funck-Prentano, J.L. (1973). Polyacrylonitrile membranes. *Proc. Eur. Dialysis and Transplant Assoc.,* **10,** 236 and *Kidney Int.,* 1975 (s2) **7,** 52

Gazzard, B.G. (1974). *Lancet,* **i,** 1301

Gelfand, M.C. (1976). *Kidney Int.,* **10,** S239

Gordon, A. (1975). Absorption of toxins. *6th Int. Congress Nephrology,* 612

Lewin, A.J. (1974). Sorbent regeneration. *Trans. Am. Soc. Artif. Int. Org.,* **20,** 130

Silk, D. *et al.* (1977). Hepatic failure and polyacrylonitrile membrane dialysis. *Lancet,* **i,** 316

Winchester, J.F. (1975). Haemodialysis with charcoal haemoperfusion. *Eur. Dialysis and Transplant Assoc.,* **12,** 526 and *Kidney Int.,* 1976, **10,** S 315

Diets in chronic renal failure

Ford, J. (1969). Nitrogen balance on chronic renal failure diets. *Br. Med. J.,* **1,** 735

Giordano, C. (1963). Exogenous and endogenous urea for protein synthesis. *J. Lab. Clin. Med.,* **62,** 231

Giovanetti, S. and Maggiore, Q. (1964). A low nitrogen diet with proteins of high biological value for chronic uraemia. *Lancet,* **i,** 1000

Huttunen, J.K., Pasternak, A. (1978). Plasma triglycerides in chronic renal failure. *Acta Med. Scand.,* **204,** 211

Kopple, J.D. (1975). Protein and amino-acid metabolism on dialysis. *Kidney Int.,* **7,** S 64

Kopple, J.D. (1977). Amino-acid and keto-acid diets for therapy in renal failure. *Nephron,* **18,** 1

Richards, P. (1975). Protein metabolism in uraemia. *Nephron,* **14,** 134

Sanfelippo, M.L. (1977). Plasma triglycerides in chronic renal failure. *Kidney Int.,* **11,** 54

Shaw, A.B. *et al.* (1965). Chronic renal failure and a modified Giovanetti diet. *Q. J. Med.,* **34,** 237

Walser, M. (1973). Effect of keto-analogues in chronic uraemia. *J. Clin. Invest.,* **52,** 678

Wardle, E.N. (1975). Serum proteins and dietary protein intake in chronic renal failure. *Clin. Nephrol.,* **3,** 114

Psychology and renal disease

Abram, H. (1972). The psychiatrist and chronic renal failure. *Am. J. Psychiat.*, **128**, 12

Brown, T. *et al.* (1974). Living with dialysis. *Ann. Intern. Med.*, 81

Raimbault, G. (1973). Psychological aspects of dialysis. *Nephron*, **11**, 252

Medical problems

Bergrem, H., Flatmark, A. and Simonsen, S. (1978). Dialysis fistulas and cardiac failure. *Acta Med. Scand.*, **204**, 191

Curtis, J.R. (1969). Maintenance haemodialysis. *Q. J. Med.*, **38**, 49

Curtis, J.R. and Williams, G.B. *Clinical Management of Chronic Renal Failure.* (Oxford: Blackwell), 1975

Evans, D.B. (1977). Dialysis and transplantation. *Br. Med. J.*, **1**, 1585

Kramer, P. (1975). Uraemic pericarditis. *Br. Med. J.*, **4**, 564

Lazarus, J.M. (1975). Cardiovascular disease and dialysis. *Kidney Int.*, **7**, S167

Lindner, A. (1974). Accelerated arteriosclerosis on dialysis. *N. Engl. J. Med.*, **290**, 697

Reichsman, F. (1972). Problems in adaptation to maintenance haemodialysis. *Arch. Intern. Med.*, **130**, 859

Bone disease

Bonomini, V. (1973). Diet, dialysis and transplantation and bone lesions. *Proc. Eur. Dialysis and Transplant Assoc.*, **10**, 324

Bordier, P.J. (1975). Renal osteodystrophy. *Kidney Int.*, **7**, S 102

Doyle, F.H. (1972). Radiology in bone disease. *Br. Med. Bull.*, **28**, 220

Ellis, H.A. (1973). Histology in bone disease, *J. Clin. Pathol.*, **26**, 83

Fiaschi, E. (1975). Calcium and phosphorus on dialysis. *Nephron.*, **14**, 163

Garner, A., Ball, J. (1966). Histology in bone disease. *J. Pathol. Bacteriol.*, **91**, 545

Goldsmith, R. (1975). Calcium and phosphorus on dialysis. *Kidney Int.*, **7**, S 118

Siddiqui, J., Kerr, D.N.S. (1971). Complications of renal failure and their response to dialysis. *Br. Med. Bull.*, **27**, 153

Foreign surface effects and dialysers

Gott, V.L. and Furuse, A. (1971). Anti-thrombotic surfaces. *Fed. Proc.*, **30**, 1679 de Laval, M. (1972). Platelet kinetics during extracorporeal circulation. *Trans. Am. Soc. Artif. Intern. Org.*, **18,** 355

Lyman, D.J. (1968). Effect of surface properties of polymers on blood coagulation. *Trans. Am. Soc. Artif. Intern. Org.*, **14,** 250

Wardle, E.N. (1972). Studies of contact activation in haemodialysis. *J. Clin. Pathol.*, **25,** 1045

14
Renal transplantation

A renal transplant was first performed between identical twins by Merrill and colleagues in 1956; there are now 2300 transplants per year in Europe (EDTA). The following are specific terms used in transplantation:

(1) *Autograft* is when the organ comes from the same individual from which it was removed.

(2) *Isograft* is when the donor is of the same genotype, as when twins exchange an organ.

(3) *Allograft* is when the donor is of the same species, but a different genotype.

(4) *Xenograft* refers to donation of an organ from a different species.

Most renal transplant kidneys are, therefore, allografts.

Technique

A transplant kidney is placed retroperitoneally in the iliac fossa opposite to the side from which it was removed, so that the renal pelvis and ureter lie anteriorly and are easily anastomosed to the right iliac vessels and to the bladder. The short ureter is implanted through a submucosal tunnel and a

391

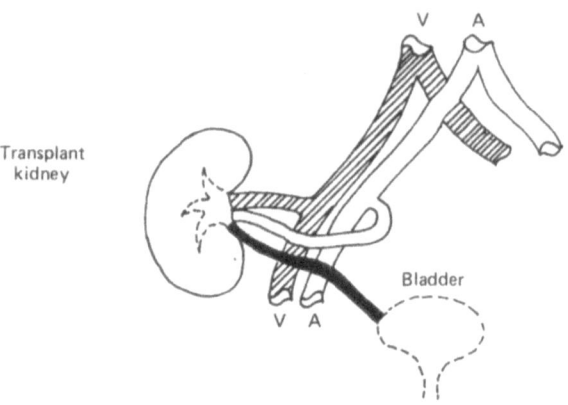

Transplant
kidney

Bladder

Figure 139.   Anastamoses of the transplant kidney

catheter is either left up the ureter for 48 h, or is placed in the bladder so as to allow freedom from straining and to permit bladder washouts (Figure 139).

Preparation of the kidney

The 'warm ischaemia time', that is the time between death of the donor and adequate cooling of the kidney, must not exceed 20 min, but a kidney can be kept in the cold for 6−12 h. In fact 1 min of warm ischaemia time does as much damage as 1 h of cold ischaemia time. The choice is between cold storage in Collin's intracellular electrolyte solution and continuous cold perfusion with cryoprecipitated plasma, plasma protein fraction or albumin. The washing removes lactic acid, and lysosomal enzymes that might be injurious, as well as any foreign cells. During the perfusion it is clearly important to supply the metabolic requirements of the kidney. Oxygen is required but there is no glucose utilization below 8 °C. A solution called 'Perfudex' is used for perfusions up to 24 h. This contains NaCl 8.0 g/l; KCl 0.4 g/l; $MgSO_4$ 0.2 g/l; Na_2HPO_4 87 mg/l; KH_2PO_4 0.2 g/l; glucose 1.0 g/l and low molecular weight dextran (40 000) 50 g/l. Some solutions contain mannitol and frusemide to maintain cellular integrity. The methyl-prednisolone that is given to a potential donor also helps to prevent injury.

The kidney is perfused with PPF (plasma protein fraction) at a pressure of 40−80 mmHg and flow rate of 100−150 ml/min at a temperature of 6 °C. With an oxygenator delivery of 95% oxygen and 5% carbon dioxide, oxygen tension of 200−400 mmHg can be obtained and the pH of the perfusate is buffered with bicarbonate so as to remain in the range 7.2−7.4. Although donor kidney perfusion has many advocates there have been recent descriptions of a *perfusion nephropathy* in which the endothelium of the glomeruli is destroyed and the glomerular capillary loops are obliterated by fibrin thrombi. Indeed it is now thought that cold stored but non-perfused kidneys may have a better immediate survival.

Condition of the donor

(1) A living related donor who volunteers a kidney must first be shown to have no renal disease or hypertension, and no transmissible disease such as hepatitis or cancer. There must be ABO compatability between donor and recipient, but the Rhesus factor can be ignored.

A renal angiogram is necessary to show that the donor organ is normal, and also to give prior information about its vascular supply. Kidneys with multiple arteries can be used but each then has to be anastomosed separately, for ligature of a renal artery branch will inevitably lead to a wedge-shaped infarct of part of that kidney.

(2) Cadaver kidneys need to be obtained from persons who are young enough to be free of arterial disease and, of course, there must be no intrinsic renal disease. There are many medical and ethical problems regarding certification of the moment of death but in respect of the donor kidney it is important to sustain the circulation for as long as possible and to ensure that the body is adequately oxygenated.

Preparation of the recipient

A recipient must be well dialysed but free of heparin, have a haemoglobin of at least 10 g% and, if a smoker, have stopped smoking for at least 1 week in order to ensure a minimum of trouble with chest infections. Six pints of blood will be needed for operative cover.

In cases of accelerated hypertension or obstructive uropathy a bilateral nephrectomy will have been performed beforehand. When anastomosis of the ureter to the normal bladder is impossible on account of a bladder abnormality, an ileal loop will have to be created.

In premeditated transplantation azathioprine (Imuran) immunosuppression will be started at a dose of 3 mg/kg at least 3 days beforehand and prednisone at a dose of 3 mg/kg. When, as more commonly happens with cadaver transplants, there are only a few hours warning, then 50 mg of azathioprine is given intravenously and 16 mg of Codelsol (equivalent to 20 mg prednisone). The object of this exercise is to damp down or prevent interaction of recipient lymphocytes with the foreign donor kidney and to suppress the formation of humoral antibodies to HLA antigens on vascular endothelium. Azathioprine is, in fact, a precursor of 6-mercaptopurine.

It is standard practice to ensure that the donor and recipient are of the same

ABO blood group and hopefully a 3/4 serologically defined HLA match should be achieved. Additionally the patient must not have cytotoxic antibodies against the donor's lymphocytes. Details of the immunological tests will be discussed shortly for, from both the clinician and patient's point of view, considerable anxiety attaches to 'graft rejection' because this is accompanied by transient or permanent deterioration of renal function.

REJECTION

Clinical signs of rejection

Rejection may occur at any time in the first year after grafting and more particularly in the first 6 weeks. It is evident as fever, malaise and tachycardia, pain and swelling of the graft kidney, and oliguria and hypertension. The urine is full of small darkly staining epitheloid cells, and some lymphocytes, and there is a non-selective proteinuria. There can be a hyperchloraemic acidosis indicative of distal tubule dysfunction, a lysozymuria indicative of proximal tubule dysfunction or even a typical Fanconi syndrome.

Of course cessation of urine flow has a variety of causes and the following also have to be carefully considered:

(1)   acute tubular necrosis—a normal feature of cadaver grafts;
(2)   ureteric obstruction or extravasation of urine;
(3)   a lymphocoele giving rise to a swelling around the kidney;
(4)   thrombosis of the renal artery or vein;
(5)   urinary infection.

At all times a rise of serum creatinine of 0.2–0.3 mg% (30μmol/l) must be taken seriously; in the case of chronic insidious rejection particularly, a slowly rising creatinine may be the only sign of deterioration.

Pathological types of rejection

Hyperacute rejection (immediate rejection)
This occurs immediately on completion of the anastomosis. There is prompt cessation of blood flow due to a combination of vascular spasm and thrombosis. The graft goes a deep purple and never passes urine. It is seen either when there is ABO group incompatability or when there are preformed cytotoxic antibodies. This latter situation means that as a result of blood transfusions or pregnancies the patient has complement-dependent lympocytotoxic antibodies to the donor lymphocytes. There is no treatment for this situation. The histology shows accumulation of polymorphs in the glomeruli. This is also the hallmark of lesser grades of 'cytotoxic antibody' (CDA) reactions.

Acute rejection (days 2–10)

The typical clinical features of acute rejection, which is basically a *cell-mediated immune reaction* caused by sensitized lymphocytes, have been described above. There is widespread interstitial oedema and gross infiltration by mononuclear cells (Figure 140). These are said to be 'pyroninophilic' as their cytoplasm is full of RNA which stains red with methyl-green pyronin. Invading host lymphocytes make contact with foreign HLA antigens and, having become sensitized, they proliferate in adjacent lymph nodes and the spleen, and when they or their progeny re-enter the graft they have a cytotoxic effect on the endothelium. So there is disruption of the venules which leads to interstitial oedema and compensatory arteriolar spasm; the peritubular capillaries are also damaged. The lymph flow may, in fact, rise from 3.0 ml/h to 60 ml/h.

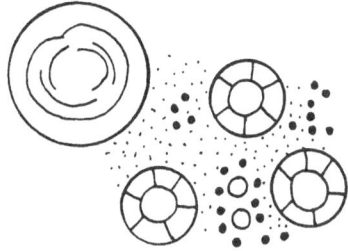

Figure 140.   Features of acute rejection

Vascular rejection (after 10 days)

The feature here is *fibrinoid necrosis of arteriolar walls* and deposits thereon, and in the glomerular capillaries, of platelet aggregates and fibrin (Figure 141). This type of rejection appears when there is humoral antibody

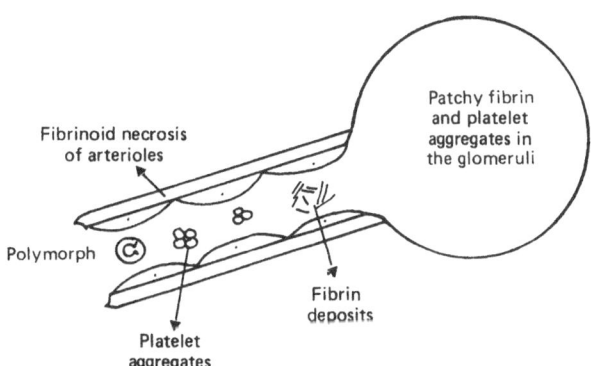

Figure 141.   Features of vascular rejection

formation to HLA antigens, so that antibody is deposited on vascular endothelium, and is detectable there together with complement by immunofluorescence. Arterioles damaged in this way contain some polymorphs. Other vessels, however, have clearly been destroyed as the result of a lymphocytic infiltration.

During rejection a kidney may become 20% longer (14–17 cm) and 40% wider (7–11 cm) than is normal. On IVU there is a prolonged nephrogram, and arteriography shows delayed arterial emptying and an inability to visualize the arcuate arteries.

Chronic insidious rejection

Instead of fibrinoid necrosis there is at this stage a *chronic obliterative endarteritis* causing onion-skin lamellation of the intima of the arteries; it involves large arteries and their interlobular branches. Fluorescence shows deposition of C3 and IgM, which reflects humoral antibody formation against HLA antigens of the donor, for it is rarely seen when there is perfect matching.

The glomeruli show a lobular or *membranous nephropathy*. There are dense deposits of amorphous material on the endothelial side of the basement membrane and in the mesangium. So there is a low grade fever, a steady decline of the creatinine clearance, and a non-selective proteinuria.

Tests for rejection

The [^{131}]iodine hippuran clearance

This measures the renal blood flow. The normal half-life of injected isotope, as measured by plasma clearance or counting over the heart, is 7–18 min but this will be prolonged to over 18 min when there is either rejection or acute tubular necrosis. This test is, therefore, a useful screening procedure but lacks specificity. The actual renogram shows a lowering of the first and second uptake phases and a reduction of radiohippuran uptake, as seen on a scintiphoto taken after 15–30 sec (page 297).

Renal biopsy and/or arteriography

These techniques yield more positive evidence as to whether there is rejection but actually they are best avoided as the complications of invasive techniques are quite significant in patients who may have to be heparinized for dialysis and who are receiving high doses of immunosuppressive drugs.

Ultrasound

The patient is scanned in the supine position, preferably with a full bladder.

Its diagnostic value is (a) in demonstrating kidney enlargement and renal cortical swelling without calcyeal dilatation in patients with acute rejection, (b) in showing dilatation of the collecting system in patients with obstruction, and (c) in demonstrating various perinephric collections of fluid as in the case of haematoma, lymphocoele or abscess formation.

Biochemical assays

A rise of serum fibrin degradation products (FDP) occurs when there is either tubular necrosis or rejection, but is clearly of little value in the postoperative period. Some claims have been made for urine FDP as an indicator of rejection but really FDP only reflect the non-selective proteinuria. A search has been made, therefore, for those enzymes of the renal tubular epithelium whose urinary loss indicates damage due to renal ischaemia. Urinary lysozyme, *N*-acetylglucosaminidase (NAG) and gammaglutamyltranspeptidase can all be used in this way. The main application is in long term follow-up and detection of unexpected rejection.

Radiofibrinogen catabolism or platelet survival studies

Acute rejection can be detected either by an increase in the catabolism of labelled fibrinogen or from a decreased survival of labelled platelets. Once again non-specific results are obtained in the postoperative period, when ischaemic acute tubular necrosis cannot be distinguished from immunological rejection, but these procedures are of value in long-term monitoring. The radiofibrinogen catabolism study is of particular value for determining long-term chronic insidious rejection.

Immunological procedures for rejection

Serum complement components show instability at the time of rejection but no specific pattern can be relied on. Many patients show a rise in serum levels and urinary excretion of heterophil agglutinins to sheep or rat red cells, but again too much faith should not be placed on the assay.

It was originally hoped that a heightened phytohaemagglutinin (PHA) responsiveness of blood lymphocytes would anticipate rejection, and to a certain extent this is so. But unfortunately almost all transplant recipients have antibodies to cytomegalovirus (CMV), and as PHA responsiveness is inversely related to the titres of such antibodies, the test can be rendered valueless.

The migration of leucocytes into a chamber containing kidney extract (as antigen) has been said to indicate sensitization prior to and during rejection (Figure 142). This test has its advocates but there are many non-specific positive and negative results. It is said that the test has greater reliability when

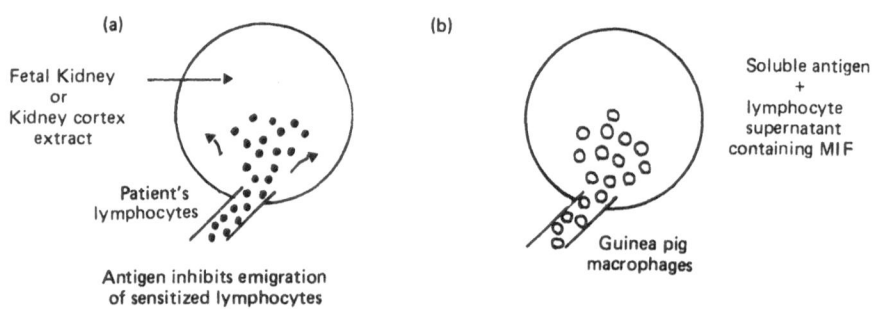

Figure 142. Leucocyte migration inhibition procedures

the supernatants from patient's peripheral blood lymphocyte cultures are incubated with soluble antigen, and are assessed by the movement of normal guinea-pig macrophages from capillary tubes into the chambers.

Treatment and prevention of rejection: immunosuppressive therapy

Preoperatively patients are given azathioprine 3 mg/kg and 16 mg of Codelsol (prednisolone).

Thereafter patients receive azathioprine 2–3 mg/kg per day and 40 mg/day of prednisone (20 mg/day in some centres but 0.5 mg/kg in others). This prednisone dosage has to be reduced by 5–10 mg every tenth day until the patient is taking the maintenance dosage of 5–10 mg/day prednisone.

Whenever there is rejection (and the distinction between rejection and acute tubular necrosis in the first days of oliguria is almost impossible) it becomes imperative to give 200 mg/day prednisone until there are signs of resolution. The alternative approach, which is now almost standard, is to give 1 g/day of Solumedrone (methyl-prednisolone) for three days and then revert to the 40 mg/day schedule. Heparin is also given intravenously by pump infusion.

X-ray radiation (200 rads/day for 3 days) and actinomycin D (200 μg/day for 3 days) are seldom used now but they are useful additional methods. Antacids are best given routinely to protect against peptic ulceration. Fungilin lozenges help to keep down *Candida* infection in the mouth.

Needle biopsy of the transplant kidney should be used infrequently. In fact many centres no longer use this procedure because of the great risk of bleeding. Always after the first week it can be assumed that there is a vascular component to rejection, so that infusion of heparin is required, followed by warfarin anticoagulation whenever there is late rejection. Platelet inhibitory drugs such as aspirin, dipyridamole, or flurbiprofen or cyproheptidine are also used.

Azathioprine has been blamed for occasional cases of jaundice and in those cases cyclophosphamide should be substituted at a dose of 0.7–1.0 mg/kg, which works out at 50–100 mg/day and, apart from gonadal atrophy, is quite safe and effective. In fact there is now some doubt whether azathioprine plays any effective role after the first 6 months of immunosuppression.

Splenectomy

Since the amount of lymphoid tissue is clearly reduced by splenectomy, this procedure was used in the early years, but no difference has been shown in the outcome of transplantation. However, patients who do have hypersplenism may develop severe leucopenia shortly after starting immunosuppressive therapy, and after splenectomy will be rendered tolerant of higher dosages of azathioprine. The outstanding problem seems to be that many of these episodes of leucopenia are, in fact, symptomatic of CMV or other viral infection and thus both the scientific merit and the ethics of the situation are in some doubt. Splenectomy always predisposes to infection and should be avoided.

COMPLICATIONS OF THE TRANSPLANT SITUATION

Infections due to immunosuppression

Fever in the transplant recipient may either signify rejection or a bacterial, viral or fungal infection. As might be anticipated, such episodes correspond to the degree of immunosuppression. They are particularly related to corticosteroid dosage, since this determines inhibition of the phagocytic capabilities of the macrophages.

Either transplant wound or urinary tract infection with Gram-negative-resistant organisms, such as *Pseudomonas* and *Klebsiella,* can be a problem. Pneumonia occurs with a whole variety of organisms, in particular cytomegalovirus (CMV) infection which can cause a perihilar interstitial pneumonitis. More commonly it presents as a fever which may go on for 2–3 weeks, and which is accompanied by a blood lymphocytosis with abnormal monocytes, splenomegaly and hepatic dysfunction that can be progressive; the overall picture resembles glandular fever. More often than not CMV is the result of reactivation of latent endogenous infection, but it may also be acquired from the graft, from blood or by spread from other patients. Typically there are intranuclear oval Feulgen-positive CMV bodies, which may be identified in the focal pneumonitis and in areas of liver cell necrosis and fatty change as the 'owl's eye' inclusions. When there is a pancreatitis or brain glial nodules, CMV is also implicated, and it often causes a haemorrhagic gastritis. The diagnosis is made by a rising titre of complement-fixing antibody and by isolation of the virus from the throat or urine.

In like manner the transplant patient may suffer from reactivation of tuberculosis, superinfection of cavities with aspergillus, or infection of the lung with other fungi such as *Candida, Nocardia* and *Cryptococcus*. The protozoan *Pneumocystis carinii* is the usual cause of 'transplant lung'. Recurrent warts, herpes simplex sores, or even herpes simplex encephalitis, and outbreaks of herpes zoster or toxoplasma all take their toll. Papova virus has been recognized as the cause of a progressive multifocal leucoencephalopathy.

Hepatic dysfunction

This has sometimes been thought to be due to azathioprine toxicity but hepatitis B infection or CMV disease is much more likely. Carriers of hepatitis B virus tend to be male, while patients with good antibody titres to HB_sAg are female. Deteriorating liver function and death in hepatic coma may sometimes occur. As to the effect on the kidney, it seems that chronic carriers fare better than other transplants but that deterioration of graft function is a feature of the female with high antibody titres and this suggests immune complex formation due to possession of precipitating antibody.

Steroid toxicity

Steroid side-effects
The usual steroid side-effects such as peptic ulceration, thinning of the bones and skin, polycythaemia and diabetes are all found in transplant recipients.

Aseptic necrosis of bone
This is a difficult problem. Pre-existing renal osteodystrophy, hyperparathyroidism, hyperlipidaemia and the total prednisone dosage are all thought to be predisposing. An early sign is a subchondral lucent crescent indicating loss of density of the epiphyseal bone (Figure 143). In weight-

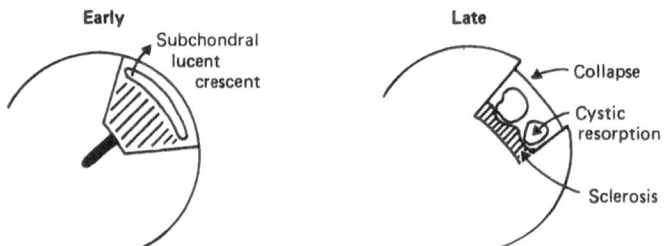

Figure 143.   Aseptic necrosis of bone

bearing joints there is subsequent loss of the normal contour of the bony surface and the development of areas of increased density and of destruction.

Ocular complications

These include steroid-induced glaucoma and posterior subcapsular cataracts. Acute herpetic keratitis or CMV retinitis can also cause trouble but alternate-day corticosteroids will reduce the incidence of these.

Hyperlipidaemia

This is a result of steroid therapy. Both the serum cholesterol and the serum triglyceride tend to correlate with the prednisone dosage.

Impairment of growth in children

This is attributable to the prednisone used after transplantation, although in the phase of chronic renal failure it is due also to a combination of the effects of acidosis, osteodystrophy, and protein and calorie restriction. A dosage of prednisone greater than 10 mg/m^2 per day is guaranteed to stop growth but children will grow at lower dosages, particularly if their bone age at the time is less than 12 years. Boys always grow better than girls.

Immunosuppression and malignancy

The incidence of lymphoma is increased some 300 times in the renal transplant recipient and there is a particular predilection for intracerebral tumours. The cytotoxic agents azathioprine and cyclophosphamide are both known to damage chromosomes and they cause both testicular and ovarian failure; it is likely too that immunosuppression favours oncogenic viruses. The usual spectrum of malignancy is not seen but rather tumours of the skin, cervix and lymphoreticular organs, so it seems highly probable that herpes viruses play a role.

Hypertension and renal artery stenosis

Hypertension is a result of the renal vasoconstriction and thrombosis that is part of acute and chronic rejection. Quite apart from this, renal artery stenosis is common, and in some centres routine arteriography is repeated at intervals. There may be stenosis in the iliac vessels of the recipient, at the suture line, or locally or diffusely in the graft artery. This gives rise to hypertension along with raised plasma renin activity, and reduction of previously good renal function.

As for the hypertension that goes with impairment of renal function due to rejection, the proportion of hypertensive patients rises during the first three months and subsequently affects about 60%. Over the years it fluctuates, so that one-third of the initially hypertensive patients become normotensive, whereas about one-third of the originally normotensive patients may end up with hypertension. Steroid-induced hypertension is occasionally seen.

Urological problems

These occur in as many as 30% of patients with renal allografts. Obstruction of the ureter or a leaking ureter is a common problem; necrosis of the distal ureter due to technical reasons, a compromised vascular supply or 'ureteric rejection' are the usual explanations. Infarction over a calyx may also give rise to a urinary leak. In order to confirm the presence of obstruction a retrograde pyelogram may be justified. Ultrasound is also helpful.

As many as 30% of renal allografts are subjected to vesicoureteric reflux, usually as a consequence of a short intramural tunnel through the bladder, or previous urine leakage and a reoperation on the ureter. It is detected by micturating cystogram. In fact the kidney seldom shows the typical cortical scar and dilated calyx of a classical reflux nephropathy, but rather some calyceal dilatation and general cortical thinning. At histology the glomeruli have the appearance of mesangiocapillary nephritis, or else of focal hyalinosis and sclerosis. Such a nephritis might arise because increased back-pressure on the renal tubular epithelium leads to entry of renal tubular antigen into the circulation causing an autoimmune Heymann's type nephritis. *E. coli* antigenaemia might also play a role.

Lymphocoeles

These are probably due to failure to ligate host lymphatics at the time of operation, but the actual accumulation of lymph may not present until months later and then the manifestations can be in a variety of ways: there may be a mass around the kidney or suprapubically or *per rectum*; unilateral leg oedema; a filling defect in the bladder on routine IVP, or recurrent urinary infection due to some obstruction. The problem lies in the differentiation from haematoma, a perinephric abscess or a urinary leak. This has to be done by needle aspiration, by IVU and cystogram, or by ultrasonography. Management should be conservative as spontaneous resolution often occurs.

Hyperparathyroidism after transplantation

Since hyperplastic parathyroid glands take time to involute, persisting hypercalcaemia after a renal transplant is not an indication for operation, unless it appears that the hypercalcaemia is so extreme as to cause reduced glomerular filtration, or that it is playing some part in aseptic necrosis of bone.

Sometimes the onset of the hypercalcaemia is delayed for more than 6 months (see also page 325).

THE IMMUNOLOGY OF TRANSPLANTATION

The histocompatability or transplantation antigens

Antigens occur on all nucleated cells, the white cells and the platelets which determine the recognition of 'foreignness'. They are glycoproteins containing some 10% carbohydrate, and occur on the cell surface and in the interior. They are called the HLA (human leucocyte antigen) system. Two approaches are used in the analysis of this complex antigen system (Figure 144).

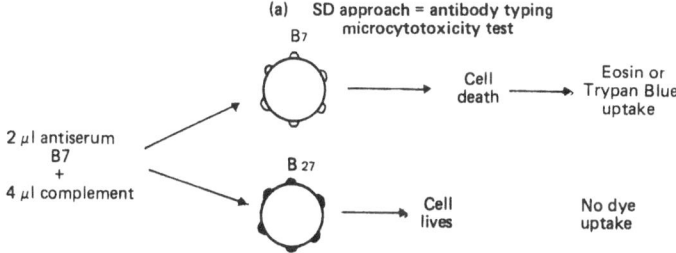

(a) Serological defined approach

Otherwise known as:-
    the dye exclusion complement dependent assay (DE-CDA) or
    ^{51}Cr release complement dependent assay

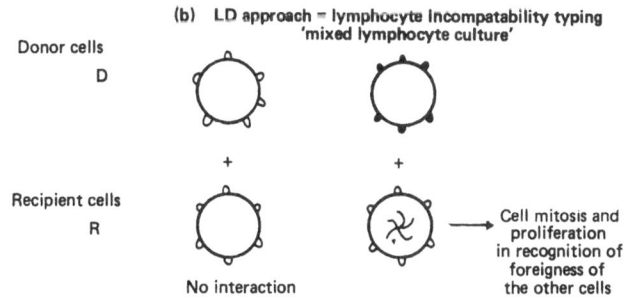

(b) Lymphocyte defined approach

Figure 144.   Approach to human leucocyte antigen analysis

(1)   *The SD (serologically-defined) approach,* in which specific antibodies are used to detect cell surface antigens.

(2)   *The LD (lymphocyte-defined) approach* which applies in mixed

lymphocyte culture (MLC), when antigens on a foreign donor lymphocyte (even though it has been killed) will cause the living recipient lymphocytes to proliferate according to their degree of incompatability.

The SD and LD systems are, in fact, determined by closely linked genes which in man form the HLA complex on chromosome 6, and in the mouse the H2 complex.

When typing with antisera it is found that each human has two antigens from a 'first locus gene' (16 or more possible antigens) and another two antigens from a 'second locus gene' (about 12 possible antigens). Such is the polymorphism of the system that another person will have a different set of antigens.

Person X   antigens B. 5.7   Person Y   antigens B 8.12 (second locus)
(donor)   A. 1.2   (recipient)   A 1.2 (first locus)

In the illustration two antigens from the first locus are identical, whilst those of the second locus differ. Therefore, if organ X is given to recipient Y, there will be immunological rejection since the degree of histocompatability is only designated as a 2/4 match. Complete identity as in the case of twins is called a full 4/4 match. It is normally preferable in renal transplantation to attempt to achieve 3/4 matching.

On human chromosome 6 there are four major gene loci called HLA-A, HLA-B, HLA-C and HLA-D. The latter is actually the MLC locus. Commonly only locus A and locus B are defined by the current sera. Human chromosome 6 can be visualized as shown in Figure 145.

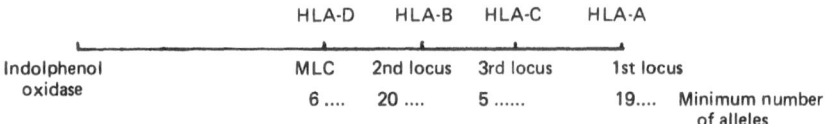

Figure 145. Human chromosome six

The *HLA antigens* and their gene frequencies are categorized in Table 45.

One would expect the various antigens to be distributed at random, but in fact some pairs occur more often than expected, for example HLA-A1 and HLA-B8; HLA-A2 and HLA-B12; HLA-A3 and HLA-B7. The genes which control these groups of antigens are, therefore, said to be in *linkage disequilibrium*—thus HLA-A1 has a gene frequency of 0.17 and HLA-B8 of 0.11, and therefore, one might predict that A1 and B8 will be found together with a frequency of 0.17 x 0.11 = 0.0187; the actual figure is 0.13 to 0.04. Linkage disequilibrium between the B and C gene loci is also extremely high.

Table 45   HLA antigens and their gene frequencies

Locus HLA-A		*Locus HLA-B*		*Locus HLA-C*	*Locus HLA-D (MLC)*
A1	0.17	B5	0.04	CW1	DW1
A2	0.32	B7	0.16	CW2	DW2
A3	0.14	B8	0.11	CW3	DW3
A9	0.10	B12	0.18	CW4	DW4
A10	0.06	B13	0.01	CW5	DW5
A11	0.04	B14	0.04		DW6
A28	0.01	B15	0.07		
A29	0.04	BW16	0.01		
AW 23, 24, 25, 26,		BW17	0.06		
AW 30, 31, 32, 33		BW18	0.05		
		BW21	0.01		
		BW22	0.02		

The HLA system controls a number of biological functions:

(1)   determination of cell surface antigens and, therefore cellular and humoral histocompatability reactions;
(2)   T and B cell cooperative reactions;
(3)   'immune responsiveness' since the HLA genes are closely related to *Ir* genes;
(4)   levels of serum complement components.

Many diseases have HLA associations. The frequency of HLA-A2 is significantly increased in patients with chronic glomerulonephritis (and DRW2 is associated with Goodpasture's syndrome). Again juvenile diabetes is associated with HLA-A1, B8 and DRW3.

The object of this brief introduction is to emphasize the relevance of the HLA system to renal transplantation. We can now review the tests and their usefulness.

The cells participating in immune reactions

The nephrologist may need a reminder that production of a *humoral antibody* to an antigen requires processing of that antigen by macrophages feeding

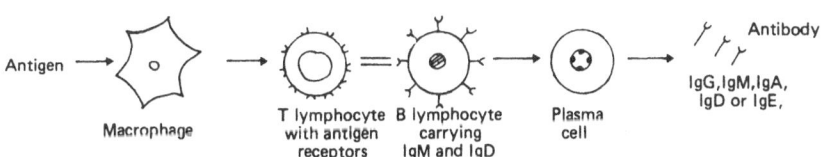

Figure 146.   Cell cooperation in immune reactions

405

information to T lymphocytes which then cooperate with B lymphocytes, which themselves are transformed to the plasma cells synthesizing the appropriate antibody (Figure 146).

In transplant rejection much damage is done by B lymphocytes which carry immunoglobulins on their cell surface. There are both 'helper' and 'suppressor' T cells. The details of their several roles are still under investigation.

For our purpose it is only necessary to be able to separate T (thymusderived) lymphocytes from the B (bursa or bone marrow) lymphocytes. The lymphocytes of peripheral blood are generally used but so also are extracts of lymph nodes. Since T lymphocytes adhere to neuraminidase-treated sheep red cells to form rosettes, after incubating lymphocytes in this way for 30 min at 5 °C, the mixture is centrifuged through Ficoll-Hypaque at 60 g for 10 min. By this means the rosetted T cells are spun down, while the B lymphocytes are left at the interface; 2-aminoethyl-isothiouronium bromide-treated sheep cells can be used as an alternative. Thereafter the sheep red cells can be lysed by incubating the rosettes with rabbit complement for 15 min at 37 °C. Thus the B lymphocytes or the T cells can be harvested separately.

Tests used in transplant immunology

The complement-dependent lymphocyte microcytotoxicity test (CDA–LMC)
Donor B lymphocytes from heparinized blood are separated on a Ficol/Triosil layer so that they are harvested from the interface. The test is then carried out in a Falcon microtest plate by adding in turn:

(a) the SD-typing serum (or the recipients serum);
(b) the donor B lymphocytes;
(c) excess of rabbit serum (used because its complement content together with rabbit IgM plays a lethal role).

The cells are incubated for 1 h and the dead cells are then identified because they will take up eosin or Trypan blue stains (the 'dye-exclusion' CDA) (see Figure 144a).

The sera used for serological definition (SD) are obtained from three sources

(1) from multiparous females, of whom 10–40% form antibodies against leucocytes;
(2) from transfused patients;
(3) from experiments in which patients are given skin grafts or transplants.

The test can be made more sensitive by using lymphocytes or other target cells (such as renal endothelial cells) that have been labelled with

^{51}Cr. It then becomes the '^{51}C release' complement-dependent assay ^{51}Cr-CDA.

This test is used

(1)   for typing of donor tissues;
(2)   as a 'cytotoxic cross-match' to detect 'presensitization'.

So if one examines the sera of transfused patients for cytotoxic antibody, it is found that (a) there are some 30% non-responders, (b) others have transient cytotoxic antibodies, or (c) that others have persistent cytotoxic antibodies.

There are, of course, problems. Presensitization is difficult to detect with a single plasma sample if there is a state of latent sensitization, and a long incubation cross-match has had to be developed to detect weak antibodies (Ting, 1973). Indeed the cytotoxic cross-match still does not prevent the failure of some 10% first grafts of either living or cadaver donors, and some 20% of second or third grafts.

Presensitization, therefore, should be looked for by several means—the CDA–LMC, the ^{51}Cr–CDA, the CML and the LDA tests (fig. 149).

The mixed lymphocyte culture (MLC)
This detects at least eight antigens which occur on the B lymphocytes and which are determined by the MLC (HLA-D) locus (Figure 147).

The performance of the test in which donor and recipient lymphocytes are mixed is facilitated in two ways (see Figure 144b). Firstly the response is made undirectional by killing the donor stimulating cells by means of mitomycin C or irradiation. Secondly, the proliferative response is accurately monitored by following the uptake by the recipient lymphocytes of tritiated thymidine.

In fact, the MLC typing takes at least 1 week but a *primed lymphocyte typing test* (PLT) may allow typing within 24 h.

The cell-mediated lympholysis (CML) test
This is for circulating cytotoxic T cells. The responding cells which appear in

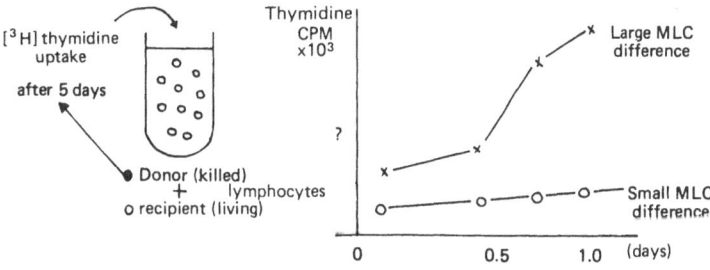

Figure 147.   The mixed lymphocyte culture (MLC) test

the MLC incubation mixture were originally noted to become cytotoxic to target B cells that are taken from the donor. Thereafter, Lightbody introduced the use of PHA-stimulated donor lymphoblasts that are labelled as target cells with $[^{51}Cr]$sodium chromate. This test is the present CML (figure 148). Regrettably this procedure means that the target B lymphocytes have to be stimulated first for 3 days in culture with PHA.

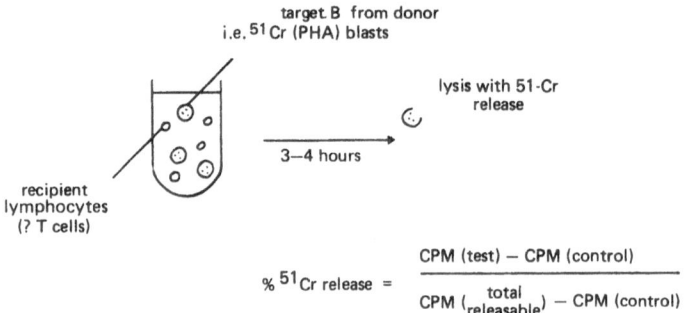

Figure 148.   Cell mediated lympholysis test

Lymphocyte dependent antibodies (LDA)
The serum of the recipient is incubated for a few hours with target cells (fibroblasts or lymphocytes for example) and the peripheral blood lymphocytes of a normal control. These serve as effector K cells, which kill the target cells when there are sensitizing antibodies in the serum of the recipient.

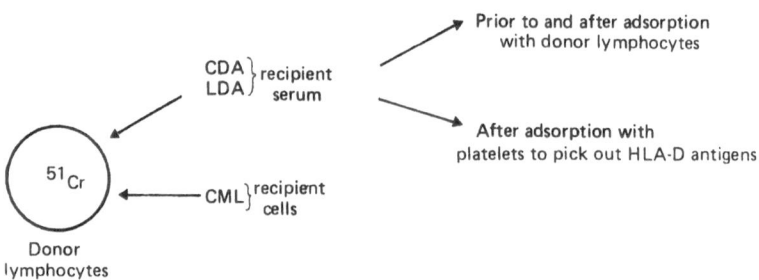

Figure 149.   Summary of typing schemes

Such a scheme is desirable as a comprehensive cross-match. Indeed because the standard CDA cannot detect lymphocyte-dependent (LDA) or cell-mediated (CML) reactions, two powerful mechanisms of allograft destruction would otherwise be overlooked.

Detection of Ir (immune response) antigens

These are the same as Ia in the mouse. They are mixed lymphocyte locus (MLC), that is HLA-D gene products, and they are detected by a standard microcytotoxicity test. B lymphocytes are incubated with antibody at 20 °C for 1 h and then with complement at 20 °C for 2 h. This is called the 20-20 test. At the same time a 5-20 test is performed by incubating B cells in serum containing potential antibody at 5 °C and thereafter adding complement for 2 h at 20 °C.

Positive reactions occur commonly in the cold incubation 5-20 tests. Indeed 50% of people over the age of 60 have cold lymphocytotoxins. They seem to appear after pregnancy or vaccinations and of course as part of SLE. In these situations the test is detecting an autoantibody.

In the transplant situation it is now clear that patients who have pretransplant antibodies that react with donor B lymphocytes at 5 °C have a much higher kidney survival rate. The beneficial effect only applies to those antibodies that react at 5 °C, but not to those that react at 5 °C and 37 °C. The former antibodies seem to represent '*enhancing antibodies*'; indeed they appear to account for a high graft survival rate even in persons who have an HLA incompatability with their donor.

Clinical relevance of transplant immunology

Lymphocyte and humoral antibody reactions

It is now certain that good HLA matching, particularly at the second B locus, correlates with a good graft prognosis. However, in addition to the SD antigen matching, LD factors are important since survival of kidneys in MLC 'weak response' pairs is 90% as opposed to only 20% when there is a large MLC difference. This confirms what one might expect, namely that rejection of an allograft involves the recognition of both cellular (lymphocyte-defined) and humoral (SD) differences. This is to say that rejection depends on the strength of the cellular proliferative response, as defined by lymphocyte disparities, and at the same time the nature of the target cell (as defined by serological differences). On the one hand there might be strong LD disparity, but poor targets on account of relative SD similarity (3/4 match). Alternatively one can have weak LD interactions but excellent targets because of SD differences (0/4). Thus one always has to allow for an interaction between the cellular and humoral systems.

Cytotoxic antibodies

The detection of presensitization is of major importance so as to anticipate and avoid unwanted rejection reactions. It should be sought by means of

[51]Cr- CDA, CML and LDA tests. It is the weak reaction requiring a long incubation that may be easily missed.

The CML test for cytotoxic T cells is being used as a monitoring process, but one has to be aware that CML becomes negative during steroid therapy. It rebounds, however, after dosage reduction, and then a positive result may predict the occurrence of rejection or a failure to respond to therapy.

Blood transfusion and enhancing antibodies

It turns out that allografts given to patients who have never received blood transfusions often do badly, compared with those recipients who have received transfusions. Patients transfused in the 3 months prior to grafting or even as a single transfusion prior to or at operation do best of all. Clearly this is a process of 'natural selection' that is not just designed to select and eliminate those who have developed cytotoxic antibodies, but is a means of developing 'enhancing' or 'blocking' antibodies. An enhancing antibody (EA) is a blocking antibody that in some way coats and protects the target cell.

Precise attempts have been made to create 'enhancing antibodies' in man. In 1970 Batchelor prepared passive enhancing antibody for a child whose kidney was donated by the mother. This was done by immunizing the father with maternal leucocytes and then preparing a pepsin digest of his antiserum in order to obtain the $F(ab)_2$ fragments.

Conversely deletion of MLC responses can be attained by using the variable region (idiotype) determinants of receptor molecules as antigen in order to generate an autoimmune response to that idiotype. The result is

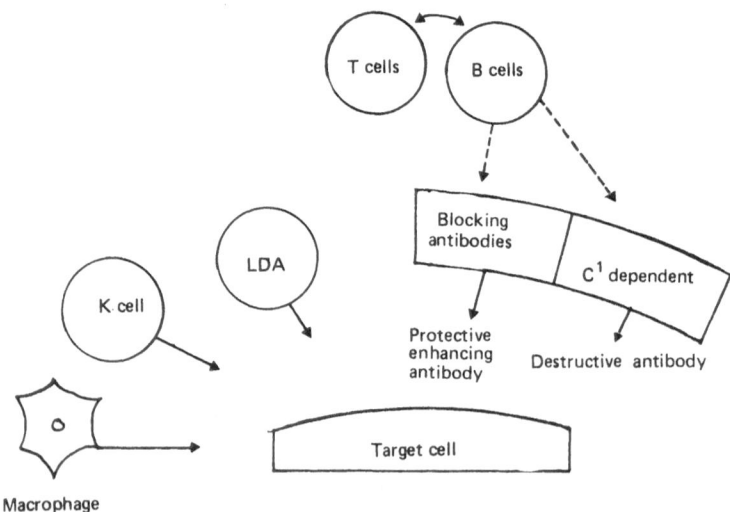

Figure 150. Complexity of immune reactions in the transplant situation

elimination of histocompatability antigen-reactive T cells. It remains to be seen whether the induction of an autoimmune response to a given idiotype will have harmful consequences.

Figure 150 summarizes the various immunological reactions that have to be contemplated in the transplant situation.

Macrophages that are armed with antibody, killer K cells and lymphocytes may all attach the foreign target cells, as also will humoral destructive antibodies, but when grafts survive, even in the face of apparent incompatabilities, the secret may depend on enhancing antibody. Indeed when rhesus monkeys with bad HLA matches are first given blood transfusions, their graft survival is enhanced. Nobody has analyzed how the HLA match of the transfused blood should fit the prospective match. There are several theoretical possibilities. Yet not all these observed phenomena may represent immunologically specific reactions. Thus gammaglobulin obtained from expressed placental tissue has been found to improve survival rates in patients with preformed lymphocytotoxic antibodies, by apparently suppressing humoral rejection. As is the case in the tolerance of the fetus by the mother in pregnancy, other proteins such as a_2-macroglobulin may play an important blocking role.

Blocking factors
The ability of patient's sera to block mixed lymphocyte reactions is currently under investigation. In fact the ability of specifically sensitized lymphocytes to kill appropriate target cells can be shown to blocked *either* by blocking anti-B cell antibodies, *or* by antigen–antibody complexes. For this type of test donor skin fibroblasts can be trypsinized to provide a suspension suitable for plating in wells. Moreover they can be labelled with ^{51}Cr so that chromium release can later be monitored. Control or recipient serum is then added, and after 45 min the control or test lymphocytes. 48 h later the number of remaining fibroblasts are counted by staining with crystal violet, or, instead the ^{51}Cr loss can be counted.

Tolerance
The goal of many transplant researchers is to find some way of inducing tolerance. Owen in 1945 had shown that twin cattle sharing a placenta are red cell chimaeras, so they will also accept a skin graft from one another. In mice tolerance can be induced up to 6 days after birth to strong histocompatability antigens by means of the injection of allogeneic lymphocytes from the donor, from whom they will eventually receive a skin graft. Brent has induced tolerance in mice by giving a preparation of donor antigen 16 days before skin grafting together with the administration of antilymphocyte serum. Such tolerance means a central failure of the immune response. For maintenance it

requires the *persistence of antigen* in the form of living chimaeric cells or periodic injection of antigen extract. Thymectomy is also required.

The ability to accept a foreign graft is actually transferable to irradiated syngeneic recipients via spleen cells of the primary graft recipient. As this suppressive effect is abolished by treatment of the transferred cells with anti-θ cell serum plus complement, a role for suppressor T lymphocytes is anticipated.

Reduction of antigenicity

Pretreatment of an allograft donor with immunosuppressive drugs has been referred to above (page 393). It is believed that this eliminates passenger leukocytes within the allograft parenchyma.

Cross-reactivity of antigens

One last point to be made briefly, since it may be a pointer to the future, is that there is some evidence that lymphocytotoxins produced in response to infection with Gram-negative organisms will cross-react with the host HLA antigens. This reminds one of the cross-reactivity between streptococcal M protein and HLA antigens. The suggestion is that some patients who are referred to as 'responders' might have been rendered so by bacterial infections. In this way infection with bacterial antigens (for example defined *E. coli* serotypes) results in presensitization and the production of lymphocytotoxins that contribute to renal allograft damage. By the same token it is possible (in theory) that enhancing antibodies could arise in similar fashion.

REFERENCES

Surgical technique

Calne, R.Y. *Renal Transplantation*. (London: Arnold) 1963
Calne, R.Y. *Clinical Organ Transplantation*. (Oxford: Blackwell) 1971
Calne, R.Y. (1974). Clinical organ transplantation. *Urology*, **3**, 171
Kauffman, H.M. (1974). Splenectomy. *Surg. Gynecol., Obstet.*, **139**, 33
Meakins, J.L. (1972). *En bloc* transplantation from children. *Surgery*, **71**, 72
Starzl, T. (1964). Adult homografts in children. *Surg. Gynecol. and Obstet.*, **119**, 106

Immunopathology

Andres, G.A. (1968). *Lab. Invest.*, **22**, 588
Andres, G.A. and Accinni, L. (1975). *6th Int. Congress Nephrology, Florence*, 722

Lindqvist, R.R. (1968). *Am. J. Pathol.*, **53,** 851
Matthew, T.H. (1975). *Am. J. Med.*, **59,** 177
Porter, K.A. (1967). *J. Clin. Pathol.*, (suppl). **20,** 518
Porter, K.A. (1972). *Int. Rev. Exp. Pathol.*, **11,** 73
Zollinger, H.U. (1973). *Curr. Top. Pathol.*, **57,** 1

Clinical aspects

Bergström, K. and Blomstrand, R. (1968). Signs of rejection. *Acta Chir. Scand.*, **134,** 476
Busch, G.J. (1971). Long term. *Medicine*, **50,** 29
Chisholm, G.D. (1969). Signs of rejection in renal transplantation. *Lancet*, **i,** 904
Kissmeyer-Nielsen, F. (1966). Hyper-acute rejection. *Lancet*, **ii,** 666

Children

Henriksson, C. (1975). *Acta Paediatr. Scand.*, **64,** 833
Lilly, J.R. (1971). *Paediatrics*, **47,** 548

Evaluation of transplants

Burrows, L. (1973). Platelets and rejection. *Transplant. Proc.*, **5,** 157
Carpenter, C.B. (1967). Complement changes. *Am. J. Med.*, **43,** 854
Collins, J.J. (1965). By renograms. *Ann. Surg.*, **161,** 428
Hall, C. (1973). Urinary FDP. *Br. Med. J.*, **3,** 204
Harris, J. (1972). DNA in lymphocytes. *Transplant. Proc.*, **4,** 659
Martin, D.C. (1974). Isotope scanning. *J. Urol.*, **112,** 2
Petrek, J. (1977). By ultrasound. *Ann. Surg.*, **185,** 441
Shehadeh, I.H. (1970). Lysozymuria, complement and heterophile antibodies. *Arch. Intern. Med.*, **125,** 850
Wardle, E.N. (1974). Fibrinogen catabolism. *Transplantation*, **18,** 508
Williams, R.J. (1974). Leucocyte migration test. *Clin. Nephrol.*, **2,** 100

Kidney preservation

Baxby, K. (1974). Assessment of kidneys for transplantation. *Lancet*, **13,** 270
Claes, G. (1974). New Gambro perfusion machine. *Transplant. Proc.*, **6,** 261
Collins, G.M. (1974). 72-hour kidney storage. *Surg. Forum.*, **25,** 275
Johnson, R.W.G. (1972). Use of PPF. *Transplantation*, **13,** 270
McCabe, R.E. (1972). Preservation of human cadaver kidneys. *J. Am. Med. Assoc.*, **219,** 1056
Opelz, G. (1976). Perfusion versus cold storage. *Transplant. Proc.*, **8,** 212

Shiel, A.G.R. (1975). Machine perfusion. *Lancet*, **2**, 287
Spector, D. (1976). Perfusion nephropathy. *N. Engl. J. Med.*, **295**, 1217

Drug therapy

Carpenter, C.B. (1969). Immunosuppression. *Arch. Intern. Med.*, **123**, 501
Dicke, H.W. (1971). Use of azathioprine. *Transplant. Proc.*, **3**, 484
Friedman, E.A. (1970). Daily or alternate day therapy. *Transplantation*, **10**, 552
Guttmann, R.D. (1975). High dose cytotoxic drug pretreatment. *6th Int. Congress Nephrology, Florence*, 748
Levin, R.H. (1964). 6-Mercaptopurine. *N. Engl. J. Med.*, **271**, 16
McGregor, R.R. (1969). Daily or alternate day therapy. *N. Engl. J. Med.*, **280**, 1427
McMillan, R. (1968). Heparin. *Lancet*, **i**, 1178
Murray, J.E. (1964). Immunosuppression, **160**, 449
Starzl, T. (1971). Use of cyclophosphamide. *Lancet*, **2**, 70
Turcotte, J. (1972). Rejection crises treated with high dose methyl prednisolone. *Arch. Surg.*, **105**, 230

Survival

Carpenter, C.B. (1976). Antibodies in the rejection or enhancement of organ grafts. *Adv. Immunol.*, **22**, 1
Clark, C.E. (1974). Cadaver kidney transplants at one month. *N. Engl. J. Med.*, **291**, 1099
Dausset, J. (1974). Serologically determined HLA antigens and long-term survival. *N. Engl. J. Med.*, **290**, 979
Festenstein, H. (1976). Improved survival by transfusions together with good matching. *Lancet*, **i**, 157
Lucas, Z.J. (1970). Early renal transplant failure with subliminal sensitization. *Transplantation*, **10**, 522
Murray, S. (1974). *Tissue antigens*, **4**, 548
Opelz, G. (1973). *Transplant. Proc.*, **5**, 253
Rowlands, D.T. (1976). Renal allografts in HLA matched recipients. *Am. J. Pathol.*, **61**, 177
Terasaki, P.I. (1971). Pre-sensitization and transplant failures (cytotoxic antibodies). *Postgrad. Med. J.*, **47**, 89

Transplant nephritis recurrence

Berger, J. (1975). Recurrence of mesangial IgA. *Kidney Int.*, **7**, 232
Berthoux, F.C. (1975). Recurrence of MCGN. *Kidney Int.*, **7**, S 323

Hoyer, J.R. (1972). Idiopathic nephrotic syndrome after transplantation. *Lancet*, **2**, 343

Hume, D.M. (1972). Recurrent glomerulonephritis. *Transplant. Proc.*, **4,**673

Lameijer, L.D.F. (1973). Recurrence of nephrotic syndrome. *Clinical Nephrol.*, **1**, 49

McPhaul, J.J. (1973). Nephritogenic mechanisms in grafts. *J. Clin. Invest.*, **52**, 1059

Milgrom, F. (1971). Immunological injury of renal allografts. *J. Exp. Med.*, **134**, 139s

Petersen, V.P. (1975) Late failure of transplants. *Medicine*, **54**, 45

Rossmann, P. (1970). Ultrastructure of recurrent glomerulonephritis. *Beitrag. Pathol.*, **141**, 213

Wilson, C.B. (1974). Antitubular basement membrane antibodies after transplantation. *Transplantation*, **18**, 447

Complications of transplantation

Aldrete, J.S. (1975). Gastrointestinal and hepatic complications. *Am. J. Surg.*, **129**, 115

Bailey, G.L. Griffiths,H.J.and Mocelin, H.J. (1972). *Trans. Am. Soc. Artif. Int. Org.*, **18**, 401

Betts, R.F. and Hanshaw, J.B. (1977). Cytomegalovirus in the compromised host. *Ann. Rev. Med.*, **28**, 103

Briggs, W.A. Hampers, C.L. and Merrill, J.P. (1972). Avascular necrosis of bone. *Ann. Surg.*, **175**, 282

Cameron, J.S. (1975). *J. Clin. Pathol. (suppl)*. **9**, 24

Eickhoff, T.E. (1973). *Transplant. Proc.*, **5**, 1233

Harrington, K.D. and Murray, W.R. (1971). *J. Bone Joint Surg.*, **53A,** 203

Hill, R.B. (1967). Death after transplantation. *Am. J. Med.*, **42,** 327

Lopez, C. (1974). Rejection and virus infections. *Am. J. Med.*, **56**, 280

Ibels, L.S., Alfrey, A.C., Huffer, W.E. and Weil, R. (1978). *Medicine*, **57,** 25

Malek, G.H. (1973). Urological complications. *J. Urol.*, **109**, 173

Myerowtiz, R.L. (1972). Bacterial infections. *Am. J. Med.*, **53,** 308

Payne, J.E. (1974). CMV and rejection. *Surg. Forum*, **25**, 273

Penn, I. and Starzl, T.E. (1973). Immunosuppression and cancer. *Transplant. Proc.*, **5**, 943

Pirson, Y. and Alexandre, G. (1977). Hepatic disease. *N. Engl. J. Med.*, **296**, 194 and *Transplant Proc.* 1975, **7**, 1

Salaman, J.R. (1974). Death after kidney transplantation. *Br. Med. J.*, **3,**736

Starzl, T.E. (1970). *Ann. Surg.*, **172**, 1

Vidne, B.A. (1976). Vascular complications. *Surgery*, **79**, 77

Immunological test systems

Boyum, A. (1968). Separation of leucocytes from blood and bone marrow. *Scand. J. Clin. Lab. Invest.*, (suppl. 1.) **21**, 97

Colberg, J.E. *et al.* (1972). The cross-match profile. *Arch. Surg.*, **105**, 237

Hasegawa, T. *et al.* (1973). Granulocyte microcytotoxicity. *Transplantation*, **15**, 492

Hattler, B.G. *et al.* (1973). Blocking antibody in sera and on the kidneys. *Transplant. Proc.*, **6**, 665

Jeannet, M. *et al.* (1970). Humoral antibodies in transplantation. *N. Eng. J. Med.*, **282**, 111

Monaco, A.P. *et al.* (1975). Enhancement of tissue allografts. *Adv. Nephrol.*, **5**, 135

Opelz, G. and Terasaki, P.I. (1978). Effect of blood transfusions. *N. Engl. J. Med.*, **299**, 799

Park, M.S. and Terasaki, P. (1977). Auto-antibody against B lymphocytes. *Lancet*, **2**, 465

Pierce, J.C. and Lee, H.M. (1974). The kidney cell cross-match. *Surgery*, **76**, 101

Quadracci, L.J. *et al.* (1973). Homograft survival and blocking factors. *Transplant Proc.*, **5**, 649

Rogentine, G.N. (1967). 51-Cr-cytotoxicity test. *Transplantation*, **5**, 1323.

Sengar, D.P.S. *et al.* (1974). HLA antigens on human kidney cells. *Vox. Sang.*, **27**, 1

Sheehy, M.J. (1975). Primed lymphocyte typing test. *Science*, **188**, 1308

Sybesma, J. Ph., Kater, L. *et al.* (1973). HLA antigens in kidney tissue. *Dialysis, Transplant., Nephrol.*, **10**, 406

Terasaki, P.I. *et al.* (1971). Pre-sensitization and kidney transplant failure. *Postgrad. Med., J.*, **47**, 89

Ting, A. *et al.* (1973). Pre-sensitization detected by a sensitive cross-match. *Transplant Proc.*, **5**, 813

Ting, A. *et al.* (1975). Lymphocyte dependent antibody cross-matching. *Lancet*, **i**, 304

Weigle, W.O. *et al.* (1975). Possible modes of suppressor cells in Immunological tolerance. *Transplant. Rev.*, **26**, 186

Yust, I. *et al.* (1974). Lymphocyte-dependent antibody in sera of multiple transfused patients. *Transplantation*, **18**, 99

Index

Index